The Buffaloes of World
and
Water Buffalo Production

Nityanand Pathak

BSc, BVSc and AH, MVSc, PhD
FNAVS, FANA, FMOBS, MAAVN

Former
Director, Central Institute for Research on Buffalo, Hisar
Director, Centre of Advance Studies and Head, Animal Nutrition Division, IVRI, Izatnagar
Project Leader and Buffalo Nutrition Expert, ITEC, SR Vietnam
Vice President, Indian Society for Buffalo Development, Hisar
Secretary, National Academy of Veterinary Science, New Delhi
President of Animal Nutrition Association, Izatnagar
President of Animal Nutrition Society of India, Karnal
Vice President, Zoo and Wildlife Veterinarians, Bareilly
President, National Academy of Veterinary Nutrition and Animal Welfare, Bareilly

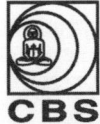

CBS

CBS Publishers & Distributors Pvt Ltd

New Delhi • Bengaluru • Chennai • Kochi • Kolkata • Mumbai
Bhopal • Bhubaneswar • Hyderabad • Jharkhand • Nagpur • Patna • Pune • Uttarakhand • Dhaka (Bangladesh)

The Buffaloes of World and Water Buffalo Production

ISBN: 978-93-87964-19-8

Copyright © Author and Publisher

First Edition: 2019

Published by Satish Kumar Jain and produced by Varun Jain for

CBS Publishers and Distributors Pvt Ltd

4819/XI Prahlad Street, 24 Ansari Road, Daryaganj, New Delhi 110 002, India.
Ph: 23289259, 23266861, 23266867   Fax: 011-23243014
Website: www.cbspd.com   e-mail: delhi@cbspd.com; cbspubs@airtelmail.in.

Corporate Office: 204 FIE, Industrial Area, Patparganj, Delhi 110 092, India
Ph: 4934 4934   Fax: 4934 4935   e-mail: publishing@cbspd.com; publicity@cbspd.com

Branches

- **Bengaluru:** Seema House 2975, 17th Cross, K.R. Road, Banasankari 2nd Stage, Bengaluru 560 070, Karnataka, India
  Ph: +91-80-26771678/79   Fax: +91-80-26771680   e-mail: bangalore@cbspd.com
- **Chennai:** 7, Subbaraya Street, Shenoy Nagar, Chennai 600 030, Tamil Nadu, India.
  Ph: +91-44-26680620, 26681266   Fax: +91-44-42032115   e-mail: chennai@cbspd.com
- **Kochi:** 42/1325, 1326, Power House Road, Opposite KSEB Power House, Ernakulam 682 018, Kochi, Kerala, India.
  Ph: +91-484-4059061-65   Fax: +91-484-4059065   e-mail: kochi@cbspd.com
- **Kolkata:** 6/B, Ground Floor, Rameswar Shaw Road, Kolkata-700 014 (West Bengal), India.
  Ph: +91-33-2289-1126, 2289-1127, 2289-1128   e-mail: kolkata@cbspd.com
- **Mumbai:** 83-C, Dr E Moses Road, Worli, Mumbai-400018, Maharashtra, India.
  Ph: +91-22-24902340/41   Fax: +91-22-24902342   e-mail: mumbai@cbspd.com

Representatives

• **Bhopal**	0-8319310552	• **Bhubaneswar**	0-9911037372	• **Hyderabad**	0-9885175004	• **Jharkhand**	0-9811541605
• **Nagpur**	0-9021734563	• **Patna**	0-9334159340	• **Pune**	0-9623451994	• **Uttarakhand**	0-9716462459
• **Dhaka (Bangladesh)**	01912-003485						

Printed at: Mudrak, Nodia, UP, India

Preface

Domestic water buffalo (*Bubalus* spp.) has emerged as an important global farm animal for nutritious food production. The two domesticated species of water buffaloes were bred to meet regional requirements of the tropical Asian countries. The dairy type Indian river buffalo (*Bubalus bubalis*) was bred for fat rich high milk production in different parts of the Indian subcontinent and swamp buffalo (*Bubalus swamps*) was primarily evolved for draught power, specially for pudding the waterlogged paddy fields. Now, dairy buffaloes are spread globally as a dairy animal of tropical and subtropical countries in all the six continents. Swamp buffaloes were introduced in Australia and made feral on the tall growing grasses of northwest Australia for meat (buffen) and harvested periodically for the export of meat and hide to Caribbean countries. The value of water buffaloes is increasing progressively. Earlier as a part of breeding, management and nutrition courses, the buffalo production science is now occupying an independent place in the syllabi of veterinary science, animal husbandary, and agriculture not only in the Indian subcontinent but also in many other countries. There are at present some books on the buffaloes but the present book has been synthesized to meet the requirements of courses on buffalo production. In preparation of different chapters all accessible published research works on buffaloes have been referred. The experience of author as a research worker and manager at the Indian Veterinary Research Institute, Izatnagar, Buffalo Breeding Institute, Song Be, SR Vietnam, and Central Institute for Research on Buffaloes, Hisar (Haryana, India), has helped to make the book of global uses.

The book has been organised in 12 chapters comprising introduction; buffaloes of the world; types and breeds of domesticated water buffaloes (*Bubalus* spp.); feeding of buffaloes; management of buffaloes, reproductive system of water buffalo: female reproductive system; semen production, processing and artificial insemination; mammary glands and lactation; milk and milk products; buffalo meat and meat products' utilization of by-products of buffalo; and economic contribution of domestic buffaloes.

In preparation of this valuable book the help received directly and indirectly from colleagues Dr LC Chaudhary, Dr SK Saha, Dr KK Baruah, and Shri HC Singh is acknowledged. Late Sushila is an inspiring force and grandchildren Ananya, Anshuman, Annuvrata, Adiya, Anuliya, Atharva, Anavartika, and Akchhita are strength. Contribution of Padmashini for line diagrams and proofreading is acknowledged.

Nityanand Pathak

Contents

Introduction

Long ago the term was used for the Asian buffaloes (*Bubalus* spp.), African wild buffalo (*Syncerus* spp.), Bison (*Bison* spp.) and Asian pseudo (*Pseudonovibos spiralis*). Out of these only main Asian buffalo (*Bubalus bubalis*) has been domesticated and developed as one of the important farm animal of economic importance for the farming community. Now, domesticated Asian buffalo has acquired almost cosmopolitan status distributed in almost all the continents. However, uptil now it has not succeeded in making consiberable presence in the north America. The main inhabited regions of domestic buffaloes are the tropical countries in both the hemispheres but due to high adaptability, it has been successfully bred and established in the subtemperate regions. The domesticated Asian (water) buffalo has established itself as a multipurpose farm animal capable of thriving in dominated natural herbage cover. The Indian subcontinent is the home-land of dairy type Indian (River) buffalo, globally famous for fat rich thick milk of high nutritive value. The other type of domestic Asian buffalo is the 'draught swamp buffalo' capable of working in knee deep muddy water fields of paddy crop. The home tract of swamp buffalo extends from Indian to Philippines, and other Indo-Pacific island region via Nepal, Bangaladesh, Bhutan, Mayanmar, Thialand, Combodia, Laos, SR Vietnam, China, Taiwan, and Korea, etc. The high adaptation capacity of domesticated water buffalo has fovoured it for finding newer homes. During ancient time domestic buffalo was almost an integral part of the nomadic families of Asia-Europe an region and in European countries. Domestic buffalo farming was introduced by Asian nomads and others. In Indian Murrah breed of dairy buffalo is a highly valuable dairy animal which has been taken to many countries for farming. In Egypt there is a 'Al Murrah' tribe and Murrah breed of buffalo has been found the needs of anthropological studies.

▶ CONTRIBUTION OF DOMESTIC WATER BUFFALO (*BUBALUS BUBALIS*)

The economic contributions of domestic water buffaloes are both direct and indirect.

The Direct Economic Contributions of Domestic Water Buffaloes

1. **Production of highly nutritious foods:** Milk and meat are the main foods produced by the buffaloes. Both foods are highly rich sources of dietary energy and balanced proteins rich on essential amino acids besides adequate supply of minerals and vitamins. Since there is no need of sacrificing animals for milk production

and sufficient milk is spared by the animals after nursing their calves, the milk of buffalo is extensively consumed even by the strict vegetarian population of India. Buffen (Buffalo meat) is the another nutritious food rich in energy and balanced complete protein. Earlier fattening of buffaloes for good quality meat production was practiced in Egytp, near east, Europe, Australia, and Latin American countries but during the last few decades buffalo fattening for good quality buffen production has also gained momentum in the Asian countries. This happened due to sparing of large number of draught buffaloes due to increasing mechanization of paddy and sugarcane farming. In these regions only spent animals were disposed for meat production about half a century ago. Even the surviving male calves of dairy buffaloes were also reared for draught purpose.

2. **Draught power:** The buffaloes are sturdy, agile, and hard working animals of high endurance. Although animal is slow in movement but preferred due to its high traction power, hardiness, ability of ploughing the water logged mudy paddy fields, longer daily working capacity, easy handling, and less expensive maintenance than the other draught animals. Preferably males of dairy breeds and both sexes of swamp buffaloes are used for working. However, female buffaloes are put to light work like ploughing and puddling the paddy fields. Only infertile and sterile females of dairy breeds are used for draught purpose in some of the countries.

3. **Manure production:** The buffaloes are continuous source of organic manure. Both dung and urine along with soiled bedding of straw, dry leaves or dry grass are used for preparation of organic manure by composting. Manure prepared from the buffalo excreta is a good source of nitrogen, carbon, calcium, phosphorus, and many minerals required for optimum crop production. Use of organic manure in the field improves soil health and water holding capacity necessary for optimum crop production. It also stimulates the movement and multiplication of earthworms in the field which increases aeration and turnover of the soil considered to improve the fertility of soil.

4. **Use of fallen buffaloes:** The carcasses of dead animals provide hide, horns, hooves and switch hairs of industrial uses. The flesh and bones are largely used in cottage industry for the manufacture of meat meal, meat cum-bone meal, bone meal, and bone ash used for supplementing the diets of poultry and pig for the supply of essential amino acids and minerals. Bone meal and bone ash are also used as fertilizers for the crops. The hide and horns are used in cottage industry as well as large scale leather manufacturing industries.

5. **Use of slaughter house by-products:** The edible carcass is the primary product of abattoir but in big industrial cities glands, blood, sex organs, and empty gastro-intestinal tracts are mostly used for the manufacture of pharmaceuticals, industrial oil, casings for stuffed meat products, and others. The residue available after the extraction of enzyme, hormones, and the other pharmaceutical products is further processed for the manufacture of animal protein supplements or manure, if not fit for animal consumption.

Indirect Economic Contribution of Domestic Buffaloes

1. **Source of power for agricultural and industrial works:** Buffalo is a most suitable draft animal for puddling the paddy field and traction of carts loaded with agricultural produce. Buffaloes are also used for haulage of industrial goods for short distance. Although slow in pace the high load pulling capacity and endurance

had made it a draft animal of choice for the transportation of grains and straw to market, and sugarcane to crushers and sugar mills. Due to low heat tolerance and heavy traffic on roads during daytime the haulage of goods form villages to mandi and other markets is done during the relatively comfortable hours of night. In most parts of northern India, it is a common seen to see the carvan of loaded carts moving in almost a constant pace and disciplined line. One, two or more lighted lanterns hang from the wheel beam of the cart. Normally, one lantern is used for 5–6 carts and maximum number may not be more than three even for 25 loaded carts. The main objective of placing lighted lentern is to give signals to other vehicles for preventing collision.

2. **Food grain production:** Buffaloes supply traction power and organic manure for crop production. The food grains and vegetables produced from the exclusive application of organic manure are considered healthy foods and fetch higher price. Increasing demand of organic foods are simultaneously increasing the price of dung manure and higher return from buffalo keeping.

3. **Buffalo as source of employment:** In large commercial farming system buffalo production needs only few persons but in small holder buffalo keeping system a large number of part-time and full time employments are generated. Various jobs generated from buffalo rearing in rural and urban areas are:
   a. Buffalo management
   b. Grazing of buffaloes
   c. Milking of buffaloes
   d. Preparation of milk products at home
   e. Marketing of raw (liquid) milk and milk products
   f. Use of milk for the preparation of khoa, chenna, paneer, srikhand, and a variety of sweets provide employment for owner, halwais, and salesman
   g. Marketing of animals on foot
   h. Fattening and meat industry provides employment for rearing, processing and marketing
   i. Hide provides jobs in leather making, leather goods manufacture, and marketing
   j. Horns provide employment to artisans in cottage industry for the making of decoration items and daily use articles
   k. Dead animal carcass and abattoir rejects are used for the manufacture of pharmaceuticals, vaccines, and diagnostics, etc.
   l. Employment in pharmaceutical industry for the manufacture of pharmaceuticals, storage, transportation, marketing, and accounting are the integral part of almost all the production system for commercial purpose.

4. **Miscellaneous contributions:** The buffalo are used for joy riding during grazing, and wallowing in running water source, and johads (Ponds for wallowing of buffaloes). In some countries buffalo bull fighting is organized at specific festivals. Sacrifice of entire buffalo, specially the yearling is practised to please specific deities. Ritual sacrifice of buffaloes was quite common in India, Nepal, and Indonesia but now it is decreasing.

▶ INDUSTRIAL DEVELOPMENT AROUND BUFFALOES

A large number of industries of various dimension ranging from small scale cottage industries in rural areas to big manufacturing houses of industrial areas are dependent on the growth and production of buffaloes. Some of the common industries around buffalo production are listed as follows:

1. **Buffalo handling articles and gears:** These include ropes, halters, whips, pegs, plough, carts and their harness, nose ring and nose string, etc. All these works required the services of artisans like carpenter, blacksmith and cobbler, etc. Greater proportion of raw materials are produced locally. Greater quantity of products is also marketed locally.

2. **Feed stuff cultivation and processing equipments:** Almost all equipments required for the cultivation of grains are also used for the cultivation of fodder. These are ploughs, harrows, leveling plank (henga or patella), tractor, trolly, dibler, sickle, and harvesting machine.

3. **Fodder and feed processing equipments:** These are chaff cutter, drier, grinder, feed mixer, pelleting machine, extruder, and feed block making machines.

4. **Feeding articles:** These include baskets, troughs, trench, etc. for offering and feeding of the buffaloes. For watering buckets, trough or trench are used in the stall feeding system.

5. **Milking and milk handling equipments:** These are milking pail, earthen milking pot (ghooncha), and metallic bucket for milking. Earthen pot (Kahantari or Nadi) and metallic can or pan for heating, boiling, evaporation, curd making, churning, freezing, and sweets making.

6. Abattoir construction and abattoir machine manufacturing industry.

7. Buffalo meat and meat products manufacturing, handling, packaging, storage, transporation, and marketing industries.

8. Hide processing industries for the manufacture of leather.

9. Leather goods manufacturing industries.

10. Horns and hooves utilization industries.

11. Hide flaying and fallen animal utilization industries.

12. Pharmaceutical and cosmetics industries.

13. **Miscellaneous cottage and household industries:** There are utilization of long and coarse hairs of tail switch for making ropes and mats; dung for making dung cake for fuel and abattoir wastes for making manure.

The long list depicts the dimension of employment generation around buffalo farming. In the land holding pattern of India dominated by small and marginal farmers and landless farming families Animal Husbandry, specially the buffalo keeping has been found to be a reasonably satisfactory source of livelihood through part-time and full time employment.

▶ **DOMESTICATION OF WATER BUFFALO (BUBALUS BUBALIS)**

Domestication of water buffalo for the production of foods and working animals was taken up much later than the domestication of cattle. This was probably due to high affinity of Asian buffaloes for water and swamp. These buffaloes spend longer part of day time in wallowing in water bodies or lying deep in mud holes. During free living wild state making gathered sufficient knowledge regarding the hostile conditions on the earth. They gradually learnt to meet their necessary requirement for survival. In the process of evolution they frequently encountered dangerous and furious wild animals and learnt protection with the use of twigs, bamboo, and pavels, etc. Initially they started living in groups beneath the natural shelters and caves and for a very long period lead nomadic life in search of food, water, and shelter. During the course of settlement some wild animals sought the proximity of humans and some of the useful species were initially lured by offering foods. These selected species were gradually tamed and then domesticated for controlled management. Among the tamed species dogs and horses are considered to be domesticated first. These were subsequently followed by cattle, sheep, and goats. Probably buffaloes were domesticated much later but hunted for food and hide in most parts of their homelands. The taming and herding of buffaloes on marshes was started so that they may be made available for food on a short notice as evident from the incidence of 'Ramayan epic' (more than 3000 BC or about 5000 years ago). It has been mentioned in couplet (doha) of Ram Charit Manas (By Shri Goswami Tulasi Das ji) that when despondent Lankapati Ravan went to awake his brother Kumbhakaran, before the lapse of his six months sleeping period, for fighting with the army of Lord Ram. On awaking Kumbhakaran came to know the rivalary of Ravan with Ram, he was shunned. He started praising Lord Ram for his kinderness, generosity and other goodness of lord Ram, Ravan was also absorbed for a moment but immediately omen time prevailed. In order to divert the attention of Kumbhakaran and to prepare him for fighting Ravan ordered for the immediate supply of thousands of pitchers of wine and enumerable fattened buffaloes for the feast of Kumbhakaran as mentioned in the following couplet of Ram Charit Manas (Pathak, 2003).

'Ram roop gun sumirat magan bhayou chhan ek
Raven mangeu koti ghat mud aru Mahish anek'

After eating buffaloes and drinking wine the Kumbhakaran roared like thunder, and drunk he marched to battlefield alone from his fort as depicted in the following couplet of Ram Charit Manas:

'Mahish khai kari madira pana,
Garja bajra ghat samana
Kumbhakaran durmad run ranga
Chala durg taji, sen na sanga'

During the period of Mahabharat epic buffalo was wild beast like wild animals such as lion, tiger, boar, bear, elephant, and apes. The domesticated animals of the era were cattle, sheep, goats, horses, ass, and mule.

There is also reference to taming boars, buffaloes and elephant for food supply and other works like extensive use of domesticated elephants in war and also for the ride of royals and rich. Domestication of several species of animals was perfected before the Mahabharat period. The advancement in Animal Husbandry can be visualize by the evidence of well cattle by Nakul and Shadev, respectively. In post epic period, Emperor Ashoka the great is credited for the systematic education and training of the veterinarians. During this period specialized Veterinary education was imparted and Veterinary hospitals were established before the start of Christian calendar for the livestock of public. Organized farming of cattle, buffaloes, goats, and sheep for milk, work, meat, and fiber production was developed. The hides and skins were used for the manufacture of leather goods, fiber for fabrics and oxen for power has been distributed in detail in the 'Kuatiliya Arthashastra' (321–186 BC). Almost all domesticated animal were grazed on the well-managed pastures. The management of heards, flocks, and pasture lands was carried by different level of workers, supervisors, and superintendents for high production and maintenance of good health of livestock.

More informations on the rearing of buffaloes are available from the medieval period. Vast area from Mesopotamia to Indo-Gangatic plains intercepted by several rives and covered by dense forest and swamps provided suitable environment for the growth of riverine buffaloes during the third millennium BC (Bats, 1937). Almost similar conditions were present along the perennial rivers and lakes, and large swamps in most parts of the tropical Asian countries and island countries of the Asia-Pacific region. These favourable conditions provided optimum environment for the inhabitation of swamp buffaloes during the pre-historic period. Several modern historians believe that the buffaloes were first tamed and then domesticated for working in agricultural operations before 2500 BC in the Mesopotamia during the period of Akkadian dynasty and in the Indus valley civilization of the Indian subcontinent extending to Harrappa, Mohenjodaro, some parts of Rajasthan, Gujarat, Maharastra, Haryana, Madhya Pradesh, and Uttar Pradesh. The evidences are available in the seals and small sculptors depicting mostly male buffaloes. On one of the seal of Indus valley excavation, now present in Lahore museum, depiction of male buffaloes on feeding through may be considered sample evidence of domestication of buffaloes. Some multi-coloured ceramics of the 'Nal Culture' of the south Balochistan depict buffaloes (Brentijes, 1969) and it is contemporary with the Indus valley civilization. A picture of holding of growing buffalo by its fore legs and a horn probably depict a fight or an attempt to control the beast. Another, scene showing watering of buffaloes in a stream by two God heroes, and the buffaloes being charged by the lions. These are considered reasonable evidences of domestication of water buffalo during 2350–2150 BC; and in the ancient Mesopotamia it was restricted to two periods, i.e. the late third millennium BC to Sasonian period during 224–651 AD (Boehmer, 1974). It has also been suggested that during both period buffaloes were introduced from the domesticated herds of the Indus valley areas (Cockraill, 1977). It means buffaloes were already domesticated in the Indus valley before 2350 BC.

Another almost contemporary river civilization existed along the Yangtze and the yellow rivers in the China during the Shang dynasty (about 1766–1123 BC). Evidences of tamed buffaloes during the second millennium BC are present (White, 1974). The importance of buffaloes in the socioeconomic and cultural life is evident from the depictions on the clay vessels, pillars, and paintings of the Shang dynasty period (Bentjes, 1969). In the north-east region of Thailand the bone remains of buffaloes stored during ploughing for paddy cultivation around 1600 BC suggested the taming of buffaloes in the south-east Asian countries during the second millennium BC (Higham and Kijugam, 1979).

Despite economic importance of the buffaloes through direct and indirect contribution of foods and work power supply since the beginning of river valley civilization in the Asian countries and Egypt, there appears to be lack of serious attempts in finding the correct period of domestication of water buffaloes and linkages among the different buffalo breeding tracts.

Till further evidences are collected, it may be suggested that pre-historic wild water buffalo (*Bubalus arnee*) was domesticated in the region of Indus valley and thereafter it extended to Mesopotamia in the west, and China in the east. Had domestication initiated in the Mesopotamia during the third millennium BC, it could have spread at least west to Mesopotamia during the said period (Epstein, 1969).

Clear genetic difference in two broad groups of water buffalo, i.e. river or dairy buffalo with $2n = 50$ chromosomes and another swamp buffalo with $2n = 48$ number of chromosomes shows the existence of two distinct ancestral strains of wild ancestor of domesticated Indian river buffalo, if the wild group in the reserved forest area near Kolhapur in Maharasthra does not contain $2n = 50$ number of chromosomes. The present

Asian wild buffalo in the forests of eastern states of India, Nepal Tarai, Mayanmar, Thailand, Combodia, Laos, Vietnam and probably in China is the ancestor of modern domesticated, tamed and ferel swamp buffaloes with $2n = 48$ number of chromosomes.

Development of several good breeds of the dairy type river buffalo (*Bubalus bubalis*, better to use trinomical name (*Bubalus bubalis ...*) in the Indian subcontinent suggests that it was the seat of domestication of riverine/dairy type water buffalo. Development of good number of well-defined breeds of dairy type buffalo, before the use of modern breeding system, shows that interest, deep involvement, and scientific approach of breeding through intensive selection to meet their area specific requirements. Some of the important breeds of riverine buffalo are the Murrah, Mehsana, Nili-Ravi, Kundi, Banni, Jaffarabadi, Surti, Nagpuri, Pandharpuri, Bhadawari, and Tarai. On the other hand, in case of swamp buffalo (*Bubalus bubalis carabaosis*) less serious efforts have been made in the past for the development of specific breeds. The swamp buffaloes are very low milk producers but some selection practice in some areas of the north-east states of India has considerably improved milk production capacity (Singh, 1978 and Tamuli, 1978).

Reasons for the Domestication of Water Buffalo (*Bubalus Bubalis*)

Buffaloes were initially domesticated for the assured regular supply of nutritious foods like milk and meat. Later on with the start of food grain farming buffaloes particularly that in swamp areas were found more useful for pudding the paddy fields than the cattle. Subsequently the main use of riverine and swamp buffaloes precipitated as dairy animal and draught animal respectively. In practice both types of buffaloes are used for milk, meat, and draught. The reasons for the domestication of water buffalo may be listed as follows:

1. Proximity of wild water buffalo with human inhabitation along the running rivers, and other perennial water sources and marshy lands for wallowing. This behaviour provided opportunity for taming and capture of docile buffaloes and young stock.
2. Water buffaloes are generally docile and easy to handle. Capture of female buffaloes in terminal stage of pregnancy and lactating buffaloes nursing the calves is quite easy. Although, nursing buffaloes normally do not allow strangers to handle their calves and turn highly offensive to the extent that in lack of adequate precaution their charging may be highly injurious or even fatal. But once her calf is restrained she will not go away.
3. Buffaloes are capable of thriving on large variety of herbages including the coarse grasses of low feeding value. Water logging and mud do not create problem for buffaloes rather they prefer wallowing for several hours.
4. Buffaloes continue grazing even during the rains and enjoy rain bath.
5. Production of highly nutritious foods such as milk and meat. These foods are rich sources of essential amino acids besides high energy value and good amount of dietary essential minerals and vitamins.
6. Buffalo is a powerful beast of high traction ability. It is preferred over oxen for paddy cultivation and sugarcane haulage.

Reasons for the Growth of Domesticated Water Buffaloes

The buffalo population is continuously growing in most countries of home tract and also in many of the other countries where buffaloes were introduced for good production. However, as diminishing trend in buffalo population has been observed in some of the European countries. The growth in buffalo population reflects the economic contribution and sustainability of the animal under the diversified agroclimatic of the tropical and subtropical countries. Some of the important reasons for the steady growth of buffaloes particularly that of dairy type riverine buffaloes are listed as follows:

1. **Requirement of local people:** In the Indian subcontinent buffalo is the main dairy animal and contributes more than half of the total milk production by different dairy animals.

2. **Temperament of the animal:** Domestic buffaloes are slow, docile, and harmless. Handling is very easy and any familiar person can handle buffaloes fearlessly. Buffaloes do not accept strangers easily and acquaintance need longer time and kind approach.

3. **Management case:** Docile nature, slow pace, and quite disposition make the management of buffaloes easier. They eat poor quality crop residues and dry roughages with equal interest. Although wheat straw feeding alone is non-sustainable but buffalo can consume up to 2% of body weight (John *et al.*, 1982).

4. **Ability of energy conservation:** Due to slow movement on grazing lands the buffaloes spend more time in eating and also loose less energy in movement for feeding. One can easily differentiate in the thriftness of cattle and buffaloes grazing the same pasture. The buffaloes on poor pasture maintain significantly better health than the cattle (Pathak, 1988).

5. **Consumer's choice:** In dairy buffalo dominant countries people have developed taste for the high fat containing buffalo milk. Recovery of ghee (clarified butter oil), Khoa (dehydrated milk), Chenna (coagulated milk clot), paneer, and curd from the buffalo milk is much higher than from the cow milk. Therefore, sweets and milk products are more popular. Mozrella cheese is the most popular buffalo milk product of west. Buffalo veal is quite popular in near east and European countries.

6. **Relative price of buffalo and cattle:** The buffaloes for milk, meat, and draught were much cheaper than the cattle of respective class. Although the difference in price between the two species is gradually decreasing, indeed buffalo for meat and working buffaloes are much cheaper in most of the buffalo breeding countries.
    In most of the countries buffen in much cheaper than most of the edible meats. In recent years, fattening of buffalo has shown an increasing trend due to increasing demand of good quality meat and sparing of sizable number of buffaloes for works. Despite extensive mechanization of agriculture, the use of buffaloes in paddy cultivation will continue as the buffaloes are more suitable for pudding paddy fields than the oxen.

7. **Utilization ability of course roughages:** The buffaloes consume wide variety of herbages and thrive better than cattle on coarse fodder. They eat fibrous crop residues like straws, stovers, and tops of sugarcane and root crops with great appetite. However, almost all dry cereal crop residues are highly deficient in most of the essential nutrients and energy, and need supplemental feeding of more nutritious feeds for survival (Johri *et al.*, 1982).

8. **Gainful utilization of by-products of buffaloes:** Different kinds of by-products are available from the live, slaughtered and dead animals and all are utilized for the benefits of mankind. The excreta and soiled wastes of slaughter house and eviscerated dead buffaloes are composed for manure making. The gastrointestinal tract is utilized for the preparation of casings and other products. Blood, glands, reproductive organs, and joint oil are used for pharmaceuticals and industrial

purpose. Hide is used for the manufacture of valuable leather and leather goods. Horns are used for the preparation of trophies, decoration pieces, fancy items, and ornaments, etc. Dressed carcass of fallen animals is used for the manufacture of meat meal, meat-cum-bone meal or bone meal, and autolized carcass is converted into manure. The long hairs of tail switch is used for ropes and mat making.

▶ GLOBAL DISTRIBUTION OF RIVER BUFFALOES

Although by origin water buffaloes are the animals of humid-hot tropics of Asia but due to high adaptability they have spread beyond 45°C latitude in the temperature zone. From Asia buffaloes spread to island countries of Asia-Pacific region, near east and Europe long back. Later on it was taken to south Africa and Americas for the utilization of natural pastures of wet regions for the production of meat and milk. Now river buffaloes can be seen in almost all the continents including the United States of America. The population of water buffalo is increasing at a very high rate of 12–13% per year. The buffaloes were first introduced in Brazil followed by Venezuela and Columbia for milk and meat production. Buffaloes are quite popular in Trinidad and Cuba and now they also paved into Canada, Mexico, Panama, Costa Rica, Guatemala, Honduras, and Belice (Zava, 2007).

In the home tract of swamp buffaloes, milch breeds of river buffalo (Murrah and Nili-Ravi) have been introduced for developing triple purpose (milk, meat, and work) breeds. The countries using Murrah and Nili-Ravi for crossing with swamp buffaloes are the China, Combodia, Laos, Philippines, Thailand, Vietnam, Indonesia, Malaysia and many other contries.

▶ ADAPTABILITY IN RIVER BUFFALOES

Buffaloes are normally under stress in hot climatic condition and undergo wallowing in cool water and mud hole for several hours to alleviate the heat stress. Despite this limitation largest number of buffaloes are found in the tropical countries of Asia and India houses about 70% percent of the domesticated water buffaloes on the earth (FAO, 2007). The dairy type river buffaloes are mostly congregated in the dry hot zone of India, i.e., Punjab, Haryana, Delhi, Rajasthan, Uttar Pradesh, Madhya Pradesh, and Maharashtra. Greater proportion of draught type swamp buffaloes is distributed in the east and north-east states of India, Nepal, Bangladesh, Mayanmar, Thailand, Combodia, Lao, Vietnam, China, Taiwan, Philipines, and other countries of Asia-Pacific region. Water buffaloes prefer grazing in the cool hours of morning and late in the evening to avoid heat of the sun. During hot hours grazing buffaloes cluster beneath the shady trees, or wallow in water and mud. Planting of trees with large canopy and housing in well-ventilated sheds provide protection from direct exposure to sun rays. The evaporative effect of blowing air produces cooling effect. Showers, rains, and wallowing provide comfortable environment by conduction (Minett, 1947).

Plastering of body with mud provides protection form direct solar radiation and produce cooling effect through the heat loss in the evaporation of moisture of mud on the body. The heat tolerance coefficient of buffaloes varies from 76 in adult animals to 85.15 in young calves below 1 year of age (Asker et al., 1952; Bhatnagar and Choudhary, 1960). The heat tolerance coefficient of Egyptian buffaloes is much less than 91, 85, 83, and 89 for the Egyptian native cattle, pure shorthorn cattle, pure jersey cattle, half bred shorthorn and three-fourths shorthorn cattle respectively. The average rise in body temperature on the exposure to direct sun had been much higher in buffaloes than the cattle. The buffaloes tethered in open during the daytime of summer season became restless in a short-time. Heat stress causes excessive salivation, cessation of rumination and exhaustion. The rise in body temperature and respiration rate of the buffaloes due to exposure in sunlight is much higher than the zebu and humpless European cattle (Minett, 1947; Badreldin et al., 1951; Askar et al., 1952). In the conventional management of collecting the grazing buffaloes beneath the tree or housed in airy sheds provides satisfactory protection from heat stress. There is no abnormal rise in body temperature (rectal), respiration rate and pulse rate. Significant rise in the body temperature and pulse rate indicates the higher susceptibility of buffaloes to direct solar radiation. The high haemoglobin content during summer has been considered as an index of good adaption ability of the river buffaloes are more hyperthermic on exposure to direct solar radiation due to black pigmentation of skin and scanty hairs on the body. The increase in body temperature is quite sharp and ranges from 0.3°C to 2.4°C depending on the atmospheric temperature and duration of exposure occurs on shifting the animals in sheds, sprinkling cold water, and wallowing (Villoz and Nguyen, 1939; Minette, 1947; Misra et al., 1963).

▶ HEAT PRODUCTION

Metabolic heat production for the maintenance of optimum body temperature is a normal physiological function of the living animals. Average rate of heat production in adult buffaloes is about 485 ±31 kcal per hour, which is equivalent to about 107 kcal per hour per square metre body surface area. The heat production rate in almost similar in buffaloes to that of crossbred cattle (Bos indicus x Bos Taurus) but significantly higher than the zebu cattle of India (Mullick and Kehar, 1952). The heat production rate in buffaloes is significantly influenced by the seasons and it is higher in winter season (524 kcal per hour) in comparison to summer season (462 kcal per hour). The change in body heat production is associated with changes in pulse and respiration rates (Mullick, 1964).

▶ BODY HEAT DISSIPATION ROUTES AND THERMOREGULATION

For the maintenance of normal physiological functions, the body produces heat by metabolism activities and also external heat enters into the body by radiation, conduction and convection systems. The body also looses heat through similar processes added by evaporation of moisture from the skin, respiratory exhalation and also through excretion (dung and urine). Like many homoeotherms, the loss of excess heat from the body of buffalo takes place by circulatory adjustments, cutaneous evaporation and increased respiration rate.

Circulatory Adjustment for the Maintenance of Homoeostasis in Buffaloes

In the warm weather vaso dilation of the skin takes place. This causes a steep change in the heat exchange gradient for the atmospheric below skin temperature. This steep change between the two temperature zones decreases heat loss form the body. Considerable increase in the blood and plasma volume of the buffalo occurs on rise in the atmospheric temperature (Table 1.1). This increase provides more space for the adjustment of absorbed heat in the summer season (Murti and Mullick, 1961).

TABLE 1.1: Mean volume of blood and plasma of various groups of buffaloes in different seasons of northern India at Izatnagar

Physiological stage/ age of buffalo	Blood volume (ml/kg body weight)			Plasma volume (ml/kg body weight)		
	Summer	Rains	Winter	Summer	Rain	Winter
Young buffaloes						
Below 12 months	67.2	59.3	59.9	45.0	43.3	40.7
13–24 months	57.1	56.5	54.2	41.3	39.2	36.6
Buffalo bulls	51.5	51.9	50.9	34.7	35.7	33.9
She buffaloes,						
Dry	56.0	48.5	51.0	38.2	35.1	33.6
Lactation	58.7	55.9	54.2	41.1	38.1	36.4
Pregnant	59.7	55.4	55.6	39.9	37.4	35.1
Overall	58.4	54.6	54.3	39.9	38.1	36.0
Relative (%)	107.6	100.6	100.0	110.8	105.8	100.0

Cutaneous Evaporation

The adaption mechanism of buffaloes to hot climatic conditions is limited by the black pigmentation of skin, which favours the absorption of infrared rays of solar radiation (Badreldin and Ghay, 1952). Therefore, direct exposure of buffaloes to sun should be avoided in the summer season. On poor pastures the frequency of mud plastering on the body increases because hungry buffaloes need longer time for grazing to fill their belly. Mud plastering also prevents the absorption of heat from the hot air and ground and helps in dissipation of heat from the body during the process of moisture evaporation of mud plaster on the body. Taking the advantage of this behaviour of buffaloes the owners of draught buffaloes use mud plastering or wet gunny bag for covering the head and body of buffaloes used for the traction of loaded cart during daytime in the summer season.

The buffalo possesses two types of sweat glands, i.e. the apocirne and accrino glands. The accrino glands are scanty in number (Hafez and shafei, 1954). Great variation has been reported in the density of sweat glands in different buffaloes. It ranges from 135 to 142 per cm^2 in the adult swamp buffaloes (Yamano and Ono, 1936). The average in calves of Egyption buffalo at birth is 124.8 per cm^2, which increases to 394 per cm^2 in the adult buffaloes (Hafez et al., 1955). Average 124 sweat glands per cm^2 has been recorded in buffalo bullock (Prusty, 1965) and 160 ±11 per cm^2 in the adult non-descript and Murrah buffaloes (Nair and Benjamin, 1963). Highly significant difference has been reported in the density of sweat glands of Murrah buffalo heifers of different age group (Table 1.2), which showed fluctuating pattern with the increase in age of the Murrah buffalo heifers (Sachdeva and Nagarcenker, 1981). The density of sweat glands in the buffaloes is only 6–7% of that recorded in the cattle of same area (Govindaiah and Nagarcenker, 1978). In the Egyptian buffaloes these glands are about one-third of the Egyptain cattle of same area (Hafez et al., 1955).

Mean heritability of the density of sweat glands has been estimated to be 0.67 0.37, which shows the scope of selection at young age among the progeny of selected sires for better homeothermy (Sachdeva and Nagarcenker, 1981).

The muzzle glands of buffaloes are the compound tubuloacinar and multilobular seromucous modified sweat glands. The glandular acini are made of myoepithelial cells and a basement membrane (Quasem et al., 1976). The presence of sweat drops on the muzzle does not require justification regarding the sweating of muzzle glands but there is doubt about the function of sweat glands on the body and their role in heat regulation (Prusty, 1973). This doubt was removed in subsequent studies. Although body surface evaporation through sweating is apparently insensible but has shown the functional characters of sweat glands in the skin of buffaloes (Joshi et al., 1968; Agarwal et al., 1983). Average sweating rate is lower in winter and highest in summer. The sweat excretion rate increases considerably with the increase in environmental temperature (Joshi et al., 1968). Average sweating rate between 37–45°C has been about 21.7 ± 2.2 g per square metre per hour in the adult Murrah buffalo bulls (Agarwal et al., 1983). Sweating is though limited but contributes in the amelioration of heat stress through the loss of heat in the evaporation of sweat. Approximately 0.58 kcal heat is lost in the evaporation of 1 g water.

Respiratory Heat Dissipation

It is observed that panting and parotid salivation increase during high environmental temperature by about 2 to 2.5 times. The buffalo has a relatively lower level of respiration rate, body temperature, and pulse rate than the cattle and shows noticeable distress in hot climate (Badreldin et al., 1951; Pandey and Roy, 1969b; Chikamune and Shimizu, 1983). The reaction of buffaloes is more vigorous in their increased rate of respiration and higher body temperature at air temperature about 74.4 8°F or 23.55°C (Goswmai and Narain, 1962). During summer months the buffaloes exhibit an increased respiration rate associated with rise in body temperature and pulse rate on direct exposure to sun light. Sudden decline in respiration rate occurs when buffaloes are removed from the sun, but fall in body temperature takes place after a latent period of about 10 minutes and pulse rate falls after about 40 minutes (Table 1.2). Respiration evaporation is more important in buffaloes than the other mechanism for the regulation of body heat balance. The rise in respiration rate during hot climate is necessary and effective in maintaining the body temperature with in the physiological limits (Kamal and Ibrahim, 1969; Pandey and Roy, 1969).

TABLE 1.2: Effect of direct exposure to sunlight and then return to shade on some physiological reactions in buffaloes

Treatments	Body temperature	Respiration rate per minute	Pulse rate per minute
Normal housing at 10 AM	38.3	36	54
Exposure to direct			
Sunlight	10 AM		
	11 AM		
	12 AM		
On return back to shade, 12 NOON			
1 PM	38.6	40	53
2 PM	38.2	32	51

▶ EFFECT OF LATITUDE AND ALTITUDE ON THE ADAPTABILITY OF WATER BUFFALOES

Both dairy type river buffalo and draught type swamp buffaloes are distributed from equatorial zone to beyond 45°C latitude in both the hemispheres.

The performance of local Mediterranean buffalo and exotic Murrah buffaloes are quite satisfactory in the European countries like Bulgaria, Italy, Romania, etc. though Murrah is a native of hot-humid tropics of India. The Murrah and other breeds of Indian dairy buffaloes are performing satisfactorily in the hot and humid –hot climate of Indonesia, Srilanka, Malayasia, Thailand, China, Combodia, Loas, S.R. Vietnam, Singapore, Philippines, etc. These buffaloes have adapted well to the high altitude of Uttrakhand, Himachal Pradesh, Nepal, Sikkim, and Bhutan. The increase in migration rate domestic buffaloes specially the dairy breeds of the Indian subcontinent to Brazil, Venezuella, and other countries of Americas show their high ability of adapting in diversified agroclimatic conditions provided they are protected from the fatal diseases and water supply is assured. Protection from extreme climatic conditions like direct solar heat higher than 35°C for longer period and chilling frost for several days. Rains and running water are the highly desirable situations for the dairy type river buffaloes of Indian origin.

▶ BUFFALOES IN MYTHOLOGY, RELIGION, AND SPORTS

Some information about the use of buffaloes in mythology, religion, and sports, etc. are presented in brief to show the closeness of this multipurpose beast with mankind since prehistorical period. India is the home land of riverine buffalo while major part of east and south aisa is the homeland of swamp buffaloes, this animal had been closely associated with the socioeconomic activities of the besides the main contribution of milk and draught power.

1. In India and Nepal, ritual sacrifice of entire male buffaloes had been quite common at the festive occasion of ' Dusshera or Durgapooja'. Goddess Durga incarnated as 'Chamunda' and killed 'Mahishasur' (means demon buffalo) at Mysore. The word Mysore is actually a distorted form of the original word *Mahish oor'* means the 'chest of buffalo'. It is believed that goddess 'Chamunda' after killing 'Mahishasur' constructed a town on his chest and named it 'Mahishoor' which in use subsequently became the present day 'Mysore'.

2. During Mahabharat period 'Pandavas' charged with the sin of homicide for murdering cousins 'Kauravas' in war. To get pardoned they required the blessings of Lord 'Shiva' but thou went in hide. In search of 'Shiva' the Pandavas reached 'Kedarnath'. The 'Shiva' took the form of a buffalo bull and mixed with the buffaloes. Some how one of the Pandavas, Bhim suspected that robust buffalo bull in the herd is Shiva. He then moved to catch him. The moment Shiva saw Bhim running to him Shiva started entering into the earth but Bhim succeeded in catching him by tail. At Kedarnath in high Himalaya the Lord Shiva is worshiped in the form of Buffalo bull with front buried in the earth and hind part on the ground.

3. Lord Shiva created 'Yamraj' the god of death from eight strong buffaloes for infusing great strength in him necessary for performing the hard job of managing the death of creatures on the earth.

4. The gesture shown by a gatekeeper of lord Shiva palace named 'Nontakara' by throwing flower on a nymph of palace angered the Shiva and he was made a buffalo 'Tarap'. The gesture was regarded misbehaviour. Later on his request for relief was considered for release from buffalo life. For this he was to be killed by his own male progeny. He was provided 5000 breedable buffaloes. One of these female buffaloes conceived but she was knowing that if she delivers a male calf, that may kill 'Tarap'. Thus, she ran away to hide herself in a cave where she delivered a male calf and

named it 'Tarapee'. The calf grew as a strong buffalo bull matching his father. The mother of 'Tarapeer' made all possible efforts for preventing encounter between father and son but failed. Subsequently, in a fierce fighting 'Tarapee' killed 'Tarap' to revent back to original 'Nantakara'.

Further survival of 'Tarapee' was dangerous for others and he was killed by the great warrier monkey king 'Bali' on the dictate of the God.

5. In the China, the founder of 'Taoism', the great philosopher monk 'Lao Tzu' left China after completing his jog on the back of a male water buffalo to west not to return again. The period of 'Laotz' is about sixth century BC (Cu-I, Tai, 1959). This shows the domestication of buffalo during the period of Taoism.

6. The albinioid specimen of carabao (swamp buffalo) is regarded as a notional symbol in the Philippines.

7. In Indonesia, Torajan community, is believed to come from Combodia in boats and settled in isolation on hills. This was a community of illiterate people of fierce nature and inaccessible for the native Indonesia. Later on this community was gradually brought into mainstream by the efforts of the European missionaries during the beginning of the twentieth century. Torajan people practice many rituals which are performed at different occasions by the specific priests. Sacrifice of buffaloes is quite common at such occasions.

The buffalo is also considered a symbol of fertility and worshiped for the maintenance of fertility in humans and worshiped. A famous 'Mabua' ceremony is organized every 12 years and the priests wearing dress decorated with buffalo horns in head dress and dance around a sacred tree.

8. Ritual sacrifice of buffalo is practiced in Laos and number slaughtered depends on the size of community for feast.

9. In Vietnam water buffalo is the symbol of prosperity and these are more precious than the common member of the family. In ancient time the name of west lake Ha Noi was *Kim Nguu* means the 'golden buffalo'. Probably due to this reason the mascot of the 22nd southeast Asian Games organized in Vietnam was a 'golden water buffalo'. The water buffalo is a symbol of power and strength of the martial race the native of Vietnam.

10. In Malaysia buffaloes are sacrificed at major sociocultural occasions for the community feast. Some of the such occasions are the laying of foundation for the construction of house. At this occasion head and legs of the sacrified buffalo are buried deep beneath the central pillar. The remaining flesh is served in community feast. However, albinoid buffaloes are considered inauspicious and they are not used for ritual sacrifices.

11. In Combodia buffaloes are used in religious functions and processions. The decorated buffalo bulls and calves suckling the dams are carved on the walls of the world famous 'Ankore batt temple' constructed during 9th to 10 century AD.

▶ BUFFALO FIGHT FESTIVALS OF DIFFERENT COUNTRIES

Buffalo fight festivals are quite common in one or the other form in most of the Asian countries in the home tract of water buffalo.

1. Organization of buffalo bullfight is quite common in Assam (India) at the festival of 'Bhogali Bihoo'. It is called 'Moh Yuddha' (fight between buffaloes). For this purpose buffalo bulls are specially reared and trained. The buffalo bulls participating in the fight festival may be from the different groups of same village or from different

villages. The 'Ahotguri' village in Naogaon district in upper Assam is famous for organizing 'Moh Yuddha' competition.

2. **Mud race of buffaloes in southern India:** This is a festival of Palakkad district of Keral and Mangalore district of Karnataka in India. The male buffaloes are yoked in pairs and driven to run in mud by the person standing on the wooden plank pulled by the racing buffaloes. This is known as 'Kambala' race. The race is competition and each participant wants to wean the race.

3. **Bullfight show at the occacion of Goberdhan pooja in India:** In greater part of India workship of mount Goberdhan is celebrated on the next day of Dipawali festival. Both cow and buffalo bulls may be used for the show. It is a nonfatal fight between the two bulls of comparable power. In the region of Rohilkhand in the northern part of India generally buffalo bulls are used for the friendly fight show. The bulls may be from the same village or different villages. Competition is also organized and prizes are distributed. A red or orange scarf is tied around the horns of winner bull. The show is witnessed by large number of villagers and necessary arrangements are kept ready for stopping the fierce fight, if occurs due to excitement during the show.

4. The buffalo fight festival of Thailand is known as 'Ko Samui' and generally organized at the occasion of New Year Day in January and 'Songkaran' in April. For this purpose buffalo bulls are raised and trained for head-on fight. It is a prize winning competition. The buffalo that turns away and run away is the looser. The fight is mostly nonfatal. The market value of winner buffalo increases many fold.

5. The annual water buffalo race festival of Thailand or Chon Buri water buffalo race. Chon Buri is a town situated about 70 km away from the Bangkok in south. It is an annual festival celebrated in the month of October before harvesting the paddy crop. This is a newer festival evolved over hundred years ago from the casual argument between the two buffalo owners of Chon Buri claiming fast racing ability and agility of their buffalo. This has now become the annual festival attracting large number of tourists from different countries to witness buffalo race. The participant join the race in group of 5 to 6 jokies riding bare back buffaloes. The total number of buffaloes may be more than 300.

6. **Water buffalo race festival of Vihear Gour village in Combodia**: It is an annual festival of Vihear Guor village of Combodia to honour the pledge made to a spirit for protecting the farm animals from dreaded diseases organize a buffalo race on the last day of the "Pchum ben" festival. This village is situated about 30 km north east from the capital city 'Phnom Penh'. It is said that more than thousand years ago large number of draught cattle used in various agricultural operations were killed by an unknown disease. Thereafter they shot the help of a sprit for soving their animals. Since then people of this village arrange buffalo race annually on a fixed date to please the spirit as per pledge made at that time. At this occasion the horns of the buffaloes are decorated by wrapping a coloured cloth. The jocky rides on bare back and excite the racing buffalo by bouncing for high speed.

7. **'Karapan Sapi' buffalo race festival of Madura, Indonesia:** The Community of Madura island in east Java of Indonesia organize buffalo race events at least three times every year particularly in the month of August, September and October. People are generally free from the agricultural works. For this purpose selected buffalo calves are raised for strength and trained for high speed for winning the race. The

owner of winner receives prize and the market value of winner buffalo increases many folds. The high caloric nutritious diets of these racing buffaloes may be made of several raw eggs and honey fortified with different kinds of medicinal herbs. Some of the towns famous for attractive buffalo race are Bangkalan, Pamekasan and Sampang.

8. **Water buffalo race on the occasion of 'Babulang' ceremony at Sarawak in Malaysia:** The 'Babulang' is the grand festival of Borneo island inhabited by the 'Bisaya' community inhabiting in Limbang of Sarawak province. At this occasion water buffaloes are put to racing competition known as 'Ratu babulang'.

9. **Buffalo fight festival of 'Do Son' in Hiphong city:** It is an annual festival celebrated on the 9th day of the eight month of the Lunar calendar of Vietnam. The race is complete in three rounds. Greater proportion of the participating buffaloes are eliminated from the final race during first and second races organized in the middle of the 5th and 8th month of the lunar calendar of Vietnam.

   For this fighting festival male buffaloes calves are selected young and raised on highly nutritious diets during growth. The animals are given rigorous training for fighting. For this purpose an experienced fighter buffalo is put against the novice. The buffaloes are used for competition at 4 to 5 years of age. The animal must appear masculine with robust disposition, broad and deep chest with well-sprung ribs, long groin, a long and strong neck and bow shaped massive horns. The feeding, management and training of these buffaloes are arranged separated and kept away from the common buffaloes.

   It is an elaborate festival. The worship ceremony is performed up to mid day or lunch time. The ceremony begins with a great procession chair carried by six strong youth followed by a team of eight singers. In the procession finally selected six buffaloes covered with red drape and reddish horn band are lead in the procession. On the fighting ground the two opposite teams stand near their flag known as 'Ngu phung' holding their buffalo opposite each other. Now a signal is given to begin. The buffaloes of both sides are brought against each other within 20 m distance. The buffaloes of either side is left free at them same time by releasing the rope tied with nose peg or nose ring. At this time a group excite their buffalo by shouting. At the end of fight time the winner buffalo is received with applause and rewarded by the leader of community.

   This buffalo fighting festival is organized annually for worshiping a water god and also for showing gratitude to martial spirit of the local people, the 'Hien Sinh' custom.

10. **Makepung buffalo race in Negara of Bali island of Indonesia:** It is an annual event of Bali island organized on every Sunday from July to October. The buffalo bulls are specially reared and trained for winning the race. For this race a pair of buffalo bulls is yoked in a chariot. Two pairs participate in each round of race on a dusty tract of about 1.5 km. The sport ground is situated in the interior part about 150 km away from the Kuta, Negara. It is a traditional race organized by Bali people (Nick, 2006).

11. **Water buffalo in folk lore of Indonesia:** In a popular folklore of Java in Indonesia the victory of Javanese queen over the king of Sumatra is nawated. The queen won with the help of an unfair fight between the buffalo bulls of the two kingdoms. To commemorate the occasion the ladies decorate the head covering part of special dress to depict the horns of buffalo. The male folk of Java also wear a head dress

decorated with the pair of buffalo horns and several varieties of medicinal herbs. These are considered to infuse power and increase the lifespan of the person.

REFERENCES

Agarwal, S P, Singh, N, Agarwal, V K and Dwarkanath, P K, 1983. Indian J. Anim. Hlth., 22; 29.34.

Asker, A.A., Ghany, M A and Raglab, M T 1952. Nature, London, 170; 457–458.

Badreldin, A L and Ghany, M A 1954. J. Agric Sci., Camb., 44; 160–164.

Badreldin, A L, Oloufa, M M and Ghany, M A 1951. Nature, London, 167, 856.

Bats, M S 1973. Indus valley civilization. Cultural Heritage of India. Ram Krishna Mission Institute of culture, Calcutta.

Bhatnagar, D S and Choudhary, N C 1960. Indian Vet J, 37, 404–409.

Boehmer, R M Von, 1974. Zeittschrift fur Ashyriologie, 64; 1–19.

Brentjes, B 1969. Zeitshschrift fur saugetierkunde, 34; 3

Chikamunl, T and Shimizu, H 1983. Indian J. Anim. Sic., 53; 595–604.

Cockrail, R W 1977. The water buffalo. FAO, Rome

Epstein, H 1969. Domestic Animal of China, CAB Pub, London.

FAO, 2007, FAO stat, Rome.

Goswami, S.B. Narian, P. 1962. Indian J. Vet Sci. Anim. Husb., 32; 112–116.

Hafez, ESE. Badreldin, A L and Shafei, M M 1955. J. Agric Sci., Camb. 46: 19–30.

Higham, C and Kijugam, A, 1979. J. Archeol Sci., 6; 211–213.

Johri, C B. Ranjhan, S.K. and Pathak, N.N. 1982. Indian J. Anim Sci.

Joshi. B C, McDowell, R E and Sadhu, D P. 1968. J. Dairy Sci. 51, 1688–1692.

Kamal, T.H. and Ibahi, 1969. Intern J. Biomet, 12: 275–285.

Minett, F.C. 1947. J. Anim, Sci., 6; 35–49.

Misra, M.S, Sengupta, B. P and Roy, A 1963. Indian J. Dairy Sci. 17; 203–215

Moran, J.B. 1973. Australian J. Agric. Res. 24: 775–782.

Mullick, D N 1964. Indian J. Dairy Sci., 17, 45–50.

Mullick, D N and Kehar, N D, 1952. Annual report, A.N. Division, IVRI, Izatnagar.

Murti, T.L. and Mullick, D.N 1961. Annual Biochem Exptl. Med., 21; 91–96.

Nair, P.G. and Benjamin, B.R. 1963. Indian J. Vet Sci. Anim. Husb., 33; 102–106.

Ou-Tai–1959. Chiense Mythology, New Larouse Encyclopedia of Mythology, Prometeheus Press, Paris.

Pandey, M.D. and Roy, A. 1969a. Indian J. Anim, Sci., 39, 325–330.

Pandey, M.D. and Roy, A. 1969b. Indian J. Anim. Sci., 39, 376–386.

Pathak, N N 1988. Feeding of buffalo,IVRI, Izatnagar

Pathak, N N 2003. Buffaloes in Ancient India, Chapter 14, Veterinary Science and Animal Husbandry in Ancient India, IVRI, Izatbnagar.

Prusthy, J. N 1965. Indian vet. J, 12; 33–37.

Quasem, M A, Mia, M A, Khan, MAB and Talukdar, A H 1976. Bangladesh Vet J., 10; 23–29.

Ranjhan, S.K. and Pathak, N N 1978. Management and Feeding of Buffaloes. Vikas Pub., New Delhi.

Sachdeva, G.K. and Nagarcenker, R. 1981. World Rev. Anim. Prod., 17(1); 41–44.

Singh, M. 1978. MVSc. Thesis, Assam Agril University Campus, Khanapara, Guwahati.

Tamuli, B C, 1978. MVSc Thesis, Assam Agril University campus Khanapara, Guwahati.

Villoz, R and Nguyen, Ngoc Minh 1939. Rec. Med., Vet Exot, 12; 147.

White, L. 1974. J. Medieval Studies, 49, 201–221.

Yamane, J. and Ono, Y. 1936. Mem. Fac Sci. Agric,Talhoku, 10; 87–136.

2

Buffaloes of the World

Basically buffaloes have been evolved as a tropical beast capable of thriving on tropical herbage of relatively low palatability, digestibility, and nutritive value for most of the other ruminant species. However, due to high adaptability Asiatic particularly the dairy type Indian (riverine) water buffaloes have spread in many countries and satisfactorily performing in the subtropical or even for design temperate agroclimatic conditions of the European countries. Asian buffaloes have high affinity for water and Indian dairy or riverine buffaloes like wallowing in water while draught type swamp buffaloes prefer lying in mud holes. The African wild buffaloes need water daily for drinking and live near the water sources but they are not fond of wallowing.

▶ TYPES OF BUFFALOES

There are two types of true buffaloes on the earth found in the tropical and subtropical zones of Asia, Asia-Pacific islands, and Africa. A pseudobuffalo has been described from the hilly forest areas of easset Indo-China region (Floffmann, 1986; Kuztentsov et al., 2001). The two major groups of true buffaloes are: (i) the African wild buffalo, syncerus species, and (ii) the Asiative water buffaloes, *Bubalus* spp. The two groups of true buffaloes are independent and so far no fertile breeding could occur despite housing eligible male and female together for several years in properly managed housing. There is no record of hybrid birth of African wild buffalo (*Syncerus* spp.) and Asiatic water buffalo (*Bubalus* spp.).

▶ CLASSIFICATION OF TRUE BUFFALOES

The buffaloes are true ruminants (pecora) of the suborder Ruminantia and family Bovidae. The two subfamilies representing true buffaloes are the: (i) Bubalina and (ii) Syncerina. The phylogeny tree of true buffaloes has been shown in Table 2.1.

▶ THE AFRICAN WILD BUFFALOES (*Syncerus* spp.)

The native African buffaloes distributed from the south bordering area of Sahara desert to south Africa are one of the large herbivorous game of Africa extensively hunted for hide, flash, and long horns (Fig. 2.1). The trophies made of buffalo horns fetch handsome amount. The bulky, robust, and aggressive beast dislikes the presence of humans and charges humans when sighted in their territory. An wounded buffalo is more aggressive (Stuart and Stuart, 1997). Probably witnessing of frequent killing of

TABLE 2.1:	Phylogeny tree of true buffaloes	
Kingdom	Animalia	
Phylum	Cordata	
Class	Mamalia	
Subclass	Ungulata (hooved animals)	
Order	Artiodactyla	
Suborder	Ruminantia (pecova)	
Family	Bovidae	
Subfamily	(1) Bufalina and (2) Syncrine	
Genus	*Bubalus*	*Syncerus*
Species	*Bubalus bubalis*	(1) *Syncerus caffer*
		(2) *Syncerus nanus*

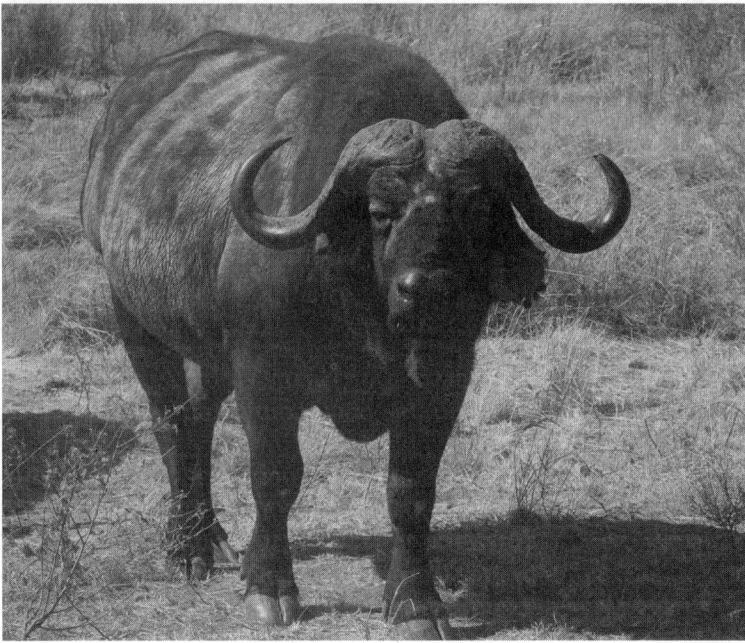

Fig. 2.1: *Syncerus* sp.

the members of their group by human hunters has infused hatred in their heart and mind for the humans. The African wild buffaloes are largest and heaviest of the other wild native ruminants of Africa but they are lighter than the two main Asiatic water buffaloes, the dairy type riverine buffaloes and the draught type swamp buffaloes and their wild ancestor *Bubalus arnee*.

▶ TYPES OF AFRICAN WILD BUFFALOES

Although there is not yet full agreement on the nomenclature of African wild buffaloes but broadly they are divided into two morphologically and genetically distinct broad species: the large size grayish black to dark black buffaloes of savannah commonly known as cape buffaloes or Savanah buffaloes, *Syncerus* caffs and another small size red to reddish brown buffaloes of forests in hilly region commonly known as Congo or red buffalo or forest buffalo, *Syncerus nanus*. The massive cape buffaloes have been further differentiated into at least three sub species, the west wild African buffalo, Syncerus caffer brachycrus, the central African wild buffalo, Syncerus caffer aequinotialis and the south African wild buffalo, Syncerus caffer caffer (East, 1999). Similarly, two subspecies of Congo or red wild African buffaloes have been described (Kington, 1997). Since it is not possible to restrict breeding among the different subspecies living in adjoining locale of wild habitat, there are different type of variants are born. It is also very difficult to closely observed their characteristics and behaviour in wild state. Such indiscriminate breeding among different subspecies has resulted in the birth of different types of unstable crossbreds. Therefore, for all practical purposes the African wild buffaloes may be classified into two widely different and distinct groups of large size cape savannah buffalo of black colour with 3 subspecies, i.e. syncus caffer brachycrus (Synerus c. brochycerus), Syncerus C. aequinoctialis and Syncerus C. Caffer predominantly found in the west, control and south parts of the tropical African savannah respectively. The S.C. brachycerus has been identified intermediate in size and also called Sudan type buffalo (buchholtz, 1990). The second major type of red to reddish brown buffaloes of smaller size have been distinguished into 2 subspecies, the red forest buffalo, S.C. nanus and another red to reddish brown colour S.C. mathewsi.

All types of African wild buffaloes are now protected animals in different National wildlife parks in many African countries. Few specimen are also available in the zoological gardens of different countries. The buffaloes maintained in the national wildlife parks are mostly species specific and after few generations it may be possible to distinctly describe the morphological and genetic characteristic of the two main species of African wild buffaloes and their five subspecies (three of Cape buffaloes and two of the Cong type African wild buffaloes). On the basis of present information gathered through several studies (Buchholtz, 1990, Nowak, 1991, Alden *et al*, 1995, Nowak, 1997, Mcdonald, 2006) have been summarized (Table 2.2) for the cape (*Syncerus caffer*) and the Congo (*Syncerus nanus*) type African wild buffaloes.

TABLE 2.2: Some characteristics of the café (*Syncerus caffer*) and the Congo (*Syncerus nanus*) type African wild buffaloes

Traits	Sex	Cape buffalo (Syncerus caffer)	Congo buffalo (Syncerus nanus)
Length (cm)		240–440	170–220
Shoulder height (cm)		75–110	50–80
Adult weight (kg)	Male	500–900 (700)	300–400 (320)
	Female	300–700 (500)	250–300 (260)
Tail length (cm)		75–110	50–80
Colour		Grayish black to dark black	Red to reddish brown
Herd size		Few hundred to more than 1000	Few, 10 to 20
Horns	Male	Heavy and large	Heavy and short
	Female	Thinner and long	Thinner and short
Habitat		Grassland with scattered shade trees and water sources	High land and forest area near water source

The colour of calf at birth and in early life is red to reddish brown. The colour changes gradually with the increase in age and turns grayish black to black in cape buffalo (*Syncerus caffer*) and remains red to reddish brown in Congo (*Syncerus nanus*) buffalo. However, in the areas of mixing of two major types several crossbreds of widely variable colour may be seen between the two extremes. The body of calf is covered with soft coat which becomes scarce with the increase in age (Buchholtz, 1990; Nowak, 1991; Kingdom, 1997). The body colour of males is darker than the females of the corresponding species. The head is broad and dome shaped in cape buffaloes and slightly convex in Congo type. The horns always emerge together and the entire crown. The horns are heavier in male than in the female (Mannuqicky, 1960; Van Zyl and Skead, 1964).

▶ GENETIC DIFFERENCE BETWEEN THE TWO MAIN SPECIES OF AFRICAN WILD BUFFALOES

Although fertile breeding occurs between the two main species of African wild buffaloes, *Syncerus caffer* and *Syncerus nanus* but chromosome numbers are different. The chromosome number $2n = 52$ is for cape type large buffalo *Syncerus caffer* while $2n = 54$ is for smaller red or Congo type buffalo. Crossbreds of two main types many contain 52, 53 or 54 number of chromosomes. Probably there is no information about the fertility status of crosses between the two species of African wild buffaloes.

So far no fertile breeding by natural or artificial method between the *Syncerus* spp. and *Bubalus* spp. has been recorded anywhere. In Vadodara zoo of Gujarat in India a fertile bull of cake buffalo (*Syncerus caffer*) was housed with fertile few Indian dairy buffaloes (*Bubalus bubalis*) for several years without any sign of fertilization.

▶ TRINOMIAL NOMENCLATURE OF AFRICAN WILD BUFFALOES

Morphologically and genetically there are two major types of African wild buffaloes. The large size beast of long horns and grayish black to dark black body colour is called cape buffalo of African Savannah, the *Syncerus caffer* with $2n = 52$ numbe of chromosomes. The second major type is the much smaller Cong buffalo of brownish red to red colour and small size horns, *Syncerus nanus* with $2n = 54$ number of chromosomes. The massive cape or Savannah buffaloes are further differentiated into at least 3 subspecies: (i) the west African wild buffaloes, (ii) The central Africa wild buffalo, and (iii) the southern African wild buffalo (East, 1999). Similarly, the cong type red wild buffaloes have been differentiated in to 2 subspecies (Kingdom, 1997). These 5 subspecies of African wild buffaloes, *Syncerus* spp. have been given trinormial names of cape (*Syncerus caffer*) and 2 subspecies of Congo (*Syncerus namus*) are genetically different with $2n = 52$ and $2n = 54$ number of chromosomes respectively. The trinomial names for cape type *S.C. aequinoctialis*, *S.C. brachycerus*, and *S.C. caffer* and that of Congo or red type *S.C. mathewsi* and *S.C. nanus* give the impression that all the five sub species belong to *Syncerus caffer* type.

Therefore, to make the identification of two major types of African wild buffaloes in trinomial nomenclature it will be more appropriate to use earlier binomial names as prefix in the trinomial system. Adoptation of rearranged trinomial nomenclature will be more specific and the name itself will provide important characteristics of the different subspecies of the African wild buffaloes (*Syncerus species*). The rearranged names of so far differentiated five subspecies may be adopted as follows:

1. The trinomial names of west African (*S.C. brachycrus*), central African (*S.C. aequinoctialis*) and southern African wild buffalo (*S.C. caffer*) will remain unchanged.

2. The trinomial names of two subspecies of Congo type red buffalo (*Syncerus nanus*) will be *S.C. mathewsi* in place of *S.C. mathewsi* and *S.n. nanus* in place of *S.C. nanus* fro the forest type and hill type of Cong type African wild buffaloes.

The African wild buffaloes have been also differentiated into three species on the basis of morphological characteristics. These are largest Cape type, *Syncerus caffer*, intermediate type *Syncerus brachycrus* and smallest red variety, *Syncerus nanus* (Buchholtz, 1990; kingdom, 1997). Some of the observed physical charachteristics of these three species are presented in Table 2.3).

TABLE 2.3: Some physical characteristics of three species of African wild buffaloes

Characteristics	Syncerus caffer	Syncerus brachycrus	Syncerus nanus
Body size	Large	Medium	Small
Height (cm)	140–150	125–140	100–125
Body weight (kg)	500–1000	350–700	520–350
Body colour	Black	Grayish black	Red to brown
Horn size	Long	Long	Short
Head	Convex	Convex	Less convex
Herd size	Large	Large	Small
Families in herd	Many	Many	Mostly single

However, this classification (Table 2.3) may not be acceptable on genetical probing because the number of chromosomes of *Syncerus caffer* and *Syncerus brachycrus* are same $2n = 52$. Since, there is clear difference in chromosome number of red buffalo ($2n = 54$) than the other African wild buffaloes ($2n = 52$), it would be more appropriate to consider cape type Savannah buffaloes as one species of genus *Syncerus*, the *syncerus caffer* (S.C.) and small size red buffaloes of Congo type as a second species of *Syncerus*, i.e. *Syncerus nanus* (S.n), the subspecies of there two major species of the African wild buffaloes may be identified as 3 subspecies of *S. Caffer* and 2 subspecies of *S. nanus*. The trinomial nomenclature of 3 subspecies of *S. Caffer* will be *S.C. brachycrus*, *S.C. aequirnoctialis* and *S.C. caffer* for the west, central and southern types respectively. *S.C. brachycrus* is intermediate in size among the 3 subspecies (Buccholtz, 1970) kingdom, 1997). The two subspecies of *S. nanus* should be *S.n. nanus* and *S.n. mathewsi* which are almost half of the cape buffaloes in body size and colour ranges from red to redish brown.

The calves of all types of African wild buffaloes are generally grayish brown to red at birth and gradually acquire the characteristic colour of subspecies during growth phase. The body colour of cape type or Savannah buffaloes and Congo type or red buffaloes differs widely. There are several types of crossbreds of the two major species and found mostly in the areas where two major groups live in neighbourhood. The body of adult buffaloes is covered with scanty short hairs. The density of body coat decreases with the advancement of age. The body colour is highly variable due to uncontrolled interbreeding among the different species and sub species. The males of all the sub-species are darker in coat colour than the females the respective subspecies (Buccholtz, 1970; Nowak, 1997).

▶ **SOCIAL BEHAVIOUR AND HERD ORGANIZATION PATTERN IN AFRICAN WILD BUFFALOES**

The informations available are more on the lifestyle of large herds of black Cape or Savannah buffaloes because they live in large herds on grazing lands. The much smaller red to redish brown Congo buffaloes live in very small herds (mostly family herds) in the forest of hilly region. The cape group of buffaloes spent more time for wallowing and grazing and Congo type small buffaloes live hidden for long-time in the forest and hills. The social organization of large herds of Cape buffaloes is based on male hierarchy.

The most dominant, robust, and aggressive adult male buffalo controls the herd but other eligible adult males also live with the herd during different periods. The large herds are differentiated into the following groups:

    i. Large groups of nursing female buffaloes with calves on foot.

    ii. Pregnant buffaloes, both pregnant heifers and buffalo cows.

    iii. Adult males that isolate from the females during the off breeding season.

    iv. The smaller groups of juvenile males from weaning to puberty.

    v. The retired males to live a hermit life under the protection of large herd.

The various factors governing the division of large herds into different smaller groups within the herd are:

    a. Herbage cows of the Savannah,

    b. **Breeding season:** Different eligible buffalo bulls form their groups of breedable females for covering during the breeding season.

    c. **Age of the animals:** The groups of weaned growing calves live in smaller groups during prepubertal stages of growth.

    d. **The habitats of predators:** The herding systems in African wild buffaloes (*Syncerus* spp.) have been evolved to provide safety and greater protection from the lions.

The Savannah herbage cover provides fodder (Sinclair, 1974) and scattered trees on the Savannah provide shade and shelter when sun turns hot during the daytime.

The Congo type red buffaloes of forest and hills live in very small herds of mostly 8–10 animals of generally same maternal group.

These are almost half of the cape buffalo in size with short, thick, and inwards curved crescent horns with blunt tips. The herd may include an adult male, few females, and followers. The groups are probably based on family system which divides on increasing the number of eligible males for breeding. The spent aged males retire from breeding and isolate themselves from the groups. Small groups of retired males live nearer to active herds for protection from the predators.

All types of African wild buffaloes are always found near the water sources preferably running water sources (Moloiy, 1973).

▶ PREDATORS OF AFRICAN WILD BUFFALOES

1. Before imposing strict restriction and providing protection under different state rules human hunters were the main predators. The large number of buffaloes were hunted for the valuable large horns used for the manufacture of trophies mounted on wood or metal. The flash was used for food and hide was used for making leather goods.
2. Lions are the natural predators of grazing beasts including buffaloes on the African Savannah and grasses of forest in hilly region.
3. Crocodiles hunt buffaloes during drinking, wallowing, and crossing the water sources. Crocodiles preferably capture old and weak, solitary animals, and young calves (Buchholtz, 1990).

4. Wild canines rarely kill young calves isolated from the herd, weak animals, and immovable injured buffaloes. Wild canines normally feed on the dead carcass and residues left by the large felines.

▶ LONGIVITY OF AFRICAN WILD BUFFALOES

The lifespan of African wild buffaloes may extend beyond 29 years recorded in a zoo buffalo. In captive habitat lifespan is 20–26 years but wild buffalo has been seen up to 18 year old (Buccholtz, 1990; Nowak, 1991). However, with the protection provided in different wildlife parks in most of the African countries may be helpful in increasing the lifespan of African wild buffaloes.

▶ DISTRIBUTION OF AFRICAN WILD BUFFALOES

The homelands of African wild buffalo extends south of the Sahara desert covering entire central African territory and northern region of the south African (Buchholtz, 1990). The African countries inhabiting mostly protected herds of the African wild buffaloes are Angola, Benin, Botswana, Burkina-Fasco, Burundi) Camerron, Central African Republic, Chad, Congo, Democratic Republic of the Congo, Cote d'Ivoire, Equatorial Guinea, Ethiopia, Gabon, Gambia, Ghana, Guinea, Guinea-Bissao, Kenya, Liberia, Malawi, Mali, Mozambique, Namibia, Niger, Nigeria, Rwanda, Senegal, Sierra –Leone, Somalia, South Africa, Sudan, Swaziland, United Republic of Tanzania, Tongo, Uganda, Zambia, and Zimbabwe (IUCN, 2004).

▶ RELATIONSHIP WITH HUMANS

African wild buffaloes consider human as enemy number one due to continuous observation of killing their herd mates with arrows and firearms for centuries. This has infused hatred for humans in the behaviour.

African wild buffalo particularly the large size and black cape buffalo is one of the 'big five' beasts of Africa also known as the 'black death'. The wild buffalo kills many people every year and the number may be up to zoo. Such high killing has been also claimed for the other African wild beasts like Hippopotamus and crocodiles (http//www.on-the-matix.com/africa/buffalo.asp.). African wild buffaloes are very dangerous and famous for notorious behaviour among all the five big games of African Savannah. Wounded buffaloes has been found to be very dangerous by the hunters. Such animals hide in tall grass and attack the hunters (http//www.safaribwana.com/ANIMALS/animpages/buffalo.htm.).

▶ RELATIONSHIP AMONG THE MEMBERS OF HERD

Informations regarding relationship among the animals of herds is more available for the Cape type living in large herds more than a thound heads (Stuart and Stuart, 1997). The male buffaloes detached from a herd often lead a solitary life or several such males for a bachelor group. Herd life is more useful than the solitary living. There is strong bondage among the members of herds and between the small herds of large herds. In herd life, there is a system of communication. The leaders of herd pass on informations regarding the search of more lush green pastures and water sources for sharing. Females of herd maintain stronger bonds and provide protection from the predators like lion (Mc Donald, 2006). If a member of herd attached by lion (s), the members of the herd quickly respond to bellowing distress calls and quickly run to save. The action is properly organized and a herd of buffalo is capable to chase away a full pride of lions for saving the herd fellow from their clutch (Mills and Hes, 1997).

When a member of herd is chased by a pride of lions or pack of canines, the members of the herd take position by clustering closer in a offensive form. The calves are collected in the middle. The herd makes all possible attempts to relieve the member caught. A distren call of calf will not only draw the attention of mother but the whole herd will move in mob for fighting the predator and risk the animal. There are recorded instances when attacking lions were forced to remain on tree for two hours. In another instance a calf could be saved from the lions as well as crocodile after aggressive attack by the herd (http//wapedia.mobi/on/African buffalo).

The forest and hill type red Congo buffaloes live in small herds of less than 20 animals and they are less exposed to predation of Savannah. The habitat of red buffaloes is inconvenient for the predators and it is difficult for them to persue and catch the prey due to provision of natural shelters of hills and forests (Kingdom, 1997). However, even in small herd of Congo buffaloes social bond is quite strong. The herd provides full protection to weaker and injured member throughout its life.

▶ MORPHOLOGICAL CHARACTERISTICS OF THE AFRICAN WILD BUFFALOES

The African wild buffaloes have been clearly classified into grayish black to dark black colour large size buffaloes with broad head and massive long horns of Cape or Savannah type, *Syncerus caffer* and small size brownish red to red colour buffaloes with very short horns of Congo region, *Syncerus nanus*. There are three subspecies of *S.caffer* and two subspecies of *S. nanus*. In addition, there are various intermediate products of crossbreeding in the open system of free living. Detail observations recorded on the morphology of two anain types (Mammericky, 1960; Van Zyl and Skead, 1964; Buchholtz, 1990; Nowak, 1991; Alden et al. 1995; Kingdom, 1997). Some of the common characteristics of all types of the African wild buffaloes may be enumerated as follows:

1. The density of hairs on the body reduces with the advancement in age and becomes sparse and short in adults.
2. The males of same group are much heavier than the females.
3. The newborn calves of all types are red to brownish red at birth which changes gradually to acquire characteristic colour at puberty.
4. The barrel shaped body provides large space for the consumption of course fodder.
5. Broad chest of well-sprung ribs provides ample space for housing capacious lungs required for the animals moving long distances in search of feed and water.
6. Horns are present in both sexes but these are longer and heavier in the males.
7. Long tail terminates in a thick switch.
8. The head is massive, short, the neck is thick and legs are stocky.
9. The long and droopy ears are fringed with long hairs on the edges.

▶ DISTINGUISHING FEATURES OF CAPE OR SAVANNAH BUFFALOES (SYNCERUS CAFFER)

1. Body colour is grayish black to dark black.
2. Horns are long and originate conjoint from poll to sides, turn slightly doorwards and then curls upwards in crescent shape and known.
3. Horns are longer and heavier in males which attract the hunters for making valuable trophies. The length of horn of buffalo bull on outer curvature may be more than 160 cm and the horizontal spread more than 90 cm.

4. The adult males are darker in colour than the females. They are mostly black.
5. In old males there may be appearance of grizzled white patches around the eyes.

▶ DISTINGUISHING FEATURES OF CONGO OR RED BUFFALO (*SYNCERUS NANUS*)

1. The body colour range from brownish red to red.
2. The animals are almost half of the size of Cape/Savannah buffalo.
3. The horns although originate conjoint on the occiput but they are much shorter, stumpy and slight sweep back from the headline.
4. Body colour turns darker with increase in age and may be blackish red in old males.
5. Horn legth is only 30–40 cm and does not form boss like that in Cape buffalo bulls.
6. In forest type two long white or pale yellow hair strips line the inner surface of the ears and extend as tufts along the edges of pina.
7. Despite very small herd size the bondage among the members of group is very strong. A weak or injured member is not left behind to suffer pain or die in isolation. Other members of the group take care till last day of life of such animals.

▶ HABITATS AND ACTIVITIES OF AFRICAN WILD BUFFALO

Consipicuous differences have been recorvded in the habitats and activities of the two distinct major types of African wild buffaloes. The large size Cape buffalo (*Syncerus caffer*) prefer of live within the limits of Savannah and does not like migration. In home range of about 126 to 10 75 square kilometres supports a buffalo population density of 0.17 to 3.77 animals per square kilometre but in the high rainfall area of east Africa with dense grass cover much small home range of only 10 square kilometre carries greater density of up to 18 buffaloes per square kilometre (Nowak, 1991). There are no signs of territory marking but affinity for the habitat even during changed conditions causing thinning of herbage cows (Buccholtz, 1990; Kingdon, 1997). The Savannah buffalo is an active animal walking for 18 hours daily. Grazing is more intensive during afternoon. Trampling of Savannah during grazing has been advantageous for the regrowth of herbages. This is probably due to dispersal of dung and urine of high nutritive value and activation of growth stimulating hormones in the plants. This supports repeated cyclic grazing in an area of 50–105 km. Average walking speed in about 5.7 km per hour but can run at the speed of up to 57 km per hour for short distance. Cape buffaloes like to live in open than resting beneath the shade of trees (Nowak, 1991). In case of disturbance caused by increased human movements the grazing becomes nocternal (Kingdon, 1997).

Congo or red African wild buffaloes are found hidden in the forest and hills and live in small herds of 8–12 and rarely up to 20 animals cinsisting of the progeny of one, two, and three breedable females. Cong buffaloes are nocturnal in habit and may also come out of the hide early in the morning and late in the evening for grazing and watering. The groups live near the water sources and enjoy wallowing in mud holes.

Observation of the daily activities were made on undisturbed herd of about 130 Cape buffaloes on the open dense grassland in Uganda for 48 hours during the wet season of rains and also for 61 hours during the dry season of scanty herbage cows at a gap of about five month. The average movement of herd was about 9.6 kilometres daily (Grimsdell and Field, 1976).

Activities of African wild buffalo has been compared with other game animals of African Savannah and cattle (Lewis, 1977). This study was conducted on limited number of different species found on the same grasslands of Kenya. The activities of African wild buffaloes in Kenya are more nearer to Kenyan cattle (*Bos indicus*) Table 2.4. However, actual grazing duration has not been mentioned which is most important aspect of activities.

TABLE 2.4: Activity pattern of common game animals and cattle in Kenya

Activities	Oryse (Oryse sp.)	Eland (Tregelaphus oryse)	Cattle (Bos indicus)	A.W. Buffalo (Syncerus caffer)
Number of animals	18	16	13	12
Diurnal activation	On the	Kenyan	Savannah	(hours/day)
Walking	1.2 ± 0.46	1.8 ± 0.55	0.2 ± 0.52	2.1 ± 0.72
Feeding	7.3 ± 0.93	8.4 ± 0.93	6.3 ± 0.84	6.3 ± 1.60
Resting (lying and/or standing)	2.7 ± 0.83	0.3 ± 0.24	1.9 ± 0.49	0.9 ± 0.57
Ruminating (Standing or lying)	0.3 ± 0.22	1.1 ± 0.73	0.8 ± 0.51	2.0 ± 1.01
Other activities	0.4 ± 0.23	0.4 ± 0.21	0.8 ± 0.15	0.8 ± 0.58
Normal activities	during	24 hours	Of a day	(hours)
Resting (Standing or lying)	5.4 ± 0.48	7.0 ± 1.25	6.0 ± 0.98	6.2 ± 0.42
Ruminating (Standing or lying)	6.4 ±	4.7 ± 0.05	5.7 ± 0.90	5.2 ± 0.78
Lying (resting or nominating)	8.3 ±	10.3 ±	8.6 ±	8.3 ± 0.89

Resting and nomination occur during the hottest period of the day which is 12 to 16 hours, i.e. noon to 4 PM in most part of the range land. During this period smaller groups of the herd are mostly seen nominating in standing or lying posture beneath the shady trees found seattered on the grassland. Grazing occurs during walking for almost 18 hours daily and it is more intensive during the dark hours of early morning and late evening grazing herds move through their native land (Nowak, 1991).

▶ **FEEDING AND WATER INTAKE**

African wild buffaloes are grazer by evolution and feeding of browse is a casual habit probably for change of taste. However, browsing on herbs, shrub, and trees may be significant due to extensive loss of green grasses caused by prolonged drought in large area reducing the scope of mass migration of wild herbivores including the African wild buffaloes. Such situation is not common in Savannah of Africa except along the sahara desert. The African wild buffaloes are non-selective grazers with a broad mouth and prehensile long tongue well-adapted for holding, biting and swallowing (Jarman, 1974), large volume of grassed. The grasses liked by buffaloes are the species of *Cynodon, Sporobolus, Digitaria, Panicum, Hetropogan* and *Conchrus* (Kingdon, 1997).

African wild buffaloes and zebu cattle spent about 52% time on grazing. An observation on a herd of 130 African wild buffaloes in the Rwengon National Park of Uganda revealed 9 hours grazing and 6.5 hours rumination daily. The cooler hours of the day are preferred for grazing and extended to night during the hot season.

An average 5.7 hours grazing in night has been recorded in the tamed African wild buffaloes penned in the night (Grimsdell and Field, 1976). The feeding time of African wild buffaloes with other wild ruminants has been compared during high and low heat load and also on good and bad vegetation. Cows on the Savannah (Table 2.5) and the percentage contribution of grasses, browse and herbs (Table 2.6) has been also observed in African wild animals (King and Health, 1975).

TABLE 2.5: Average feeding duration of African wild buffaloes and other games on the African Savannah (hours per day)

Animal species	High heat load		Low heat load	
	A	B	A	B
African wild buffalo	4.4 (18.3)	5.2 (21.7)	7.1 (29.6)	7.5 (31.3)
African zebu cattle	4.5 (18.8)	5.4 (22.5)	6.7 (27.9)	8.0 (33.3)
African eland	5.1 (21.3)	5.1 (21.3)	9.2 (38.3)	9.2 (38.3)

Note: A = good grass cow, B–Bad grass cow
Figures in parenthes are percentage time.

A significant increase in grazing time occurs due to low heat low and low grass cows in African wild buffalo and zebu cattle, but African elands are not affected by grass cows.

TABLE 2.6: Percent composition of the diets of the game animals feeding on natural herbage

Type of herbage	Afican wild buffalo	Zebu cattle	Oryse	Eland
Grasses	91	88	83	21
Browse	7	7	7	51
Herbs	2	5	5	28

Protein supply in the diets of African wild buffaloes has been estimated from the gross analysis of the ratio of leaf, sheath and stem of the grasses present in the numen content of the killed buffaloes during grazing. The protein was estimated in the similar samples collected from the protected and grazed area of the same pasture. In the Serengeti area of Tanzania the quality of diet was good during the wet season from November to July. Average protein in dry matter of grass cover is highest 10% in the dry matter of March which gradually decrease to 5.2% in July. Thereafter the protein level falls to sub-maintenance level, i.e. about 2.2% of dry matter in the month of October. The fall in crude protein content of leaves consumed during grazing. Both sex and age of the buffaloes influence herbage intake. Protein deficiency is not an induced but a normal natural effect of the region, which is regulated by many factors like distribution of rainfall, heat load and other climatic factors. Competition of African wild buffaloes increases with other herbivorous wild animals on the grasslands of river basins during the fodder scarcity of dry season.

The shortage of more nutritious leafy protein of grass cover in the dry season for longer duration in the area is a major cause of mortality of adult buffaloes. Good growth of grass is round the year on the slopes of the 'Menu' mount and buffaloes have access to swamp pastures in the dry season. But high grazing intensity due to heavy accumulation of buffaloes at the rate of approximately 51 heads per square kilometre grass cover keeps the standing grass cover low due to repeated grazing. The crude protein content remains in the range of 8 to 10% of dry matter through out the year; and the population of buffaloes is regulated by the quantity of available grazing an not by the quality. Mortality of adult buffaloes of advanced age regulated by deficient fodder supply of sub-maintenance quality limits the population of buffaloes. The size of buffalo population in the eastern region of Africa is related the annual rain precipitation. In the dry zone buffalo population is related with the availability of permanent water sources, and the grass density of riverine and swamplands. Grazing occurs mainly during cooler hours and in night with circadian rhythm and shorter cycle with synchronized herd behaviour. In this area there is little seasonal changes in grazing time but some increase occurs in the rumination duration during the summer season (Sinclair, 1974).

African wild buffaloes daily need water for drinking and also for wallowing. Water drinking is more common in early morning and late in afternoon (Stuart and Stuart, 1997). Wallowing in mud holes is quite common and frequent. Buffaloes like to live for long hours in mud. The mud has cooling effect and formation of a layer on drying provides protection from sun heat as well as insect bites. African wild buffaloes maintain good relationship of mutual benefits with many insectivorous birds like Oxpecker and Egrets pick-up biting insect infesting the buffaloes (Buccholtz, 1990). The birds get food and the buffaloes are releaved of ectoprarasites. The birds also get plenty of insects coming out of hides in grass cover due to movements on the pasture and prehensing the grasses.

▶ BREEDING AND REPRODUCTION

Since African wild buffaloes could not be domesticated, it has not been possible to make detail observations on the breeding and reproduction. However, sporatic observations have been made by several studies in the homeland and confinement of zoological gardens (Vidlar et al., 1963; Grimdell, 1973; Buccholtz, 1990; Nowak, 1991; Alden et al., 1995; Kingdon, 1997; Mills and Hes, 1997; Stuart and Stuart, 1997). Considerable variations have been found among different observations, indeed these are quite useful for breeding and reproduction management in the lately arranged habitat of large National Wildlife Parks in most of the African countries.

Although African wild buffaloes can breed and reproduce throughout the year in favourable agroclimatic conditions found in some small pockets of African Savannah, but in majority herds mating and calving are seasonal and closely influenced by rainfall (Nowak, 1991). The rainfall favours growth of pasture that improves the nutritional quality of grasses capable of supplying adequate nutrients. Buffalo heifers first conceive at 3 to 4 years of age and deliver calf at 4 to 5.5 years of age after a gestation period of 310 to 346 days in different living environment.

Mating season is somewhat variable in different areas which extends from March to May (Kingdom, 1997) and calving occurring during January to April (Mills and Hes, 1997). In an earlier record maximum calving has been reported from April to June and again in January and then July to September, which indicated mating during February to April and June to August.

After puberty oestrus cycle is repeated at an interval of 23 days until conception and oestrus duration is 5–6 days. Single calf is born at a time and twinning is an extremely rare event (Buccholtz, 1990; Nowak, 1991). Intercalving period in about two year (Kindom, 1997). Body weight of calves at birth is about 40 kg red buffalo of Congo region and in Cape or Savannah buffaloes 55–60 kg (Buceloltz, 1990). The female is oestrus attracts several eligible males but only the dominant one mates and remains with the female till the termination of oestrous period.

A study in two different populations of Cape buffaloes with 10.8 and 2 buffaloes per square kilometre area, the mean age at first calving was similar 5.5 years but calving interval was 18 and 24 months respectively. Mean conception rate in females below 5 years of age was 63 and 48 percent, and annual birth rate was 66 and 50 per 100 of eligible females respectively. However, growth rate of calves was not affected by population density. Season and population density also have no significant effect on the sexual maturity of male calves (Grimsdell, 1973).

Mating between male Cape buffalo with female Asiatic river buffalo has resulted nonfertile (Labanov, 1978). The number of chromosomes are $2n = 54$ in long buffalo (*Syncerus nanus*), $2n = 50$ in Asiatic dairy type river buffalo (*Bubalus bubalis*), and $2n = 48$ in draught type swamp buffalo (*Bubalus bubalis*). The estimated frequency of the genes responsible for semilethal and undesirable traits is 0.05 to 0.2% (Osterhoff et al., 1970).

▶ **FOOD PRODUCTION AND OTHER PRODUCTS**

African wild buffaloes had been one of the most wanted games of the Africa. The carcar data of random shot 117 adult buffaloes were comparable with the other wild bovine of Africa. Average weight of buffaloes 550 kg yielded 49.4 percent carcass of 290 cm length and 77.8 cm width. A carcar of about 250 kg weight yielded about 168 kg deboned meat. About 80% of the deboned meat was suitable for the preparation of biltong (strips of sun dried meat). Average yield of biltong is about 33.7% due to 66.3% dehydration losser (Young and Van Den Heaver, 1969).

Slaughter data on a single male buffalo reared in captivity form one month of age to eight and half years have provided very useful carcass characteristics. The buffalo attained about 686 kg body weight at maturity at 5 years of age. The body length from poll to root of the tail was 263 cm and height at shoulders 155.6 cm. Body weight at the time of sacrifice was 682 kg which yielded 376.6 kg carcar and 280 kg offals with 55.2% dressed yield. Loss in weight due to slanghter was 4.2% of body weight. The carcar yielded 74.6% lean meat, 10.9% dissectable fatty tissue and 14.5% bones and ligaments (Van Zyl and Skead, 1964). The valuable by-products are horns, hide, hooves, and switch of the tail. All the by-products are utilized in different cottage industries and long, massive horns fetch handsome amount after mounting to make shield.

▶ **ASIAN WATER BUFFALOES (BUBALUS SPP.)**

The Asian water buffalo is separate genus with four species. The water buffaloes (*Bubalus* species) are at present found in the following four forms in their native lands and translocated countries distributed in almost all the continents of both hemispheres.

1. **Wild water buffaloes:** Probably two types of wild water buffaloes (*Bubalus arnee*) were exhisted before domestication in the wet tropical region of Asia, which were ancestors of dairy type riverine buffalo with $2n = 50$ number of chromosome and another with $2n = 48$ number of chromosomes is the ancestor of draught type swamp buffaloes. The ancestor of riverine buffaloes lived in the wet region of north and west parts of the Indian subcontinent. It is most likely that ancestor of riverine buffaloes lived in the wet region buffalo is now extinct, is that present in the wildlife reserve of Kolhapur in Maharashtra does not contain $2n = 50$ number of chromosomes.

The ancestor of domesticated swamp buffaloes are still found in central, east and north east regions of India, Nepal, Bangladesh, Myanmar, Thailand, Laos, Combodia and China. Large herds of wild swamp buffaloes are quite common (Fig. 2.2) in Kaziranga and Manas wild life sancturies and other adjoing areas. Groups of wild swamp buffaloes (*Bubalus arnee*) may be seen grazing during dawn and dusk, and wallowing in water or lying in mud holes during the hot hours of the day.

There is no inhibition between the wild, feral and domestic buffaloes. Breeding interaction is quite common and domestic female buffalo in oestrum after eloper with the wild buffalo bull to return back after 2–3 days. Similarly, wild buffalo female in oestrum and away from the herd sometimes lured lay the domestic male buffalo to join the group of domestic buffaloes (Ranjhan and Pathak, 1978).

2. Feral buffaloes: The domestic swamp buffaloes that escaped to domestic herd to live in wild again are not common in Asia. However, domestic swamp buffaloes translocated from Asian region have been made feral in swampy region of Australia. The groups of domestic swamp buffaloes were introduced from. In beginning three small herds of domestic swamp buffaloes were introduced during 1826 at Melville Island, 1827 at Reffles Bay and 1838 at Port Essington. The later two places are the part of northern territory. These groups of domestic swamp buffaloes were made free to find habitat for survival when settler abandoned the places (Tulloch, 1970). The buffaloes survived and multiplied on the swampy grassland until drawing the attention of hunters. The casual hunting subsequently became feral buffalo farming. Now, the buffaloes are maintained in the limits of fenced grasslands and harvested at intervals for exporting edible flesh (buffen) and processing hides for leather and leather goods manufactor, and horns for making trophies and decoration articles.

3. Tamed buffaloes: These are semi-domesticated buffaloes reared on exclusive grazing. The animals are let loose in the morning after milking but young calves up to 4–5 months of age are retained in an enclosure of bamboo or wood. Small herds of buffaloe go alone without cowboy for grazing and wallowing. The buffaloes return at dusk and then left for resting after milking. This system was common along the Brahmaputra river and its tributaries in upper Assam which is changing to grazing by cowboys and housing in enclosures during the night.

4. Domesticated buffaloes: These buffaloes are kept in well-defined management systems evolved according to resources and the requirements in different regions. The owners range from small holder group keeping 1 to 10 buffaloes, medium group possessing 11 to 50 buffaloes, big farmers having 51 to 200 buffaloes and large farmers owning more than 200 buffaloes. The large herds of buffaloes are reared under systematic management for commercial production. There is great variation in the management of dairy buffaloes in India and Pakistan. The system is almost completely for extracting milk with the application of all known technological methods without consideration of effects on the health of animals. This system is prevalent in and around the heavily populated towns and cities where demand of liquid milk is very high and turnover of money is very fast. Cruelty it frequently encountered with the buffaloes in such system and most of the calves are intensely starved and neglected to die before 5–6 weeks of age.

▶ ASIATIC WILD BUFFALOES

Three distinct species of Asian wild buffaloes are still found on the grasslands, swamps, forests, hills of tropical, and subtropical Asian countries with main seat of origin in Bharat (India). This is called *Bubalus arnee*. The domesticated form of *Bubalus arnee* are present widely distributed in two genetically different forms of riverine buffalo (2n = 50 chromosomes) and, swamp buffalo (2n = 48 chromosomes) chromosome numbers of existing Asian wild buffalo, *Bubalus arnee* are 2n = 48 similar to that of domesticated swamp buffaloes. This shows that the wild ancestor of riverine buffaloes. This shows that the wild ancestor of riverine buffaloes is now extinct. Studies of fossils may help in finding the ancestor of riverine buffalo.

The other two dwarf species of the Asian wild buffaloes, tamaraw or Mindoro dwarf buffalo (*Bubalus mindorensis*) is present on the Mindoro island of the Philippines. The second species of comparable size but somewhat different morphology is the dwarf buffalo present on the Sulawesi island of the Indonesia and called 'anoa' (*Bubalus depressicornis*). Two strains of anoa have been identified. These are lowland anoa (*Bubalus depressicornis*) and mountain anoa (*Bubalus quarlesi*).

▶ PROPOSED ZOOLOGICAL NOMENCLATURE

Trinomial nomenclature system may be more useful for the identification of species. Adoption of trinomial system of nomenclature will also help in differentiation of the riverine and swamp types of Asian water buffaloes (Table 2.7). The nomenclature of tamaraw and anoa may be again changed in future on the basis of genetic analysis.

TABLE 2.7: Proposed names of Asian buffaloes in trinomial system

Common	Present zoological name	Proposed zoological name
Water buffalo	*Bubalus* sp.	Bubalus spp.
Riverine buffalo	*Bubalus bubalis*	*Bubalus bubalis bubalis*
Swamp buffalo	*Bubalus bubalis*	*Bubalus bubalis swampis*
Tamaraw	*Bubalus mindorensis*	*Bubalus bubalis mindorensis*
Lowland Anoa	*Bubalus depressicomis*	*Bubalus bubalis depresicornis*
Mountain Anoa	*Bubalus quarlesi*	*Bubalus bubalis quarlesi*
Wild swamp (Present)	*B. arnee*	*B. arnee swampis*
Wild riverine (Present)	*B.arnee*	*B. arnee bubalis*

▶ ASIAN WILD BUFFALO, BUBALUS ARNEE (*B. ARNEE SWAMPISH*)

Asian wild buffalo (*Bubalus arnee*) is one of the large bovids known today. Except for the large body size, aggrossiveners and lack of affinity for humans there are not much difference between the Asian wild buffaloes (*Bubalus arnee swampish*) and the domestic swamp buffaloes (*Bubalus bubalis swampish*). The body size and horn shape vary between the Asian wild buffaloes are denoted with the name of the country prefixed like Indian wild buffalo, Thai wild buffalo, Combodain wild buffalo, Chinese wild buffalo, Vietnamese wild buffalo, etc. Almost all known herds of Asain wild buffaloes except the not yet analysed herd to Kolhapur wildlife park contain $2n = 48$ chromosome, the number present in the domesticated swamp buffaloes of different countries.

Synonyms of the Asian Wild Buffalo (*Bubalus Arnee*)

The synonyms used for the wild ancestor of the modern domestic swamp buffaloes are the wild water buffalo, wild Asian buffalo, wild Asiatic buffalo, Ama bhainsa, Buffalo arni, Buffalo d'Eau, Indian wild buffalo, Buffalo de'Inde, etc.

Distribution

Habitation of largest number of Asian wild buffalo (*Bubalus arnee* or *Bubalus Bubalis arnee*) is *Bharat Bhumi* (Indian territory). The presence of wild buffaloes has been marked in the tropical forests of Gujarat, Maharashtra, Madhya Pradesh, Chhatisgarh, Orissa, Jharkhand, West Bengal, Sikkim and Assam with largest herds in the wildlife sanctuaries of Monas and Kaziranga. Asian wild buffaloes are also found in the Nepal, Bhutan, Myanmar, Thailand, Combodia, S.R. Vietnam, Laos, and probably in southern region of China, Srilanka, and bordering area of Bangladesh with Indian. Although genetically all Asian wild buffaloes of *Bubalus arnee* or *Babalus bubalis* arnee are one species but there are some phenotype variations due to geographical differences (Ranjhan and Pathak, 1978). Despite crossbreeding with the domesticated buffaloes of the inhabitants along the forests in India, Nepal, and Bhutan, unadulterated herds still exist on the swamps in open plains of deep forest areas. Such pure population of Asian wild buffalo may be also living in the forest along the Thailand, Combodia, Vietnam and Laos in the eastern part of Asia.

Wetland is essentaial for the inhabitation of Asian wild buffaloes. They prefer grass cover near rivers, swamps, lakes, and other perennial for several hours during hot period of day is an inherent habit. It is an endangered species (14 CN, 2009).

▶ DESCRIPTION OF THE ASIAN WILD BUFFALO

Probably Asian wild buffalo (*Bubalus bubalis arnee*) is the largest wild bovine on the earth. It is a heavy black to grayish black beast of massive, compact and strong body, broad head, and long horns. The males are heavier than the females of same herd. Although scattered information are available on the description of Asian wild buffaloes. In recent years more informations have been collected on the shape and size of the Asain wild buffaloes (Choudhurt, 1994; De Silva et al., 1994; Heinen, 2002; Heinen and Kandal, 2006). The shape, size, and other morphological characteristics of Asian wild buffaloes have been summarized in Table 2.8.

TABLE 2.8: Summary of morphological characteristics of Asian wild buffalo (*Bubalus bubalis arnee*)

Attributes	Descirption
Body weight	700–1200 kg in males
	500–900 kg in females
Height	170–200 cm. About 80% i.e. 136–160 cm in females
Body length	250–300 cm in males and 200–250 in females
Colour	Greyish to dark black. Males are larger than the females
Chevron	One or two.
Tail	Long and tapering with bushy switch.
	Switch may contain white hairs.
Horns	Long, broad and massive in males
	Long, narrows in females
	Shape is variable. May be hook like, pinscher like, sickle shaped or Crescetric and evnerge from either side of the occiput with large gap between the poller side of the base of two horns.
Horn span	May be up to 185 cm and maximum length of a horn has been recorded a little less than 2 meters.
Markings	Fine white lines around the nose and mouth and spectacles around the eyes. White stockings are common on knees.
Barrel	Long and broad.
Chest	Broad with well sprung ribs.
Calf	At birth light brownish grey and gradually becomes darker with increase in age.

▶ REPRODUCTION

The Asian wild buffaloes are seasonal breeder. Maximum mating occurs during wet climate of rainy season and calving occurs at the end of rainy season and beginning of dry season.

The homeland is covered with plenty of lush growing grasses to supply nutrition for rearing the calves. The time of mating and calving differs among the different zones and has close linkage with the rainy season. The reproduction traits may be summarized in the Table 2.9.

TABLE 2.9: Some reproduction traits of Asian (Indian) wild buffalo (*Bubalus arnee*)

Age of puberty	18–24 months
Gestation length	300–340 days
Age at first calving	30–36 months
Calving interval	About 2 years
Weaning of calf	At 6 to 12 months
Birth rate	1 calf. Twinning is perhaps not yet reported.
Mating and calving rate	About 50–60% per year

▶ BEHAVIOUR AND SOCIAL ORGANIZATION PATTERN

1. Adult males and females live in separate groups and competent bull joins breedable females only during the mating season.
2. Juvenile males over 2 years of age form a bachelor group. The emergence of leader is decided by friendly spar among the bachelor males.
3. Eldest female leads the family groups of few generations with their nursing and yearling calves and heifers. The family group size within the herd may be 6–15 and rarely more.
4. Orphan calves are easily adopted by the another lactating mother in the group.
5. The calves are kept in middle during grazing and movement.
6. Early morning and late evening is the grazing time. Night grazing is common in the cultivated fields along the forests.
7. Hot hours of day is spent wallowing in mud pits or water near the bank of river.
8. Wallowing in mud and rubbing the body with tree removes ectoparasites.
9. Plastering of mud on the body provides protection from the biting insects and also from heat of sun rays. Drying of mud plaster on the body has cooling effect.
10. Duration and depth of wallowing depends on the intensity of solar heat. During very hot season only nostrils and tips of horns may be visible.
11. Buffaloes live on open grasslands in or along the forests.

▶ PREDATORS OF THE ASIAN WILD BUFFALO

Some of the common predators of Asian wild buffaloes are the Bengal tiger (*Panthora tigris*), leopard (*Panthara partus*), wild dog or 'dhole' (*Cuan alpinus*) and group of jackals, hyena and wolf on the ground surface, and crowdiles in the water and swamps. Young calves are often engulged by the pythons. Wild buffaloes dislike human being and consider than predator. The herd of females with suckling calves on foot are extremely attentive and highly ferocious. An interference may be fatal for the stranger (s). During nonmating season adult males lead a solitary life. Such males should not be believed. They are highly unpredictable and can charge without showing any reaction (Heinen, 2002).

▶ **MAIN THREATS**

1. Shrinking of habitat due to increasing enchroachment on the habitat for cultivation.
2. Pollution of species by interbreeding with domestic water buffaloes along the neighbourhood.
3. Poaching for horns, hide, and sometimes for meat also.
4. Occurrence of fatal infectious diseases. In the past rinderpost alone has killed larger proposition of wild buffalo population in Bharat (India) and Sri Lanka (Chouchary, 1994); De Silva et al., 1994).

▶ **CONSERVATION OF ASIAN WILD BUFFALO**

The herd of Asian wild buffaloes in different Asian countries have been classified as endangered and critically endangered species listed in red book of 14 CN (Hedges, 1995; 14 CN, 2006). Some of the important wildlife sanctuaries and National Parks providing protection to Asian wild water buffalo (*Babalus arnee* or *Bubalus bubalis arnee*) are listed as follows:

1. Kaziranga National Park, Assam, Bharat.
2. Manas National Park, Assam, Bharat.
3. Indravati Wildlife Sanctuary, Madhya Pradesh, Bharat.
4. Koshi Tappu Wildlife Reserve in southeast Nepal.
   Crossbreeding between wild, feral, and domestic buffaloes of Koshi Tappu wildlife reserve area is continuing from centuries but distinct population of wild buffalo in pure genetic form remains in the reserve and conservation is showing about 3.5% annual growth (Muley, 2001; Flamand et al., 2003).
5. Ruhuna National Park and adjacent reserve in southeast Sri Lanka.

In addition of protected areas small herds may be seen scattered in other countries of south and southeast Asia. However, feral buffaloes are found in many parts of their native land. Translocated swamp buffaloes have been made feral long back. In Australia feral buffaloes are useful from controlling the wild growth of grass on swampy land and also provide nutritious commercial value.

▶ **MINOR ASIATIC WILD BUFFALOES ANOA AND TAMARAW**

In the islands of Asia-Pacific region two dwarf buffalo species are found. Anoa is present in the hilly forest of Sulaweri island of Indonesia and Tamaraw is present mountains of the Mindoro island of Philippines. Population of both species is quite small and there are not found out of their homeland expect few animals in zoological gardens. It is also believed that Tamaraw were plenty on the greater island of Luzon. Both the species are listed in the red species (14 CN, 2006).

▶ **TAMARAW (*BUBALUS MINDORENSIS* OR *BUBALUS BUBALIS ININDORENSIS*)**

The Tamaraw or dwarf buffalo of Mindoro island is one of the two dwarf buffalo species facing extinction but now protected in its homeland. Although national animal of the Philippines is caraboo or swamp buffalo (Philippines Independence Day Celebration, 2007), the Tamaraw is also considered equally important animal of Philippines as evident from its impression on the one-Peso coins minted in 1980 to 1990 (Breithaupt, 2003). In 2004, an act was proclaimed wide no. 692 for celebrating 1st October as Tamaraw conservation day (a holiday) in the province of Occidental Mindoro for reminding the people of Mindoro the importance of conservation of Tamaraw and its habitat.

▶ DESCRIPTION OF TAMARAW

Tamaraw (*B.mindorensis* or *Bubalus bubalis mindorensis*) is a dwarf buffalo possessing many distinguishing features from the Asian wild buffalo (*B. arnee* or *Bubalus bubalis arnee*). It is a small animal of compact body covered with more dense coat. The short horns extend backwards and slightly upwards along the short neck. Little sexual dimorphism is seen from thicker neck in males (Heude, 1888). The animal has been described by few workers (Heude, 1888, Huffman, 2007) as presented in Table 2.10.

TABLE 2.10: Summary of morphology of Tamaraw (*Bubalus bubalis mindorensis*)

Body length	200 cm
Height at shoulder	10–105 cm
Length of tail	60 cm
Body weight of adult females	200–300 kg
Body coat colour	Dark brown to grayish
Limbs	Short and stocky
Skin of nose and lips	Black
Length or ear (pinna)	13.5 cm
Horns shape	Roughly V-shaped, short and black with flat surface and triangular base.
Horn length	35–51 cm

The Tamaraw is a shy animal and avoid the presence of mankind. It is very diffcent to sight and follow the animal for observing its habits and behaviour (Nowak, 1999).

▶ HABITAT AND FORAGING

Tamaraw lives in highland forests and prefers open grassland with shady tress. Later on some changes occurred in the habitat due to human enchroachment of upland forests and some animals moved to lowland grass cover. They graze talahib or kasaunja (Saccharum spontaneum). The animal is diurnal but may become nocturnal due to extensive human activities during daytime (Fuentes, 2005).

The adults are solitary animals. Adult male and female may be seen together only for few hours for mating. However, hierarchy is maintained by adult breeding females with few nursing and juvenile followers. Solitary adult males are usually aggressive (Nowak, 1999).

The Tamaraw like wallowing in mud holes and this behaviour has been probably adapted for protection from the insect bites (Mc Millan et al., 2000).

▶ REPRODUCTION

Little information is available on the reproduction of Tamaraw. Average life is considered 20 years but may live up to 25 years. Average gestation period is about 300 days and female delivers one calf that follows her up to 4 years. Adult females live with nursing young and 1–2 follows. Intercalving period is about 2 years (Fuentes, 2005).

▶ CONSERVATION

Tamaraws are now housed protected in the following areas by the government of Philippines.

1. **Tamaraw conservation Program: Mount Ig list—Baco National Park in Mindoro occidental:** This programme is implemented by the government and private organizations and also the students of the far eastern university.
2. The Mindoro's endangered treasure of the Haribon Foundation followed by the Philippines endangered flagship species.
3. Ceasation of Mindoro buffalo slaughter by Mangyan dwellers for blood.
4. The Bangkok, Thailand International Union for the Conservation of species (14 CS) established a pool farm at Rizal, Mindoro occidental.

▶ PRESENT HABITATS

Mt. 1 glist-Baco National Park, Mt. Calavite,
Mt. Aruyan-Sablayan-Mapalad Valley,
Mt. Bansud-Bongabong-Mansalay and
Mt. Halcon-Eagle Pass.

October is the special month for the conservation and protection of Tamaraw in Philippines.

▶ ANOA *(BUBALUS DEPRESSICORNIS OR BUBALUS BUBALIS DEPRESSICORNIS)*

On the island of Sulawesi (Celebes) in Indonesia two subspecies of anoa, i.e. lowland anoa (*Bubalis depressicornis*) and mountain anoa (*Bubalus quarlesi*) have been reported (Anoa, 2000). However, there apperars to be little information on the distinguishing features of the two subspecies. So far more informations have been collected on the biology. Behaviour, habitat and distribution, etc. of the lowland anoa (*Bubalus bubalis depressicornis*) from its homeland Anonymous, 2001; Huffman, 1999; Massicot, 2001; Melisch, 1995; Nowak, 1999; O'Brien et al., 1996; Pangua, 2001; and Parker, 1990) and zoological parks (Jones, 1993 and Thomback, 1983).

▶ DESCRIPTION OF ANOA *(Bubalus bubalis* depressicornis OR *B. Depressicornis)*

Anoa is the smallest buffalo species in the world. It is exclusive native of Sulawesi island of Indonesia. Extensive hunting for horns, meat, and hide have reduced the population and now it is among the threatened species in red listing of IUCN (2006).

The body of Anoa is covered with a thick and soft coat of yellowish brown colour. The coat colour gradually change to black skin sparsely covered with dark brown to black hairs. The colour of legs down the knee and hock joints is grayish to yellowish white. In some animals hairs may be present on the throat and neck. The body is stocky and sloping from sloonlders to group. The general features of adult lowland anoa may be summarized in Table 2.11.

Only one calf is delivered at the end of the gestation period. Anoas do not live in groups except that nursing females may be seen sometimes with two successive followers.

TABLE 2.11: Morphology of ANOA

General appearance:	A short bovine with compact body, thick neck sloping from howl to shoulders and a faint chevron. The delicate legs are short and thin.
Body measurements:	Body length, 170–190 cm (68–76 inches)
	Heart girth, 170–190 cm (68–76 inches)
	Height at wither 80–100 cm (32–40 inches)
	Tail length, 25–40 cm (10–18 inches)
Body colour:	Body contains scanty hairs of grayish to yellowish white colour. The coat is generally dense and lighter is colour below the knee and hock joints.
Body weight:	Maximum 300 kg but generally much less than 300 kg
Gestation length:	270–305 days
Age at puberty:	2–3 years
Nursing period:	6–9 months.

There appears to be lack of precise informations on the habitat, behaviour, and biology of the highland forest anoas.

REFERENCES

Alden, P.C, estes, R.D, Schh itter, D and Mc Bride, B. 1995. National Audubon Society Field Guide to African Wildlife. New York Cham.

Anonymous, 2001. http://www.org/educate.com/anoalowland.html.

Breithaupt, Jan 2003. http://ecoport.org/ep?Search type = polb and Polb ID = 32573

Buchholtz, C. 1990. Cattle in grezimek Encyclopedia of mammals. (Ed. S P Parker, Mc Grawhill, Vol. 5, 360–364, New york

Chowdhury, A. 1994. Animal Genetics, 28; 103–115

De Silva, M, dissanayake, S and Santiapillai, C. 1994. Oryse 28, 70–73.

East, R. 1999. African antelope Database 1998. 14CN, SSC Antelope Specialist Group, Switzerland and Cambridge, U.K.

Flamond, J.R.B., Vanlan, D., Gairhe, K.P., Duong, H. and Barker, J.S.F. 2003. J. South Asian nat. Hist.1; 65

Fuentes, Art 2005, http://wwwharibon.org.ph/index.php?q=node/view/130.

Grimsdell, J.J.R. 1973. J Reprod. Festl. 19; 303.

Grimsdell, J.J.R. and Field, C.R. 1976. East African Wildlife J., 14; 339.

Heinen, J.T. 2002. Biological Conservation, 101; 391–394

Heinen, J.T. and Kandel, R. 2006. J. Bombay Natural History Soc., 99; 173–183

Hende 1998. Wildcattle conservation.org.

Huffman, B. 1999 and 2007 http://www.ultimateungulate.com/anaolowland.html.

Huffman, R.S. 1986 Mummalia, 50; 391

14 CN 2004, 2006, 2009. http://www.incnredlist.org.

Jarman, P.J. 1974. Behaviour, 48; 215

Jones, M. 1993. International zoo yearbook, 32; 159–169

Kingdon, J. 1997. The kingdom field Guide to African Mammals. Academic Press, San Die.

King, J.M. and Heath, B.R. 1975. Wild Animal Res. No. 16; 23

Lweis, J.G. 1973. J. agric, Sci, Camb, 89; 551

Kuznetsov, G.V., Kulikov, E.E., Petrov, N.B., Ivanova, N.V., Lomov, A.A., Naturwissenschaften, 88; 123.

Macdonald, D.W. 2006. The Encyclopedia of Mammals. Oxford University Press, Oxford.

Maloiy, G.M.U. 1973. Nutr. Abst. Rev. (1975), 45; 932, Abstr. 8109.

Mammarick, M. 1960, Animal Breed. Abst. (1963) 31, 316, Abstr. 1803.

Massicot, P. 2004. http://www.animalinfo.org/species/artiperi/bubaarne.htm.

Melisch, R.1995. Iryse, 29; 224–225

Mills, G. and Hes, L. 1997. The Complete Book of Southern African Mammals. Struik Publisher, Cape Town.

Nowak, R.M. 1991, 1997. Walker Mammals of the World. The John Hopkin's University Press, Baltimore.

O'Brien, T. and Kinnaird, M. 1996. Oryx, 30; 150–156.

Osterhoff, D.R., Young, E. and Ward-Cox, I.S. 1970. J. Southern African Vet. Med. Assoc., 41; 33.

Pangua, M. 2001. Anoa http://www.gwdg.de/cetsaf/absolventen/p3 /mpangau. htm.

Philippines Independence Day Celebration. National Symbol. 123 independence day.com.

Ranjhan, S.K. and Pathak, N.N. 1978. Text Book of Buffalo Management. Vikas Pub. Hse. Pvt. Ltd., New Delhi.

Sinclair, R.E. 1974. East African Wildlife J., 12; 291

Stuart, C. and Stuart, T. 1997. Field Guide to the Large Mammals of Africa. Struik Publisher, Cape Town.

Thornback, J.1983. Wild Cattle, bison and buffalo, their status and potential, 14 CN.

Tullock, D.G. 1970.Australian J.Zool., 17; 143–152

Vanzyl, J.H.M. and Skead, D.M. 1964. Anim, Breed. Absr. (1966), 34; 558, Abstr. 3293.

Vidler, B.O., harthorn, A.M., Brocklesby, D.W. and Robertshaw, D. 1963. East African Wildlife J., 7; 322.

Young, E. and Den Daever, L.W. 1969. J. South African Vet. Med. Assoc., 40; 83.

Types and Breeds of Domesticated Water Buffaloes

Asia is the homeland of water buffaloes (*Bubalus* spp.) comprising of dairy type riverine buffalo of the Indian subcontinent and draught type swamp buffaloes distributed from eastern parts of India to China and island countries of Indo-Pacific region. So far accepted zoological name of both types is *Bubalus bubalis*, though there is clear genotype as well as phenotype differences. The number of chromosomes of riverine buffalo is $2n = 50$ and that of swamp buffalo is $2n = 48$. However, due to fertile breeding between the two types producing $2n = 49$ prompted biologists to put two genetically different types together. Due to close genetic proximity between the riverine and swamp buffaloes, it would be more appropriate to use trinomial nomenclature as proposed in Chapter 2. Thus, the zoological name of dairy type riverine buffaloes with $2n = 50$ number of chromosomes will be *Bubalus bubalis bubalis* (*B.b bubalis*) and that of swamp type with $2n = 48$ number of chromosomes will be *Bubalus bubalis* (*B.b swampis*).

DAIRY BUFFALO OR RIVER BUFFALO OR INDIAN BUFFALO (*B.B.BUBALIS*)

The riverine buffaloes originated in the Indian subcontinent and developed for high milk production of higher milk fat content. Due to easy handling, high adaptability and capability of utilization of course herbage of wetlands riverine buffaloes were taken away by various nomadic groups and others to west. The Indian dairy buffaloes taken away to west probably included the mixture of breeds predominantly found in western parts of India.

The available breeds of dairy type reverine buffaloes are now generally differentiated into two major groups: (i) riverine buffaloes of the Indain subcontinent, and (ii) Medetarrean dairy buffaloes.

1A. **Dairy buffaloes of Indain subcontinent:** The other names are river or riverine buffalo or Indian buffalo. More than 90% of the riverine buffaloes are found in the Indain subcontinant and in India and Paskistan. Several breeds have been developed in different regions.

1B. **Dairy buffaloes of near east and Europe:** The dairy buffaloes of near east, Europe and Cancation region are the descendents of Indian dairy buffaloes which were carried by nomadic groups followed by the invaders from the west and north-west countries through western border of the Indain subcontinent. Probably buffaloes taken away at different times, were the mixture of coiled horned animal of Murrah group and Sickle horned animals of Surti and associated types. Since, many breeds are observe in the dairy buffaloes of west, it appears that different breeding system or initially indiscriminate breeding was followed.

2. **Swamp buffalo (B.b swanpis):** Although *Bubalus carabanesis* name has been often used in the Philippines but is has not yet been widely accepted. Swamp buffalo has been primarily evolved for working in knee deep water of paddy fields. However, in some parts of India and some other countries it has been developed as a dual purpose animal for work and milk or a triple purpose animal for work, milk and meat production. The swamp buffaloes of northeast states of India like Assam and Manipur produce substantial quantily of milk for 8–9 months (Pathak unpublished 1975; Singh, 1978; and Tamuli, 1978). The swamp buffaloes of Orissa, China, Thailand, and some other countries have been evolved in different breeds. Breeds of swamp buffaloes have been named mostly on the name of locality, phenotype or behaviour, etc.

▶ DAIRY OR RIVER BUFFALOES OF THE INDIAN SUBCONTINENT

This group includes the largest number of dairy buffaloes distinguished in well-defined breeds of different shape, size, behaviour, and productivity. The agroclimatic conditions, more specifically the type of herbage cover and availability of perennials water sources were the main criteria for the selection of production traits. In the home tract of dairy buffalo males were least liked in many areas but utilized for pulling heavy cart loads in sugarcane growing areas. However, in recant years, value of males has significantly increased due to increasing demand of buffen (buffalo meat) fetching remunerative price from fattening of the earlier neglected male calves of dairy buffaloes in India.

The dairy buffaloes of the Indian subcontinent may be differentiated into three distinct groups on the basis of the horns. These are Murrah group of partial or complete coiled horns, sickle shaped horns of different size and massive caliper horn decorating the occiput as crown.

Murrah Group of Dairy Buffaloes

Coiling to completely coiled horns are the characteristic feature of this group. The homeland of this group extends from western parts of Delhi, Uttar Pradesh to Punjab, Haryana, Rajsthan and Gujarat in India and Punjab and Sindh provinces of Paskistan. The breeds in Murrah group are Murrah, Mehsana, Jaffarabadi, Nili-Ravi, and Kundi. Later on Banni breed of Kutcch region has been included in this group. Godawari breed of buffalo of Murrah group has been evolved from the interbreeding of local buffalo with Murrah buffaloes translocated from the native land. Body colour of all breeds except Nili-Ravi breed contains five to seven white markings like blazed face, white limbs below knee and hock joints, white switch of the tail and walled eyes. Jaffarabadi buffaloes are jet black like Murrah and also possessing five to seven white markings like Nili-Ravi. Specimen of brown coat colour not uncommon in Murrah group of buffaloes.

Dairy Buffaloes with Sickle to Sword like Curved Horns

These are medium size dairy breeds of river buffaloes found in Gujarat, Maharashtra, Uttar Pradesh, Bihar, Chhattisgarh, and Karnataka. The horns emerge on either end of poll and extends backwards curving upwards in sickle shape on the distal end. Horns are thicker and heavier in the males. In the Pandharpuri breed very long, tapering and corrugated horns extand posteriorly along the body and in most of the animals may grow beyond withers. Curvature of the horn is inverted shallow bow shaped with tips upward and outward. One to two white chevrons are present in some of the breeds. Body colour is variable in different breeds and it is black to grayish black in most of the breeds but copper colour in Bhadawari breed of Uttar Pradesh. Various breeds of the group are Surti, Nagpuri, Marathawada, Bhadawari, Tarai, and South Kanara.

Crown Horned or Calliper Horned Buffalo

This is a stocky compact animal of strong and short limbs with massive caliper shaped horns. The horns emerge at either side of poll and grow semilunar in line with the occiput. Although milk yield is low but chromosome number (2n = 50) is like other riverine breeds. The representative is Todabreed of Nilgiri in Tamil Nadu.

Not yet Properly Described Riverine Breeds of Buffalo

It is a common practice to use the term non-descript for the herds and flocks of farm animals found in the remote areas. Although many such herds are represented by large population of morphologically identical animals. Some of the herds of considerable number of identiacal riverine buffaloes may be seen in the diara land of river Ganga and Ghaghra and some other rivers in the eastern Uttar Pradesh and northwest Bihar, Timpathi area of Andhra Pradesh, Mysore, and surrounding in Karnataka, coastal area of Ramnathpuram district in Tamil Nadu and Thiruvananthapuram in Kerala state. The dairy breed evolved from the interbreeding of Murrah or Delhi buffalo and local swamp of buffalo of earlier Assam (before the formation of the smaller states in the region) for several hundred years. Even today herds of domesticated buffaloes of Assam and sister states contain members of n different chromosome number, i.e. $2n = 50, 49$, and 48 representing riverine, riverine X swamp and swamp type respectively. Murrah group of dairy buffaloes were probably introduced by the Mughals during their march to east and later on by the Britishers and Indian traders in dairy business. Such ignored herds need proper description and their ancestral linkages.

▶ MURRAH GROUP OF RIVERINE BUFFALO (*BUBALUS BUBALIS*)

$Xn = 50$ number of chromosomes in riverine buffaloes of western region clearly shows that present day wild arnee (*Bubalus arnee*) with $2n = 48$ number of chromosomes is not their ancestor. Excavation of the region will reveal the existence of wild river buffalo in the western region of the Indian subcontinent. The recognized breed of Murrah group are the Murrah, Mehsana, Nili-Ravi, Jaffarabadi in Indian and Kundi and Nili-Ravi in Pakistan. In recent Godawari from Andhra Pradesh is in the process of joining the group. Another breed in Murrah group may be the 'Diara' buffalo breed on the diara land of river Ganga, Ghaghara (Saryu) and their tributaries in the eastern part of Uttar Pradesh and northwest parts of Bihar.

Murrah

This is a famous milk breed and now bred as a multipurpose animal for milk, meat, draught, and industrial by-products not only in India but also in many other countries from Asia to America. The consumers preference for buffalo milk in Indian subcontinent is the main reason for the growth of dairy buffalo rearing stalls (Khatalls) exclusively for milk production in the urban and peri-urban areas of the big cities, towns, and densely populated industrial areas. Good milch buffaloes of high yielding capacity have been extracted from the breeding tract for many decades to terminate in slaughter houses after dying. The calves are killed by starvation within 3–4 weeks of life. This practice has caused great damage in depleting the milk production trait of the breed. In order to protect the destruction of this valuable breed state governments of Haryana and Punjab have banned the movement of female Murrah buffaloes out of the state and have also started to give awards of different denomination for the conservation of buffaloes (Fig. 3.1) yielding more than 20 litres milk daily and their progeny.

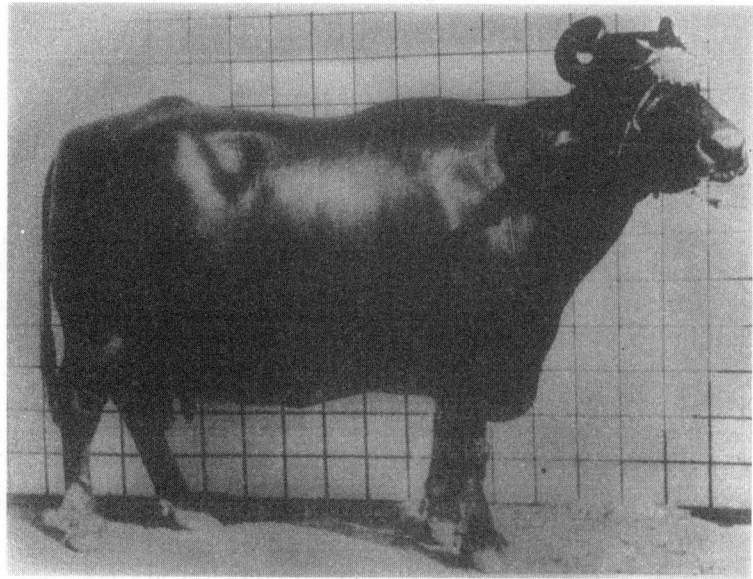

Fig. 3.1: Murrah female

Due to high milk production of high milk fat content, docile nature, easy management, and high adaptability in diverse management Murrah breed has not only spread in the Indian subcontinent but also has crossed the boundry of the continent and reached in many countries of Europe, Africa, and America.

Description

The Murrah buffalo is a large size massive animal of jet black colour (Figs. 3.1 and 3.2). The neck is fine and conical with broad base fusing with brisket. The characteristic horns are tightly coiled and in some animals require cutting of tips to prevent penetration in the head. The head is broad dorsally and slightly convex in the bulls and less convex is the females. A cushion of short hairs is present on the head and in some animals a white star is present. Long tapering tail continues in the switch of long and coarse hairs which may also be an admixture of black and white hairs. However, there are unwanted but acceptable traits. The short face is broad dorsally and narrower blunt with wide oral and the eyes are black, bright, and active. The eyes are prominent in females and slightly shunken in the Murrah bulls. The short and thin ears are placed just below the horns, and nostrils are wide apart.

Fine and smooth neck fuses dorsally with shoulder and ventrally with brisket. The slightly convex wither is tapering posteriorly. The chest is broad with well sprung ribs and long barrel is voluminous for acorn dating adequate amount of fibrous feeds. The brisket is prominent and may be bulging in healty animals of advance age due to deposition of fat. Some of the common characteristics of Murrah buffaloes are summarized in Table 3.1 and details are given by Ranjhan and Pathak (1994).

TABLE 3.1: Some physical characteristics of Murrah buffalo		
Characteristics	Male	Female
Body weight (kg)	600–1200 (750)	400–800 (550)
Body length (cm)	150–168 (159)	129–168 (149)
Height and withers (cm)	132–142 (137)	127–145 (136)
Heart girth (cm)	213–239 (226)	193–257 (225)
Tail length (cm)	117–142 (129)	114–135 (124)

Mehsana

The name has derived from the native district Mehsana of Gujarat. It is said that this breed has evolved from continuous interbreeding between Murrah and Surti (Oliver 1938) but is does not appear to be true because none of the member of Mehsana herd ever possesses even broken chevron which is characteristic for the Surti buffalo. Actually Mehsana breed is a medium size member of Murrah group of buffaloes. The phenotypic traits are quite similar to Murrah breed except the coiling of horns in very loose and often wide open, face is longer and body is less massive (Fig. 3.2). The colour is black, body is deep and low set. Sexual dimorphism is apparent ad males are heavier than the females. This breed is mostly concentrated in Mehsana, Banaskantha, Sabarkantha and Gandhinagar towns of Gujarat. Every year large number of females in early lactation and terminal month of gestation are taken away by the dairy stall owners of Mumbai, Pune, and other thickly populated cities. Greater number of such buffaloes finish in slaughter houses and their calves are subjected to fatal under feeding from elimination in the first month of life.

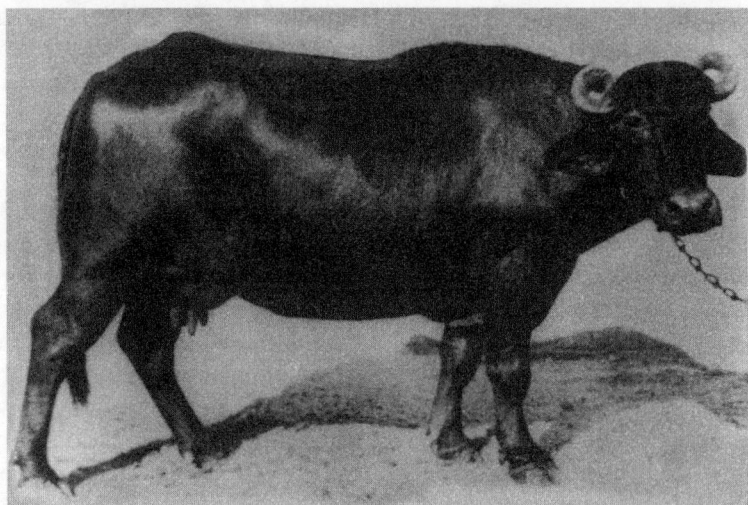

Fig. 3.2: Mehsana buffalo

Description

Mehsana buffalo is a medium size animal of north region of Gujarat bordering Rajsthan in north and Kuchchha in west. Physical appearance is quite comparable with the Murrah breed. The head is like an inverted wide mouth conical flask with shallow depression on the poll. Single loose coiled horns are short and black. The eyes are a little protruded and short nose bridge is straight. The medium size ears are just below the horns with front facing hairy inner surface. Long neck gradually widen posteriorly to fuse with the shoulders and brisket. The neck is massive in males and fine in females. Chest is wide and deep with well sprung ribs and long barrel is capacious. Wider hind quarters make the body wedge shaped in the females. The Naval flap is almost fused with abdomen in females and small blunt triangular in males. The physical measurements (Kaura, 1952) presented in Table 3.2 may be considered for revision on the basis of recent observations (Pundir et al., 2000).

TABLE 3.2: Some physical measurement of Mehsana breed

Physical traits	Male	Female
Body weight (kg)	500–650 (580)	350–600 (500)
Body length (cm)	130–137 (133)	107–142 (137)
Height and withers (cm)	127–137 (132)	112–142 (132)
Heart girth (cm)	178–185 (182)	183–218 (198)
Tail length (cm)	97–102 (99)	76–135 (124)

Mehsana breed may be more suitable for the feed scarcity areas due to smaller body size and satisfactory milk yield. It needs revised description and selective breeding.

Zaffrabadi/Jafarabadi/Jafari

This is heaviest breed of river buffalo found concentrated in the Gir forest area of Gujarat state of India. The buffaloes could survive the threat of Gir lion due to their long and massive drooping horns curling at the end (Fig. 3.3). This type of horns provide protection to larynx and windpipe from choking by the strong canines of lions. The buffaloes live in big groups on grazing land and form a circle around the youngers and challenge the predator in well-coordinated manner. This breed is mostly reared by the 'Maldhari' families' Gondal Ashram in Gujarat is maintaining an elite herd of Jaffarabadi buffaloes. Two adult bulls at the Ashram weigh about 1300 and 1400 kg and a female weighing about 1200 kg produced 32 kg milk of more than 8% milk fat content or peak yield and lactation period lasted over 300 days. Locally this breed is also called Gir and Bhavanagari buffalo. Some of physical traits of this breed recorded long back (White and Mathur, 1966) are presented in Table 3.3. However, there is urgent need of complete description of this highly valuable breed.

TABLE 3.3: Average measurements of Jafarabadi buffalo

Traits	Male	Female
Body weight (kg)	655	590
Body length (cm)	167.64	160.02
Height and withers (cm)	142.24	139.70
Heart girth (cm)	190.50	187.96

This breed is well-adapted to grazing and some animals yield more than 20 kg milk daily during the peak period. Lactation yield may be more than 2000 kg on optimum management. The breed is recognized by its distinct feature of large and rough head, convex crown, drooping broad, and long horns curled outwards and inwards on the

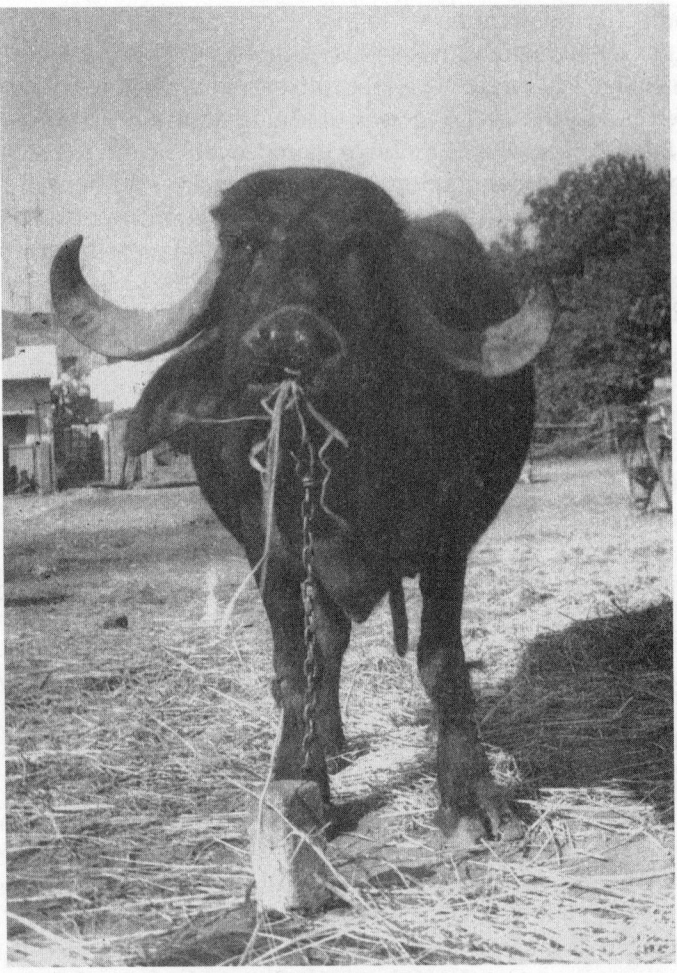

Fig. 3.3: Jaffarabadi bull

distal end (Figs 3.5 and 3.6). The skin and coat are jet black in most of the animals but good number of animals resembling Nili-Ravi in 5–7 white markings like blazed face, White limbs, walled eyes and white switch of the tail are also found. This is a strong point for clubbing Murrah, Nili-Ravi and Jafarabadi together. This breed has been developed for milk and meat production in Brazil and Venezuela.

Nili-Ravi Buffalo

This is an important breed of old Punjab. At present its number is much more in Pakistan. For the improvement of this breed a research centre of Central Buffalo Research Institute is working at Nabha in Punjab. The two almost identical breeds Nili and Ravi were made Nili-Ravi during 1938 and described as a variety of Murrah (Oliver, 1938) but this was not accepted and Nili-Ravi remained a separate breed (Kaura, 1952). However, the two were made Nili-Ravi in 1960. Earlier this breed was maintained at Military Dairy Farms of India which were replaced by exotic and crossbred dairy cattle.

The physical appearance and production of Nili-Ravi breed is similar to Murrah breed and this breed is differentiated by prominent 7 white markings like blazed face, part or complete white limbs below knee and hock joints, complete or partial walled eye and white switch of the tail. Sexual dimorphism is apparent and bulls are much heavier than the females (Fig. 3.4). Shape of horns is quite variable and may be tight sickle like but always thick. The face contains more coarse hairs than the body. Almost all characteristics of dairy breed is present in the animal. For selection lactation yield should be more than 2000 kg in 305 days. Some of the body measurements are given in Table 3.4.

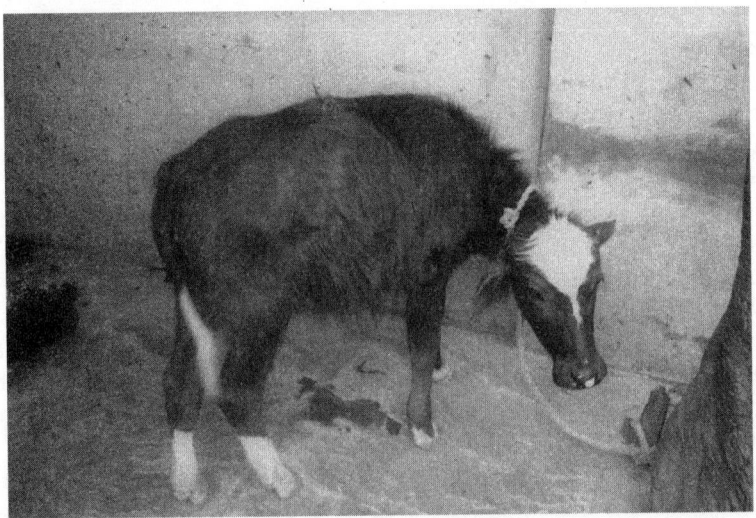

Fig. 3.4: Nill-Ravi buffalo

TABLE 3.4: Some body measurements of Nili-Ravi breed

Measurements	Male	Female
Body weight (kg)	600–1200 (800)	400–800 (600)
Body length (cm)	150–168 (159)	129–168 (149)
Height and withers (cm)	132–142 (137)	127–145 (136)
Heart girth (cm)	213–239 (226)	193–257 (225)
Tail length (cm)	117–142 (129)	114–135 (124)

At present pure Nili-Ravi buffaloes with clear seven white markings are bred at the Nabha research station of Central Institute for research on buffalo in India. Pure Nili-Ravi breed is also multiplied and used for the upgrading of local buffaloes in China. The average milk yield of Nili-Ravid buffalo breed in China has been reported 2262.2 ± 663.9 kg and that of F1, F2, and triple crossbred between swamp, Murrah, and Nili-Ravi had been 2041 ± 540.9 kg, 2325.0 ± 994.41 kg, and 2294.1 ± 772.1 kg respectively (Yang and Zhang, 2006).

Kundi Buffalo

It is an important dairy buffalo of Pakistan mostly found in the wet region of paddy cultivation area in Sindh and Baluchistan in the vicinity of Sindhu river (Indus river). The buffalo is lighter in size but comparable in milk production with Murrah and Nili-Ravi. Majority of animals are jet black but like other breeds of Murrah groups, brown animals are also found. Rare occurrence of gray colour or albinoid specimen is not uncommon. Specimens with white markings but not blazed face like Nili-Ravi are preferred in some areas.

The preferred white markings are a prominent star on forehead, all white hooves, white switch of the tail and wall eyes. Sexual dimorphism is seen as adult breeding bulls are heavier from 550–600 kg and that of females from 300–400 kg with milk yield 1700–2200 litres (Shah, 1994). Thus, this may be considered as a highly efficient dairy breed of riverine buffaloes.

Banni Buffalo

It is newly described breed of Murrah group of riverine buffaloes reared for livelihood through milk production under the extensive through milk production under the extensive and semi-intensive system of buffalo production. About 33% buffaloes are found in the Kuchchh region followed by Sabarkantha, Surendranagar, 1 Kheda and Banaskantha housing more than 35,000 buffaloes. Substantial number of Banni buffalo is also found in Anand, Gandhinagar, Rajkot, Vadodara, Surat, and Panchmahal districts of Gujarat state in India as per the 2009 census report of the Directorate of Animal Hurbandry, Ganghinagar. Limited observations recorded during the last few years (Sing and Branhakshtri, 2005; Chavan, 2006; Sing, 2007; Singh and Pachasara, 2007; and Mishra et al., 2009) have been reviewed by Singh et al. (2010). The informations on morphology and production traits of this new breed may be used until finalization of the description of Banni breed.

Some organization like Banni Breeder Asociation of Maldhari (Banni Pashu Uchharak Maldhary Sangathan), S.D. Agricultural University, Sardarkrushinagar, Hodka Paryatan and Sahjeevan are working for the protection and development of Banni buffalo as a valuable dairy animal of Gujarat. At present extensive production system is followed in the Banni area. The buffaloes are milked once daily in the morning. The animals are reared on exclusive grazing and some amount of concentrates available in the house or local market is offered at the time of milking. In other areas semiintensive system is followed. The grazing herd move with eligible buffalo bulls for natural breeding.

Description of Banni

The Banni breed is a typical dairy animal of Murrah group with wedge shaped body, fine skin and well-developed mammary apparatus. The crown is almost straight with a shallow depression in the middle. The face is long with straight bridge of nose and broad muzzle with wide nostrils. The eyes are black, bright, and prominent. The horns are tight coiled like Murrah in most of the animals but double curling is not uncommon. Medium size ears are lightly fringed. Moderate neck is narrow, smooth and without develop. The chest in deep and wide with well sprung ribs and barrel is capacious. Medium size bonned legs terminate in strong sure foot hooves of black colour. The colour of hoof is a consipicuous difference from Kundi breed. The skin is black, soft and pliable with scanty scattered black hairs. A small population may be grayish brown to copper colour as observed in many breeds. There is no record of albinoid specimen in any known herd. Long tail terminates in black switch. However, in few animals white hairs on forehead star on lower part of limbs and switch of the tail may occur.

The udder is well-developed and normally dish shaped of almost equal size quarters with moderate size conical teats of slightly lighter colour than the skin of body. The measurements of body show sexual dimorphism (Table 3.5).

TABLE 3.5: Body measurements of Banni buffalo

Attributes	Calves (0–3 month)		Adult animals	
	Male	Female	Male	Female
Height at withers (cm)	84.3 ± 1.18	87.2 ± 1.06	137.6 ± 1.89	137.3 ± 0.3
Heart girth (cm)	97.9 ± 2.24	99.5 ± 1.58	214.0 ± 5.10	203.7 ± 0.60
Paunch girth (cm)	102.9 ± 2.98	107.3 ± 2.11	228.0 ± 6.44	217.8 ± 3.08

The reproduction performance fails to prove the myth of delayed maturity and delayed breeding. The reproductive performances are comparable with the good breeds of dairy cattle and milk yield is quite satisfactory (Table 3.6).

TABLE 3.6: Some reproductive and production traits of Banni buffalo

Performance traits	Value
Age of foirst calving (months)	40.3 ± 0.25
Calving interval (months)	12.2 ± 0.08
Service period (days)	72.7 ± 1.39
Peak milk yield (kg/day)	14.74 ± 0.33
Days to attain peak yield	38.04 ± 2.92
Milk fat percentage during	
Early lactation	5.43 ± 0.01
Late lactation	7.66 ± 0.21
Over all average	6.65 ± 0.11

Although random sampling of milk yield does not demarket the peak yield (Table 3.7) but the pattern of milk secretion is showing the sustainability of milk production. The rate of decline in the daily milk yield indicates the advantage of dairying for small holders earning livelihood from the marketing of fluid milk.

TABLE 3.7: Milk yield pattern of Banni buffaloes

Month	Daily milk yield (l)	Monthly milk yield (l)
1	12.97 ± 0.30	388.44 ± 9.08
2	12.66 ± 0.32	376.37 ± 9.71
3	12.01 ± 0.36	358.59 ± 11.70
4	11.01 ± 0.35	332.96 ± 9.99
5	10.39 ± 0.33	316.28 ± 9.18
6	9.90 ± 0.31	294.35 ± 8.89
7	8.16 ± 0.33	249.74 ± 9.17
8	7.53 ± 0.26	236.93 ± 8.70
9	6.64 ± 0.42	
Overall	10.78 ± 0.11	327.87 ± 3.47

Although number of lactating animals during different months was variable but may be considered quite satisfactory for justifying the good dairy ability of the breed. A well-design long-term study on large number of animals for successive three or more lactations will provide more valuable information about the production traits of Banni buffalo.

7. Godawari Buffalo

This is a dairy type riverine buffalo breed of Murrah group and has been evolved from interbreeding between local and Murrah followed by random selection of high milk yield. The milk production potential of now stable Godawari breed is comparable with the production of Murrah. The animal is concentrated in the delta region of Godawari river in Andhra Pradesh. This is a medium size wedge shaped animal of compact body. The colour is mostly black and scanty coarse black to brownish hairs are present on the body. The head is slightly convex, face is narraw, eyes are bright and nostrils are moderately wide. Loose curled horns are falt and moderate in size. Deep chest is capacious due to well sprung ribo. Barrel is long and capacious for holding large rumen and back is straight with broad rump. Medium size udder is linked with tortuous milk vein and teats are cylindrical in majority of buffaloes. Long tapering tail extends below hock joint to terminate in a black and white or white switch of long and coarse hairs. Daily milk yield is still quite variable and ranges from 5 to 8 kg and lactation yield 1200 to 2000 kg. In the agroclimatic condition of Godawari delta breeding is quite regular and inter-calving period is less than the buffaloes of dry-hot zone of northen part of India. This breed is most smitable for the region and scope of economic growth of buffalo breeders is quite bright due to establishment of buffalo meat production industry at Hyderabad.

II. RIVERINE BUFFALO GROUP OF SICKLE SHAPED HORNS

The buffalo breeds of this are small to medium size animals of gray, grayish black, copper colour, and black colour. The characteristic features of this group of buffaloes are the posteriorly extending sickle shaped horns of different size. The horns take the shape of sickle due to shallow upward turning to end at blunt pointed tips. The horns are mostly flat and carries shallow depressions of different size. These depressions or rings were earlier used for the assessment of age of buffaloes. The dairy buffaloes of this group are found in Uttrakhand, Uttar Pradesh, Bihar, Madhya Pradesh, Rajsthan, Gujarat, Maharashtra, Chhattisgarh, Karnataka, and Kerala in India.

Surti or Suratic Buffalo

This medium size buffalo is another pride of Gujarat which was described first time by Dave (1940) and presented in Bullentin No. 86 (1960) of the Indian Council of Agricultural Research, New Delhi. The home tract of Surti buffalo spreads between the Sabarmati and Mahi rives and typical Surti predominates the buffaloes of Kaira and Vadodara districts. This breed forms the basis of cooperative dairies of the region. Surti buffalo is one of the main source of subsidiary income and success has resulted in increased number of buffalo rearing per family during the past 4–5 decades. Women flock of farming families are mostly responsible for the management of buffaloes including the marketing and health management. Some other names like Deccani, Gujarati, and Nadiadi have been earlier used for the Surti breed. Generally lactating females and their surviving followers are maintained by the farmers. A few selected males are maintained by the 'Vaghari' community for the breeding of buffaloes against payment. Considerable number of Surti buffaloes are also found in the neighbouring states like Rajsthan in the north and Maharashtra and Karnataka in the south, west part of Madhya Pradesh and also in Bangladesh.

Description

Surti is a light frame animal of medium size and stout short limbs with stocking on knees. Body colour ranges from black to brownish gray. White chevson is characteristic for the breed. The number of chevson is normally two, one just across the jowl and another in front of brisket. However, one, incomplete formed or branches chevson may also be seen occasionally. The limbs below knee and hock joints are mostly light grayish black to grayish brown. The horns are black. The bright and round prominent eyes show intelligence. A white streak is mostly seen over the eyebrows. Medium size and slightly droping ears are reddish in colour and may contain fringe of white hairs on lower border. Horns show the sexual dimorphism being heavier in males than the females. The horns emerge from the sides of skull and extends backwards along the neck and then turns upwards to form the shape of sickle or shallow hook. In few cases horns may run slightly downwards and then gradually upwards to end in shallow hook. The head is moderately broad and round between the horns with long nose bridge and broad nortrils.

The long neck is thinner and clean in female and massive in bulls without dewlap. Chest is broad with well sprug ribs and brisket in more prominent in aged animals. The shoulders bland smoothly with the body. Medium size wedge shaped barrel is quite suitable for the animals. The bulls are robust and heavier with broad shoulders and massive hips. The hind quarters are wide, deep and straight, and loins are broad. Wide apart pin bones and hook bones show capacious pelvic cavity. Prominent hocks are sturdy. The tapering and flexible tail is fairly long and terminates in a white or black and white switch (Fig. 3.5).

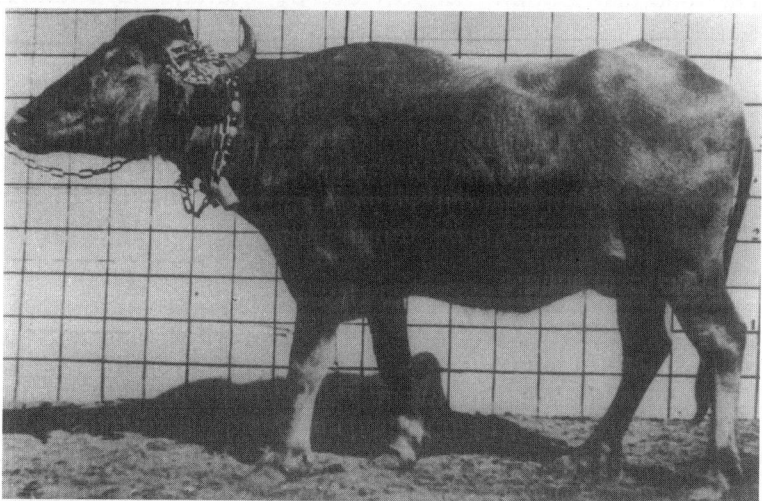

Fig. 3.5: Suratic buffalo

The mammary system is well-developed. The udder is generally dish shaped with medium teats of almost equal size. Several twist provides plenty space for the development of udder. The tortuous milk veins are prominent and capacious. The skin is pliable, smooth and soft than the skin of body. The body contains sparsely distributed black, grayish black or grayish red hairs. Body coat may be reasonably dense in animal translocated to colder climatic condition. The measurements of male and female adult Surti as per ICAR (1960) are given in Table 3.8.

TABLE 3.8: Physical measurements of adult Surti buffalo

Physical traits	Male	Female
Body weight (kg)	480–700 (590)	350–500 (450)
Body length (cm)	137–155 (143)	124–147 (138)
Height behind wither (cm)	118–140 (131)	118–131 (124)
Heart girth (cm)	175–197 (185)	177–211 (191)
Tail length (cm)	79–94 (87)	71–89 (89)

Surti buffaloes produce highly nutritious milk rich in milk fat (8.9%) and 4.06% milk protein (Vyas and Patel, 1974). Lactation milk yield ranges from 1700 to 2000 kg in a lactation period of about ten months. The animals are regular breeder and quite suitable for the owners of low economic group. An attempt of crossbreeding may destroy a promising breed of buffalo well-adapted for the home tract and other comparable agro-climatic conditions.

Nagpuri Buffalo

This is a medium size breed of Bidarbh region of Maharashtra and well-adapted for thriving on the scanty herbage cover and coarse fodder of the relatively dry agro-climatic conditions (Fig. 3.6). The synonyms of the breed are Berari, Durnathli, Ellichpuri, Gauli, Marathawada and Varadi. In recent years the buffaloes of Marathawada region has been described as a separate breed on the basis of some morphological difference. This breed was first described by Oliver (1938) and subsequently more informations on performance and distribution was provided by Kaura (1952) who has observed phenotypic variations justified for further description. The sequel is the separation of Marathawada as a separate breed.

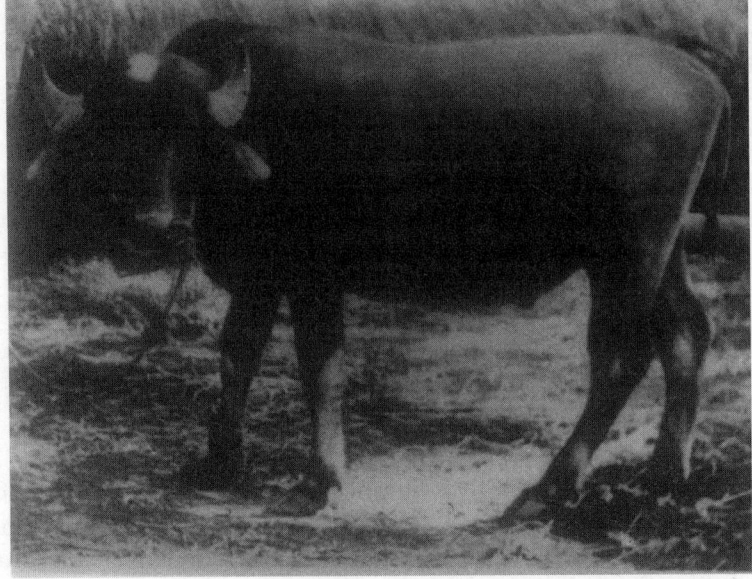

Fig. 3.6: Nagpuri buffalo

The Nagpuri is a medium size buffalo of compact body and strong sure footed legs. The animal is suitable for thriving in rough terrain of hills and forest and move in groups to keep predators away on grazing range. The colour is black with scanty hairs on the body. White markings may be found on the face, legs and switch of the tail. The variation in body weight has been shown in the records of Hadi(1966) showing body weight range from 320 to 400 kg while Whyte and Mathur (1966) have reported average 522 kg for Nagpuri bulls and 408 kg for Nagpuri females.

The face is long and narrow like an inverted cone and prominent nasal bone is strong. The fine and longer neck fuses with the shoulders dorsally and heavy brisket ventrally. Long horns may rich up to the withers and heavier in bulls than the females. The horns erupt a little posterior on the dorsolateral sidewards and than turning upwards to make the shape of the shallow sickle. Average size of Nagpuri buffalo is presented in Table 3.9.

TABLE 3.9: Average measurements of adult Nagpuri buffalo		
Physical traits	Male	Female
Body length (cm)	172	142
Height behind withers (cm)	142	132
Heart girth (cm)	211	206

Nagpuri buffaloes are reared in Nagpuri and adjoining areas of Madhya Pradesh, Chhattisgarh and Andhra Pradesh.

Marathawada Buffalo

This smaller strain of earlier described Napuri buffalo was identified as a separate breed by Rife (1957) and Hadi (1965) at Aurangabad in Maharashtra. This is mostly a black colour animal of compact body, dairy conformation and 320 to 400 kg body weight. The sickle shaped horns usually extend up to shoulders and these are heavier in males. Concentration of this breed is more in Aurangabad, Beed, Jalna, Latur, Nanded, Osmanabad, Parbhani, and some parts of Akola and Buldhana districts of Maharashtra. (Padghan et al., 2008). Average milk yield of high fat content is 960 kg per lactation. The pH of milk ranges from 6.29 to 6.79 (average 6.54). Acidity as lactic acid percentage is 0.514 (0.12 to 0.19) and specific gravity is 1.31 (1.027 to 1.035 Padghan et al., 2008).

Pandharpuri Buffalo

This is also known as Dharwari buffalo. This buffalo breed is more common in the area of Ahmadnagar, Kolhapur, and Sholapur but also found in neighbouring area of Andhra Pradesh and Karnataka. It is a medium size breed of long and compact body. This is a hardy breed capable to thrive on poor herbage cover of dry areas. The face is long and narrow with narrower frontal bone. The nose bridge is straight and veins are prominent on the nasal bone. Very long, narrow and semilunar curved with prominent grooves or extent backwards and upwards at the distal part. The length may exceed back level in many animals (Fig. 3.7.). The neck is long and narrow. The long tail extends below the hock joint to terminate normally in a white switch. Body colour is mostly black but lighter black animals are also found. The animal is mostly docile, easy to handle and can be milked 3 to 5 times at short interval for door to door sale of fresh drawn milk. Medium size udder is normally dish shaped and somewhat posteriorly placed.

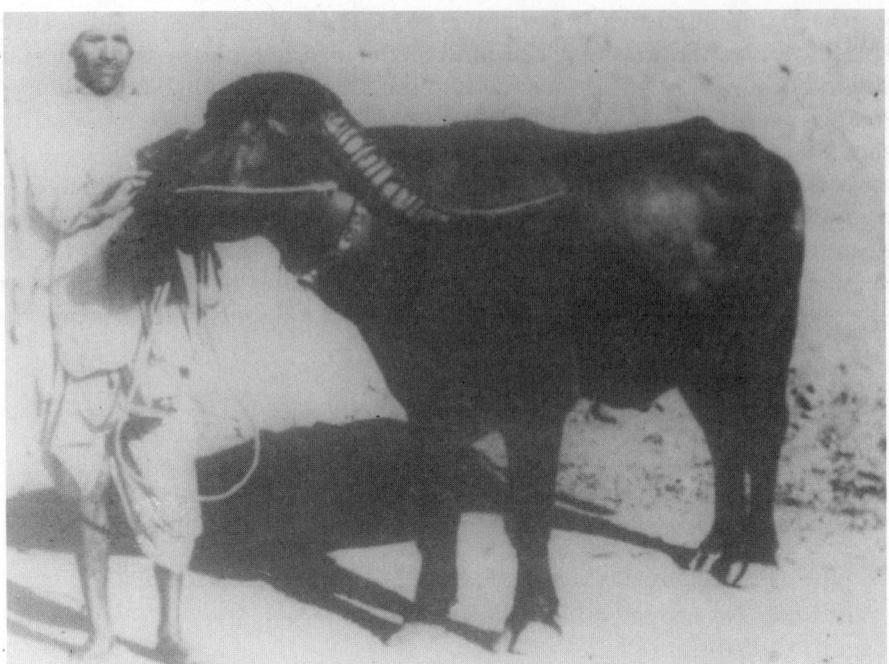

Fig. 3.7: Pandharpuri buffalo

Bhadawari Buffalo

The name 'Bhadawari' was derived from. The erstwhile 'Bhadawar' state, the home land of the breed. Earlier this breed was maintained at the government livestock farm, Bharari near Jhansi. At present this breed is maintained at the Indian grassland and fodder Research Institute, Jhansi (author is responsible for the unit established as part of Network project on Buffalo Breeding of ICRA) and another at Veterinary College, Mathura and third at a research station of Chandra Shekhar Azad University of Agriculture and Technology in Etawah district of Uttar Pradesh. The number of this breed has decreased and now few animals may be seen scattered in Agra, Mathura, Etawah and Jhansi districts of Uttar Pradesh and Gwalior, Guna, Shuvapuri, Bhind, Morena, and Datia districts of Madhya Pradesh. The popularity of this breed has lowered due to low milk yield.

Bhadawari, is a light to medium size buffalo of variable brownish colour commonly described as copper colour (Kaura, 1952). The body is narrow in front and wide behind. The legs are short an shout. Sure footed hooves are hard and black. The hind quarter is a little higher than the fore quarters. The head is medium and crown is slightly convex or flat between the horns. The horns are medium in length, flat, corrugated and turn upwards at distal end in sickle shape. The face is short and narrow with prominent nose bridge. The ears are short and the eyes are bright, active and prominent in females. Medium size neck is thin in females and massive in bulls. Two (sometimes one) V-shaped chavsons are present on the neck. The chast is capacious with well sprung ribs (Figs 3.8 and 3.9). Long and tapering tail reaches below the hock to end in a grayish white switch. Dish shaped udder is moderately developed and pinkish colour small teats are squarely placed. Some physical measurements of adult buffaloes are presented in Table 3.10.

TABLE 3.10: Some physical measurements of Bhadawari buffalo

Measurements	Minimum	Maximum	Average
Body weight (kg)	300	550	425
Body length (cm)	122	155	139
Height at withers (cm)	122	140	130
Heart girth (cm)	160	206	192
Belly girth (cm)	183	226	204

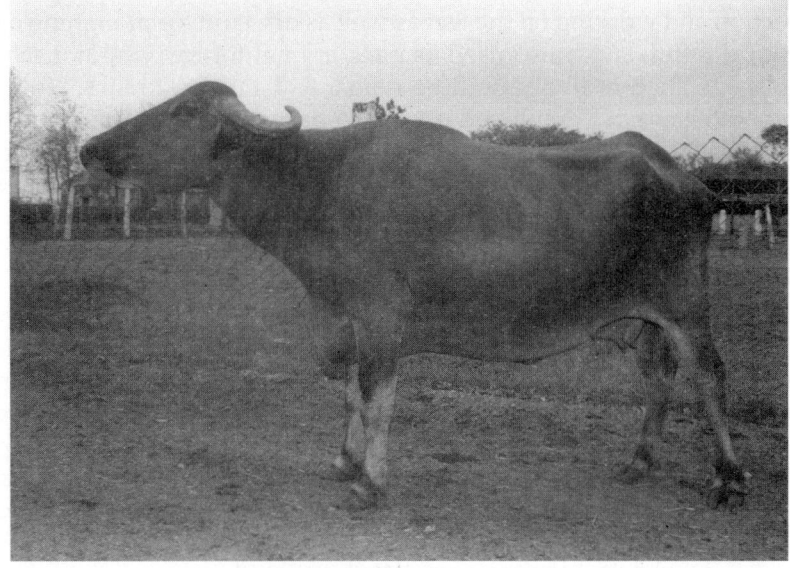

Fig. 3.8: Bhadawari female

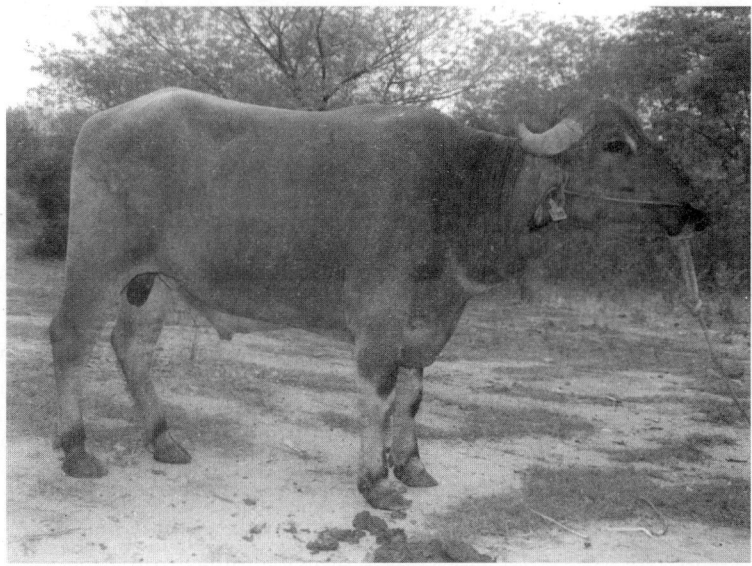

Fig. 3.9: Bhadawari male

This breed is capable of thriving on coarse roughages of dry and hilly region and produces high quality milk containing 7–8% butter fat which may be more than 12% in some rare animals. The breed is being conserved and bred for improving dairy characteristics.

Tarai Buffalo

This is a breed of medium size sturdy and hardy riverine buffalo of Himalayan Tarai. The animals are found in Tarai region of Uttar Pradesh and Utarkhand in India and the adjoining border area of Nepal. This breed has been evolved as a dual purpose animal for milk production and working on the wet as well as dry land for ploughing and pulling cart load. Some animals are also used as pack animal for carrying household goods from one place to another by the shifting nomadic 'banjara' families. Now in greater part of the native land of Tarai breed extensive use of Murrah semen has helped the upgrading of this breed resulting in higher production but spoiled the purity of breed to greater extent. Selection would have been a better approach for the improvement of milk production protential of the breed.

Description

It is a buffalo of long and compact body, short limbs with stock on knee and surefooted hooves (Kaura, 1952). Body colour ranges from jet black to grayish black and grayish-convex for head and prominent nasal bone. The muzzle is thick and darker in colour than the body, and always remains wet in healthy animals. The black eyes are bright. The colour of fore legs may be lighter than the body colour. Stockings are present on the knee. The tapering tail is moderately long and switch of the tail is usually white. The horns are heavier in males. These runs backwards along the neck and turns slightly inwards at the tip in shape of a shallow sickle. The dorsal surface is corrugated by shallow depressions. Although it is not difficult to find pure specimen but in larger area it has been crossed with Murrah due to which different types of buffaloes of Tarari × Murrah crosses are now seen particularly in Pilibhit, Bareilly, Moradabad, Rampur, Bijnore, Naivital and Hardwar districts of Uttar Pradesh and Uttarakhand.

South Canara or Kanara Buffalo

This breed belong to riverine type but due to selection for agricultural works for very long period, it has suffered great deterioration in dairy characteristics. This breed has acquired the characteristics of draught buffaloes. The synonyms used for the breed are Kanaras, Kanarese, and Malabari. This breed was spotted by littlewood (1936) and has been described by Ramesha et al. (2010 personal communication).

This breed is found in greater number in the Bantwala, Belthangadi, Mangalore, Puttur, and Sulya talukas of Dakshina Kannerda district and Karkala, Kumdapura, and Udupi talukas of the Udupi districts. This breed has been developed as a draught animal. A few selected robust buffalo bull calves are specially reared and trained for the buffalo race competition celebrated after the harvesting of paddy crop. The buffalo race is known as 'Kambala'. Both sexes are used for working. The males are used for heavy works and female for light works.

Description

This is a medium size hardy breed of compact body with well-developed shoulders and hind quarters. The limbs are boned and hooves are strong. Body colour is black to light black in females and working males but jet black in buffalo bulls and the males reared for 'Kambala' race. Moderately long, flat, and curved horns grow backwards, sidewards, and downwards along the neck region. Females yield small amount of milk of high fat content. Some of the major physical measurements (Ramesha et al., 2010, personal communication) are presented in Table 3.11.

TABLE 3.11: Some physical measurements of adult South Canara buffalo

Attributes	Female	Male	Breeding bulls
Body length (cm)	124.4 ± 1.85	126.6 ± 1.01	129.6 ± 1.28
Height at withers (cm)	128.0 ± 1.37	130.5 ± 1.25	135.2 ± 1.15
Hearth girth (cm)	212.0 ± 2.69	207.0 ± 3.11	229.6 ± 4.43
Face width (cm)	23.0 ± 0.26	23.0 ± 0.31	23.2 ± 0.37
Tail length (cm)	97.5 ± 1.05	94.5 ± 1.25	95.0 ± 0.99

Toda Buffalo

This is a medium breed of compact body and small bonned legs 'Toda' tripe of Tamil Nadu in Nilgiri region. The body is long and massive. The face is short and wide with broad and prominent forehead covered with hairs. The horns are variable in size but typical caliper shaped mounted as semilumar arch on the head. The horns are annulated and heavier in males than the females. As usual withers and dewlap are rudimentary. The chest is broad and deep with well sprung ribs. There is dense growth of course hairs along the crest like the mane in bison. Hair growth extends up to back. The colour is grayish black to gray with stockings on knees and chavaron on neck. The males of same group are heavier than the females. Average height of adult Toda bulls at withers is 160 cm and body weight 400 kg and that of adult female is 150 cm and 380 kg respectively. This is a tamed breed maintained on grazing. The animals are collected in evening for resting in night. Although this is a member of riverine group but milk yield is very low (2–4 kg daily) and lactation length losts for 6 to 8 months. Fat content in milk may exceed 8%. The milk of Toda buffaloes is more liked due to characteristic flavoured taste (Little wood, 1936). The number of this breed has significantly decreased and now protective measured are being taken for the conservation of this breed.

Sambalpuri/Gowadoo/Kimedi Buffalo

Although this breed has been named after the place of rearing, i.e. Sambalpur in Odisha (Orissa) but homeland is Bilaspur district of Chhattisgarh state. Author could not gather information on its chromosome number but from the high milk yield this breed appears to be a member of riverine group of buffaloes of sickle to sword type horn group. This may be a variant of Nagpuri breed also prevalent in Nagpur and adjoining area of Chhatisgarh. This is a large size docile animal with long lactation period of 10 to 12 months and some rare animals continue to yield but small quantity of milk only once in morning for another few months. However, this information is provided be the owners and not recorded at a farm. This breed have skin and hairs black and rarely gray or brownish gray specimen may appear in the herd. In good management and feeding milk yield may range from 2270 to 2720 kg in the lactation period of 330 to 360 days (Cockrail, 1974). Sickle shaped horns are medium to long size and sometimes length is long and extended laterally that it becomes difficult to use a pair to put yoke for pulling plough cannot tolerate sun heat for longer time.

▶ DAIRY BUFFALOES OF NEAR EAST AND EUROPE

Buffaloes entered in the countries of near east and Europe during the beginning of twentieth century. The animals were carried from the dairy buffalo tract of the Indian subcontinent primarily for milk production form the utilization of coarse grasses of the swamps and other wetlands some people also believe that a wild buffalo was present in the swamps of Egypt before the beginning of modern calendar. The morphology of modern dairy buffaloes of near east and Europe shows that the modern dairy buffaloes of this region have been developed from the interbreeding of Murrah, Nili-Ravi, Jaffarabadi, Kundi, Surti, etc. in different ratios. This is evident from the appearance of specimens with chevron, gray skin, piebald skin or very rarely alberviods. The present differences in the morphology and productivity among the buffaloes of near east and Europe is the result of variations and selection of production traits because of the difference in utility of buffaloes. In the near east countries the buffaloes were developed as a triple purpose animal for milk, meat, and draught whereas in many European countries the main purpose is milk production specially for the preparation of 'mozerella' cheese and males are fattened for buffveal and buffen production.

The buffaloes of this group have been identified is some breeds but mostly there are named after the country of breeding like Egyption, Irani, Bulgarian, Romanian, and Italian, etc. the another system of defining these buffaloes is based on the areas of their concentration like Anatolian, Causasian, and Mediterranean buffaloes. The buffaloes of high growth rate ranging from 600 g to more than one kilogram daily and high milk yield of more than 2500–3000 kg per lactation with some exceptional high yielder up to 4500 kg per lactation have been developed in Bulgaria (Peeva, 2010).

Anatolian Buffalo

This is a medium size dairy buffalo of Turkey found in wet region of Black Sea north of Anatolia. The skin is black but grayish black and rarely grayish brown animals are also found. Body is covered with long hairs which are more dense during the winter season. The body is wedge shaped with capacious barrel and broad chest due to well sprung ribs. The bowned limbs are strong. The tail of variable size mostly terminates into switch of long and coarse white hairs. Medium size horns are sickle shaped extending slightly backwards and upwards forming variable curvature. The horns are thick at the root and blunt pointed. White marks may be seen on forehead and face.

There is considerable variation in the body measurements of buffaloes ranges form 350 to 900 kg and height at withers 124 to 139 cm (Cock rail, 1974). Lactation is highly variatiable and ranges from 6 to 9 months, and milk yield 700 to 1100 kg with 6.6 to 8.1% fat content. Milk composition may be considered as a indicator of high concentration of Mehsana, Surti and Nagpuri buffaloes.

Caucasian Buffalo/Azeri Buffalo

This breed of buffalo was introduced in Iran from western parts of the Indian sub-continent before the modern calendar, i.e. about 9th century BC as evident from the presence of Engraved buffalo skulls. This is a dairy breed but also used for meat and work with some riders on the slaughter. Greater concentration of this breed is found on the marshy herbages along the Kura river valley and along the Caspian Sea coast extending in Armenia, Azarbaizan, Georgia, and Iran. Husbandry is highly variable and animals are herded in open during summer and housed indoor during the winter season.

The size of buffaloes reared in hilly region is smaller than the animals bred in lowland. The caucasion buffaloes are dark gray and body coat is generally black but may be also blackish brown in few animals. Density and size of hairs on body increase during the winter season. The calves are mostly grayish brown at birth and gradually turn darker to characteristic colour with the increase in age.

Adult males with 137 cm height at withers are taller than the 124–133 cm height of females. Body weight ranges from 390 kg to 618 kg in both sexes. Milk yield of caucasian buffaloes varies significantly among the herds of different areas. This is generally due to breeding and management variations. Milk yield ranges from 750 kg to more than 1700 kg (Cockrail, 1974). Animals reared on farms generally produce more milk than the animals on grazing.

Egyptian Buffalo

Like other buffaloes of near east and Europe the Egyption buffalo has also evolved from the interbreeding among the Indian dairy breeds introduced during 6th to 7th century by different means. There may be some relationship of 'Al Murrah' nomadic tribe of Egypt as the most popular dairy breed of Indian riverine buffalo is the Murrah. The description of various Egyption buffaloes indicates that these are the decendenty of Murrah, Nili-Ravi, Jaffarabadi, and Surti as indicated by the appearance of characteristic traits like chevron, wall eye, heavy size, and high milk yield. Although it is a common practice to describe Egyptian buffaloes as a single breed but three variants (Cockrail, 1974) need detail study for concluding the actual status. These variants or breeds are the Beheri and Menoufi of the lower region and Saidi of the upper region.

The wedge shaped body of large size animal is an important morphological trait of dairy buffalo. The males are heavier than the females.

Kuhzestani Buffalo of Iraq and Iran

This is a large dairy breed comparable with Murrah, Nili-Ravi, and Jaffarabadi breeds of India. The name has been adopted from the Kuhzestan province of Iran. The appearance of chevron and shape of horns also indicate the presence of Surti blood in the breed. Some selected large males measure 148 cm at withers and weight 800 kg whereas selected large size females are 141 cm at withers and weight 600 kg (Moiohi and Borghese, 2005). However, wide range in height 134 to 143 cm and body weight 360 to 300 kg have been reported by Cockrail (1974). The buffaloes are kept outdoor on pasture for most of the time and housed in night in paddocks having a roof of coarse grasses or palm leaves. Females resist milking in presence of strangers. Adult buffalo bulls are aggressive beast difficult to handle. Lactation period ranges from 6 to 9 month and lactation milk yield 1300 to 1800 kg but may be up to 2500 kg in some selected animals of Iran. Common skin colour is slate black but gray and grayish brown are also found. Some specimen with wall eye and white areas on the head, lego and tail might be due to presence of Nili-Ravi in the initial lots migrated from the Indian subcontinent. Medium size horns are semicircular sickle shaped. Long tapering tail extends below the hock joint and switch may be black, black and white or white. Long ears are drooping.

Mediterranean or European Buffaloes

These are generally high milk producing dairy type buffaloes evolved from the inter-breeding of dairy breeds of Indain subcontinent and brought by nomads intruders, and later on due to increasing demand of 'mozzarella' cheese. Morphologically Mediterranean buffaloes are quite comparable. However, Bulgaria and Italy have evolved better stock by selection. The countries rearing buffalo in Europe are Albania, Bulgaria, Greece, Hungry, Italy, Macedonia and Romania. Small herds are also maintained in Germany and United Kingdom.

The buffaloes are mostly heavy animals. The mean body weight of adult females ranges from 545 to 600 kg and that of males from 665 to 800 kg in different European countries being largest in Bulgaria and Italy (Borghese; 2010).

The animals are black, blackish gray or grayish brown and covered with moderate to dense coat of same colour. The medium size horns are found in different sickle shape. The base is wider and inwards turn tips are blunt pointed. These may be white hairs on head and switch of the tail. The buffaloes are mostly raised for milk and males are fattened for buffveal and buffen production. The udder is well-formed and almost inform teats are cylindrical. Lactation period ranges from 7 to 10 months and milk yield 900 to 2000 litres in different breeding and management conditions. Since demand of buffalo milk and milk products specially the mozenella cheese is increasing internationally the breeding of Mediterrean buffaloes is likely to increase and area of distribution may also in sease. This will also help in the development of buffalo meat industry at least until it becomes possible to produce only females.

▶ SWAMP BUFFALO (*BUBALUS BUBALIS SWAMPIS*)

The proposed trinomial nomenclature may be suitably modified by conscience among the buffalo breeding countries if the proposed nomenclature is not convincing. One thing has to be kept in mind that despite fertile interbreeding the two are different species and crossbreed with $2n = 49$ chromosomes is not yet made stable for multiplication.

The swamp buffaloes are normally draught animals by evolution but in some countries specially in some parts of India, Nepal, and Bangladesh it has been developed by selection as a satisfactory milk producing animal (Singh, 1978 and Tamuli, 1978). Swamp buffaloes are domesticated animals in Asia and Indo-Pacific Island countries.

Swamp Buffaloes of the Indian Subcontinent

These are multipurpose animals breed for work, milk production, and manure production. Meat production is secondry and is showing an increasing trend due to sparing of substantial number of male buffaloes replaced by increasing mechanization of agricultural operations. Some of the swamp buffalo breeds of India have been developed for satisfactory milk production in the region of Odisha (Orissa), north parts of West Bengal, Sikkim, Assam, and Manipur (Littlewood, 1936; Narayan Reddy 1939; Pathak, 1975; Ranjhan and Pathak, 1978; Singh, 1978; Tamuli, 1978; Bidhar et al., 1986; Das and Patro, 1988; Samal, 1988; Sethi et al., 2007, 2009). Two breeds of swamp buffaloes have been also described in Nepal (Rasali, 1997).

▶ CHILKA BUFFALO

Although mythological informations claim that curd prepared from the milk of Chilka buffalo was served to Lord Jagannath by Manika during the Kanchi war. This medium size buffalo thriving on the coarse herbages of swamp and submerged plants of Chilka lake and adjoining area is an important source of livelihood without any considerable input on feeding. Detail study has been conducted on this breed in recent part (Sethi et al., 2007). The name of buffalo has been derived from the prot world marine lake 'Chilka' which is the major source of fodder for this breed. Samal (1988) has listed this buffalo as 'Parikud'. The most peculiar behaviour of this buffalo is the feeding on submerged plants is the Chilka lake. The wallowing buffaloes can be seen diving in water for 1–2 minutes and then emerging out of water with mouthful herbage for chewing and ingesting. This process is repeated in quick succession (Personal observation of author). The animal is well-adapted for thriving and performing in the area of saline water sources. The taste of milk is also slightly salty and presence of higher content of salt in milk is considered to favour longer selflife than the milk of other buffaloes.

It is a medium size breed of black colour but about 10–11% animals may be brownish black to grayish black. The calves are mostly grayish to brownish black to birth and gradually acquire characteristic colour. The chest is broad and deep, and barrel is moderately developed. The face is narrow with flat forehead and straight nose bridge. Medium size horns emerged slightly sidewards and grow upwards with variable sickle shaped curvature, slightly pushed backwards, and shallow corrugation. Medium size ears are placed horizontal below the horns and possess fringe of hairs. Medium size tail runs down the hocks to terminate in switch of coarse hairs and body colour.

In recent years elaborate information have been collected on the distribution, characteristics and productivity of Chilka buffalo (Dash et al., 2007), which has been summarized in Table 3.12.

TABLE 3.12. Some important traits of Chilka buffalo

Characteristics	Male	Female
Body weight (kg)	353	341
Body length (cm)	123	121
Heart girth (cm)	173	171
Height at withers (cm)	126	124
Tail length (cm)	72	72

The udder and milk veins are less prominent but teats are well set on dish shaped udder. Daily milk yield ranges from 1 to 3 kg and lactation yield is 400 to 500 kg during 8–9 months of lactation period. Milk is highly nutritious and contains more than 8% milk fat and more than 17% total milk solids.

The males are good draught animals and used for ploughing and haulage of agricultural produce and other goods. Only retired animals, sterile females and surplus males are disposed for meat production.

Kalahandi Buffalo

This group of buffalo was described by Littlewood (1936) and named 'Pedakimedi' but subseqnently Narayan Reddy named it 'Kalahandi' due to its highest concentration in Kalahandi district of Odisha (Orrisa). The breed has been described in more detail by Das Kornel and Patro (1988) and recently by Dash et al. (2009).

The colour ranges from gray to ash gray and it appears to be the effect of selection due to greater demand of light colour draught animals in the Gunpur and Parlakimundi areas. These colour dominate in Kalahandi buffaloes of hill areas but in plain areas black colour is preferred. The sparcely distributed hairs on the body are grayish to grayish brown. Legs below knee joint are lighter in colour. Majority of calves are light gray to brownish gray and gradually acquire characteristic colour while approaching puberty. The muzzle, switch of the tail and hooves are black in more than 90% animals. The males are robust and naval flap is prominent.

The face is small with flat forehead and straight nose bridge. The animals is docile in locality but becomes alert with head extended curiously in the presence of strangers. Medium size ears are placed horizontal below the horns and lighter in colour. Average length of adult from poll to muzzle is about 50 cm. The horns are medium to large in size and extend slightly sidewards, backwards, and curving upwards in shape of sickle. These are somewhat flat and lightly corrugated. The distal one-third of horns turn inwards opposing each other. Sometimes horns are so long that it requires special skill for putting yoke on the neck of such animals. The horns of males are thicker and shorter than the females. The bowel shape udder with uniform cylindrical teats is visible laterally in lactating animals. The tapering tail runs below the hock and terminates in a switch of coarse hairs of black colour but may be gray in few buffaloes. These are apparent differences between the physical traits recorded by Das Kornel and Patro (1988) and Sethi et al., (2009). Since later study included larger number of animals, the physical characteristics have been summarized in Table 3.13.

This is a moderate milk producer yielding 2–4 kg daily on almost exclusive grazing. Sometimes dry crop residue, rice milling by products and Kichen left over are supplemented. Milk fat is more than 8% and total solids are more than 17 percent.

TABLE 3.13: Some characteristics of Kalahandi buffalo

Characteristics	Male	Female
Body weight (kg)	374	351
Body length (cm)	124	122
Height at withers (cm)	126	124
Heart girth (cm)	177	172
Birth weight (kg)	23	22
Age at puberty (days)	1085	1153

Koraput/Parlakhemundi/Manda Buffalo

This is a hardy animals of medium size comparable with Kalahandi buffaloes and found in the hilly area of Koraput district. And also found in the adjoining area of Andhra Pradesh. This breed is also known as Parlakhemundi or Ganjam buffalo. It is also a true swamp buffalo with $2n = 48$ number of chromosome (Bidhar et al., 1986). This breed was described by Narayan Reddy (1939). The important feature of this buffalo breed is the presence of an arch like curved red ring of 8–9 cm width across the chest. The sharp eyes are surrounded by a broad red margin around the lids. Common colour is brown to gray with yellowish stockings on knees fetlocks. The face is short with flat forehead, straight nasal bone, small muzzle, large jaw, and wide nostrils. The short and light neck is adapted for grazing in jungle. The back is straight and chest is well-developed with strong collar bone and ribs. The legs are short and bouned. The average values of body length, height at withers, and heart girth are 165 cm, 132 cm and 196 cm respectively. These are very good working animals capable to tolerate solar heat for several horns. Light colour working buffaloes are preferred by the farmers. Milk yield is satisfactory for almost zero input on feeding and management. There is ample scope of developing this breed as a triple purpose animal of the area for the purpose of fat rich milk production, work, and meat production from surplus animals besides the yield of valuable organic manure, and hide horns and bones for industries.

Jerangi Buffalo

It is a small breed of comparatively dry hilly region. This is also known as 'Harina buffalo due to light weight, small size, thinner legs, and active habits. The animal is found in Jerangi hills of Odisha and adjoining hilly area of Ganjam and also in Vishakhapattanam in Andhra Pradesh (Narayan Reddy, 1939). Its height rarely exceed 114 cm at withers. The face is short and narrow, chest is compact, barrel is small and tail is thin and short extending about 46 cm. Jerangi buffaloes are reared on exclusive grazing. The males are an excellent working animal for ploughing and carting. Females provide 1–2 kg milk after nursing the calf. Since this buffalo is black, its heat tolerance is low and has been found reluctant to work in hot solar exposer. Small and conical horns grow slightly backwards and upwards to terminate almost straight and blunt pointed.

Dhenukanal Buffalo

This breed has been listed by Samal (1980) and has been described comparable to Sambalpuri buffalo but smaller in size. The horns are large. Daily 2–3 kg milk yield may be considered quite satisfactory for zero input feeding management.

Kujang Buffalo

This is an animal of wet Kujang area of Cuttack district in Odisha. The medium size buffalo is black in colour and reared exclusively on grazing on the herbages of swampy area of Mahanadi. Due to lack of transport facility and herding in river basin greater proportion of milk is used for ghee making. The residual curd is consumed and ghee is sold in the nearby markets Kujang and Kendrapada. Milk yield is quite satisfactory and may be even more than 3–4 kg daily in some of the animals. The buffaloes may be seen submerged in the river and ponds during hot sun. Males are purchased for work in paddy fields. Buffalo meat is mostly eaten by the migrants of Bengal region.

Bheda Buffalo

This is a breed of Bheda area of Coastal Balasore district of Odisha reared on grazing. This breed also tolerate brackish water and can feed on submerged plants of the stagnant coastal area and swamps. The animals are also reared in Bhadrak. These are relatively larger medium buffaloes of black colour. Earlier ghee making was quite popular but due to increasing demand and quick gain liquid milk is sold in local markets. The population is decreasing due to increasing use of land for crop production (Samal, 1988).

Albinoid specimens are frequently found in most of the swamp buffalo breeds of Odisha but pie bald animals are rarely seen. These breeds are the result of mostly natural selection. However, these are scope of developing these breeds into satisfactory farm animal of economic importance for the people inhabiting at remote place in hills and forest.

Sikamese Buffalo

This is a medium size black buffalo found in Sikim and neighbouring areas of West Bengal and eastern region of Nepal. The animal is reared for milk, work, and meat. In forest area they graze in group and fight together with the predators. These animals like lying in mud holes and plaster mud on body for protection from solar heat.

Assamese Group of Swamp Buffaloes

Earlier Assamese buffalo has been mentioned as a single type also known as Mongoor (Ranjhan and Pathak, 1978). However, later observations have shown consipecuous differences among the buffaloes of different parts of Assam and other northeast hill states of India. The buffaloes reared for milk production along the Brahmaputra are the mixture of swamp buffaloes and riverine buffaloes in different ratio and animals with $2n = 48, 49$, and 50 can be observed. Indeed, pure herds of swamp buffaloes of various type can be identified easily on the basis of morphological conformation and distribution. The most important aspect of economic importance for various Assam group of buffaloes is their evolution for milk production also in addition to draught. The milk yield of swamp buffaloes of Assam (Tamuli, 1978) and lower region of Manipur (Singh, 1978) is quite high and comparable with many breeds of dairy type riverine buffaloes.

Goalpara Buffalo

This is a medium to large size grayish black to albinoid buffalo of Goalpara district of lower Assam. The upper part of horns is cylindrical in young calves which becomes almost triangular and corrugated in adult animals. Both sexes are used for ploughing but only males are used for pulling carts. The area extends in the adjoining Tura town of Meghalaya and also Bangladesh. Young calves are lighter in colour at birth. Owners do not allow handling of young calves specially the albinoid calves by strangers. They believe that touching by stranger is mostly fatal for the calf. The animal becomes furious to stragers and often charge if not properly tethered (Author experienced during survey in 1975). The territory of this buffalo may be found on the other side of river Brahmaputra. However, adulteration of native buffalo with Murrah group of buffalo cannot be ruled out in the north part because the route has been used for time immemorial for communication with the west and other parts of the country.

Swamp Buffalo of Assam

Swamp buffaloes of Assam are quite variable in different parts of Silchar are generally larger and sturdy with large size thick and corrugated angular caliper shaped horns. Although a centre for research on the description and development of swamp buffaloes of Assam was included in the network project on buffaloes during the last phase of ninth plan period on the initiation of the author, there appears to be generation of little specific information on the swamp buffaloes found in different regions of the Assam extending from the border of West Bengal and Bangladesh in west to Mezoram, Nagaland, and Manipur in the east and Arunachal Pradesh and Bhutan in the north. Therefore, the limited observations made by the author during survey in 1975 and the study of Tamuli (1978) has been used for the description of Assamese swamp buffalo or Assamese native buffalo (Fig. 3.10).

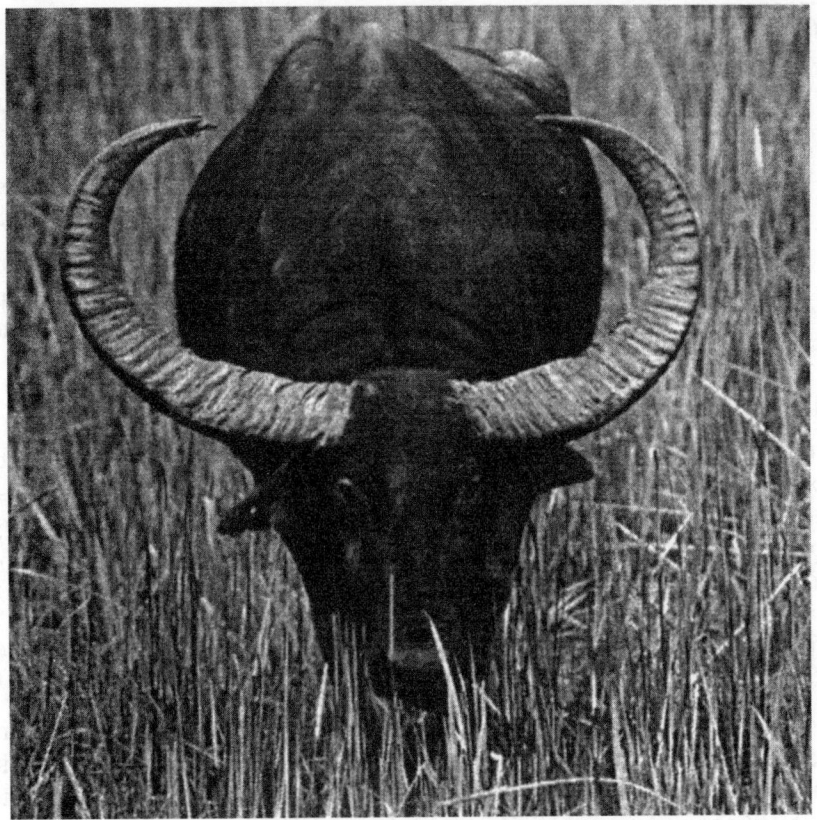

Fig. 3.10: Assamese swamp buffalo

It is a large size animal of variable morphological characteristics. The horn pattern of buffalo has been described as medium size spirocerus and large size macrocerus but on closer observations the horn pattern may be differentiated in heavy caliper shaped horns growing slightly sidewards and than backwards, upwards and inwards in semilunar shape with broad base, more or less triangular body and gradually narrowing inwards turned blunt pointed ends. The second is hook shaped light, flat, and corrugated horns emerging on either end of skull and growing upwards with gradual short deflection and narrower upper quarter turning inwards. This type has been named spirocerus. The third type of very large size and narrow horns normally growing sidewards, slightly downwards and then gradually upwards to turn inwards at the teminal end. In some buffaloes the horns grow downwards and deflected sidewards. There are also good numbers of buffaloes with long horns growing backwards and inwards.

The buffaloes are not tethered and herded at a place near the village. Only 2 to 4 buffalo bulls are kept for breeding in small herds of 70–100 females. Nursing buffaloes do not allow handling of their calves for at least one month even by the herdsman living with them. The calves after one month of age are separated and housed with other calves in a safe encloser of bamboo and thatch shed. Lactating females and those in last trimester of pregnancy are housed tethered separated from rest of the buffaloes.

Mean values of some production and reproduction traits recorded by Tamuli (1978) are summarized in Table 3.14.

TABLE 3.14: Mean values of some production and reproduction traits of Assamese swamp buffalo

Lactation number	Milk yield (kg)		Lactation length (days)	Dry period (days)	Intercalving period (days)
	Daily	Lactation			
First	1.79	460	257	242	-
Second	2.22	577	260	290	521
Third	2.62	691	264	275	572
Fourth	3.11	845	272	264	558
Fifth	3.02	800	265	280	556
Sixth	2.44	643	264	-	566

Manipuri Swamp Buffalo

The large size domesticated swamp buffaloes kept in valley along the swamp and water are medium size animals of large body, smaller legs and short face. Some of the characteristics of Manipuri swamp buffalo reported by Singh (1978) are summarized in Table 3.15.

TABLE 3.15: Characteristics of the adult Manipuri swamp buffalo

Characteristics	Male	Female
Body weight (kg)	545.0	482.0
Height at withers (cm)	136.4	125.3
Body length (cm)	139.5	127.6
Heart girth (cm)	232.0	215.5

The colour is grayish brown to grayish black but good number of albivoid and sporadic cases of piebald are also found. The eyelids and muzzle are pinkish in albivoid animals. There is no colour prejudice in Manipuri. The production, performance, and milk quality are comparable. The animals are grazed on wetlands during the day and tethered in the night. The animals are hostile for strangers. Unlike swamp buffaloes of Assam, there is normally no chevron in the typical Manipuri swamp buffalo and presence of some faint chevron in sporadic cases may be due to accidental crossing with wild or Assamese swamp buffalo. The massive horns are large, some what triangular, corrugated, broad at base, gradually extending sidewards, backwards and then bending inwards with blunt pointed tips in the shape of a caliper. There is little variation in the shape and size of horns. Tail extends below the hocks. Body coat is denser than the swamp buffalo of Assam. Calves are lighter in colour at birth and gradually turn darker to acquire characteristic colour at puberty.

Some economic traits of Manipuri swamp buffalo of 'Loktak lake' area reported by Singh (1978) have been summarized in Table 3.16.

TABLE 3.16: Economic traits of domestic Manipuri swamp buffalo

Attributes	Range	Average
Lactation length (days)	206–274	248
Lactation milk yield (kg)	670–1325	1038
Dry period (days)	100–275	189
Milk fat (%)		
Early lactation	6.78–7.55	6.99
Mid lactation	7.88–9.00	7.92
Late lactation	8.00–10.00	9.24

Good number of domestic Manipuri swamp buffaloes have been observed lactating up to tenth lactation and constitute about 2% of lactating buffaloes (Singh, 1978). Some of the characteristics of adult females are presented in Table 3.17.

The lactation yield of Manipuri swamp buffalo clearly shows the potential of milk production and scope of development of swamp buffaloes of wet zone of Assam and northeast states as a multi purpose animal for milk, meat, and draught. Low milk yield in swamp buffaloes of Assam and most parts of Odisha appears to be the effect of once day milking only in the morning before letting loose for grazing with calves during the daytime.

TABLE 3.17: Production and reproduction traits of Manipuri swamp buffalo

Calving number	Total animals	Lactation length (days)	Calving interval (days)	Lactation milk yield (kg)
1	10	199	-	946
2	103	238	413	990
3	102	242	437	1054
4	91	243	428	1094
5	45	230	453	1071
6	45	229	437	1031
7	23	222	436	1032
8	13	200	418	949
9	11	252	444	832
10	9	238	434	763

Lime Buffalo of Nepal

It is considered to be the descendent of wild arnee buffalo of Indo-Nepal border. The town 'Bhainsalotan' at the Bihar-Nepal border denotes the 'mud wallow' preferred for wallowing by swamp buffaloes. So far there appears to be no information on the domestication of 'Lime' buffalo but it is reared in most parts of the hilly region of Nepal. The herds of 'Lime' are moved to high hill for grazing on lush growing alpine pastures during the summer season. Such buffaloes are also found in the neighbouring states of India in the mid Himalayan to higher altitudes.

This is a medium size animal of grayish brown to grayish black colour possessing normally two chevsons (one behind jaw and another in front of brisket) of white or yellowish white hairs. Small ears extend horizontal and contain fringe of soft hairs on the edges and posterior surface. Small sickle shaped horns run backwards along the neck and curve facing each other at the distal end. Average body weight of adult female is 400 kg and height at withers is 115 cm. The legs are short and sturdy, and the colour is lighter below knee. The lactation length extends almost for a year and lactation yield is about 875 kg milk of 7% fat content (Rasali, 1997).

Parkote Buffalo of Nepal

It is a long horn domesticated buffalo of the Nepal Tarai. The genotype of the buffalo has changed considerably in the lower region along the Indian border due to frequent mating with Tarai and Murrah bulls of riverine Indian buffaloes. Morphological this buffalo appears to be a member of riverine group but Karyotyping is necessary for the establishment of its type.

Parkote is a medium size buffalo of black colour or slate black colour. The head is prominent and nasal bone is straight, the eyes and muzzle are black. Small and bonned legs do not have any markings. In summer, animals move to higher zone for grazing. Average body weight of adult female is 410 kg and height at withers is 114 cm (Rasali, 1997). Lactation performance is similar to Lime buffalo of Nepal. The long horns are sword shaped with inwards turned blunt pointed tips. The horns are flat and corrugated, and grow backwards or downwards and backwards deflected laterally.

▶ **DOMESTICATED SWAMP BUFFALOES OF OTHER ASIAN COUNTRIES AND INDOPACIFIC ISLAND COUNTRIES**

The swamp buffalo of Bangladesh is comparable with the Goalpara buffaloes. The buffaloes of Myanmar are probably not yet properly described but they resemble with the large breeds of swamp buffaloes bearing posteriorly growing almost caliper shaped triangular heavy horns. This strain is found in upper parts of Assam, lower parts of Thailand and Combodia with some differences due to breeding and selection. Some of the incomplete defined breeds of swamp buffalo of Thailand are Kwaitui, Kwai kam, Kwai glapp, Kwai jawn. The large size 'marid' is considered to be introduced from the Myanmar. Proportion of albinoid buffalo is more than 30% in the north but less than 5% in the central and south parts.

The two strains of combodia are the long horn 'Krabey beng' of the jungles of upland and short horn 'Krabey len' of the lower region. Albinoids are quite common. 'Bahnar' type buffaloes of strong legs and large hooves are preferred for working in paddy field of Mekong valley in Laos. The Vietnami swamp buffaloes are concentrated in the central and lower wetland. The animals are very heavy and few adult males may weigh even 1000 kg. There may be three or more strains of swamp buffaloes in Vietnam which were seen during extensive tour of Author in different parts during 1982–84 while working at Buffalo Breeding Centre, Song Be about 90 km away from the Ho chi Minh city.

In China many strains of native swamp buffaloes have been differentiated (Yag and Zhang, 2006). The 18 strains or breeds distinguished in different parts of China are Binlu, Cruizhou, Dechang, Dehong, Diandongnan, Dongliu, Enshi, Fuan, Fuling, Fuzhong, Haizi, Jianghan, Shanghai, Wenzhou, Xanlin, Xilin, Xinglong, and Xinyang. The classification is mostly on the basis of morphological differences among the buffaloes of different regions.

The seven breeds or strains of Indonesia are Aceh buffalo, Binanga, Java, Kalang, Moa, Pampangas and Spotted Sulaweri buffalo (Triwolanningshi et al., 2006).

Initially introduced as domesticated swamp buffalo during nineteenth century from Asian countries were released free after few years to trun feral. Now feral swamp buffaloes are periodically harvested for meat and leather production industries.

Both riverine and swamp buffaloes have gained importance for milk and meat production in West Indies and many other countries of South America like Brazil and Venezuela. Small herds of buffaloes have been also introduced in some states of United States of America and also in Germany. The increasing demand of buffalo milk and low fat-low cholesterol meat of buffalo will further increase the popularity of buffaloes. However, indiscriminate breeding more create problem of maintaining purity among the breeds.

More intensive studies are required for the identification and description of breeds of swamp buffaloes of different countries. Although consipicuous differences particularly in the colour, horn type, limb conformation and upper may be noticed, but there apperars to be one or two strains with long triangular deflected caliper shaped horns from the east parts of India to other countries of Asia and Indo-Pacific region. Such similarities may help intracing the route of dispersion of buffalo and linkages among the people of different countries.

REFERENCES

Bidhar, G.C., Pattanaik, G.R., Rao, P.K. and Patro, B.N. 1986. Buffalo Bulletin, 5(3); 54–56.

Borghese, Antonio 2010. Proc. Intern. Buffalo Conf., New Delhi, pp. 31–39, February 1–4.

Cockrill, Ross W. 1974. The husbandry and health of the domestic buffalo. F A O, Rome.

Das, Kornel and Patro, B.N. 1988. Buffalo Bulletin, 7 (2); 35–38

Dash, S.K., Sethi, P.C. and Ray, P.C. 2009. Buffaloes genetic Resources of Orissa-Kalahandi. Orissa Liverstock Resource Development Society and OAUT, Bhubaneswar.

Dave, C.N. 1940. Poona Agriculture College Maggine 32, 97 ICAR 1960. A brief survey of the important breeds of Cattle in India. Misc. Bull. No. 24 ICAR, New Delhi.

Kaura, R.L. Indian breeds of liverstock (including Pakistan breeds). Prem Publisher, Lucknow.

Little wood, R.W. 1963. Livestock of south India. Govt. Press, Madras.

Macgregor 1940. Thesis on buffalo. Royal Veterinary College, London

Mishra, B.P., Tantia, M.S., Bharani Kumar, S.T. and Vijh, R.K. 2007. Genetics and Molecular Biology, 30; 1097–1100.

Narayan Reddy 1939. Madras Agric. J., 27; 50

Oliver, A. 1938. A brief survey of some of the important breeds of cattle in India. Misc. Bull. No. 17, ICAR, New Delhi.

Padghan, P.V., Jaglekar, N.V., Thombre, B.M., Khandare, N.O. and Jinkurkar, A.S. 2008. Indian J. Anim. Res; 42–66.

Pathak, N.N. 1975, Survey of Assam and Meghalaya. Reports Assam Agril uni. Campus, Khamapara.

Peeva, T. 2010. Buffalo News letter 4; 6.

Pundir, R.K., Singh, D.V., Sahana, G., Dare, A.S. and Nivsarkar, A.E. 2000/Characterization of Mehsana buffalo. Dudhsagar Research and Development Assoc., Mehsana, Gujarat.

Ramesha, K.P. 2010. Personal communication.

Ranjhan, S.K. and Pathak, N.N. 1978, 1994. A Text bool of Buffalo production. 1st Kuth Ed., Vikas Pub. Hse. Pvt. Ltd., New Delhi,

Rasali, D. P. 1977. Proc. 4th global conf. on Conservation of Domestic Animal genetic resources. Rare breeds International 168.

Rife, D.C. 1959. The water buffalo of India and Paskistan. International Cooperation Administration, Washington, D.C.

Samal, Brundaban, 1988. A short history of Veterinary Medicine and Animal Husbandry in Orissa. Panchshila Publication, Bhubanerswar.

Sethi, B.P., Dash, S.K. and Ray. P.C. 2007. Buffalo genetic resources of India-Chilka. Orissa Liverstock Development Soc. And Chilka buffalo Promotors Soc., Bhubaneswar.

Singh D. 1978. Thesis on Manipuri buffalo. Assam Agrili uni., Khanapara Campus, Guwahati.

Singh, K.P. 2000. Technical folder on Banni buffalo. S D A U. Sardar Krushinagar, Gujarat.

Singh, K.P., Chaudhary, A. P. and Patel Jatin V. 2010. Proc. International Buffalo Conference, New Delhi, 1–4 February.

Singh, K.P. and Panchsara, H.H. 2007. Proc. National Symp. on role of An GR in rural livelihood security. Birsa Agril. University, Ranchi.

Tamuly, Bhupan Chandra, 1978. M.V. Sc. Thesis on buffalo. Assam Agril. Uni., Khanapura Campus, Guwahati.

White, R.O. and Mathur, M.L. 1966. Indian Dairyman, 18, 161–180.

Young, Binghuang, Liang Xianwei, Zhang Xiufang 2005, Shi Jiazhuang, 10; 22–26.

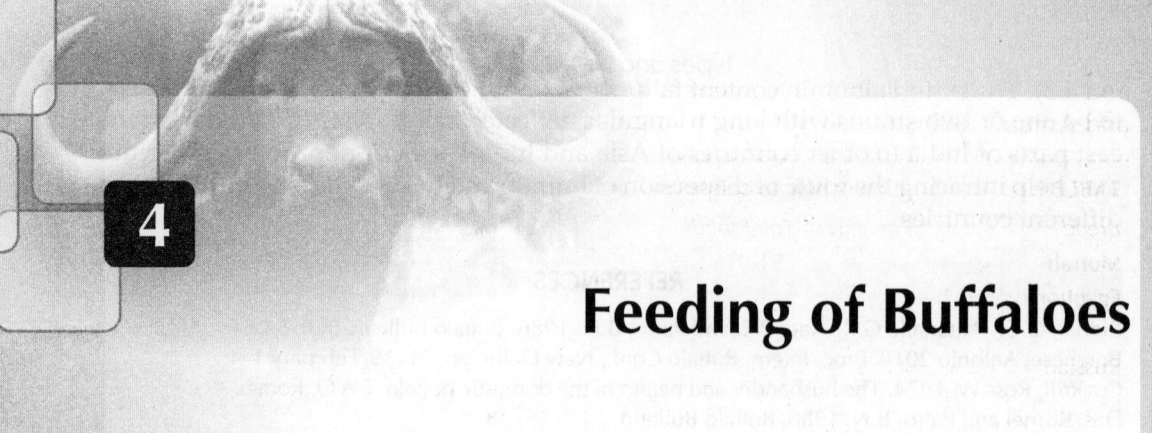

Feeding of Buffaloes

▶ FEEDING OF BUFFALO CALVES

Production of healthy replacement stock is the main aim of feeding the young calves. High plane of nutrition in early life supports higher growth and earlier onset of puberty. The numinoreticulum of buffalo calves is nonfunctional in early life and digestive processes are almost similar to that of simple stomached animals. The stomach capacity of buffalo calf at birth is about 2–3 litres depending on the size of animal. Colostrum, the first lacteal secretion after birth is the natural food of newborn calf, and it must be fed to all newborn calves as early as possible and preferably before 8 hours of birth. It is benefical to feed colostrums with in 1–2 hour of calving (Ganovski, 1979).

▶ COLOSTRUM

Colostrum is the first milk secreted by a mammalian species immediately after the birth of newborn. The composition of colostrums is different than the normal milk. It contains higher percentage of protein, fat, vitamins and minerals (Tables 4.1 and 4.2), which are in most proper mixture to supply the immediate requirements of newborn calves (Raafat et al., 1974; Ganovske, 1979). Colostrum cotains about 12.20% milk fat, 3002 IU vitamin A activity and 50 mg carotenes per kg, which are much higher than 6.12–7.66% fat, 630–1030 IU vitamin A and 22.4–37.8 kg carotenes per kg of normal milk (Soliman and Soliman, 1974). Colostrum fat contains exceptionally high content of unsaturated fatty acids (about 33.9) including polyunsaturated fatty acids (Arumughan and Narayanan, 1982). The concentration of manganese, copper, iron, and zinc is very high in the first milk, which decreases sharply to normal values by fifteen milking (Ghuionna De Maria, 1978). Only few amino acids are observed in the initial colostrums, which decrease up to 39 hours of calving and increase thereafter. All the twelve free amino acids are detected after 75 hours of calving (Table 4.3; Nofal et al., 1974). The high globulin content of colostrums provides passive immunity against many diseases in the early life of 3–4 months. Efficient absorption of globulins occurs only in the early few hours of life, which necessitates the feeding of sufficent colostrums viz., about one litre in first feed in within 4–8 hours of birth. Colostrums contains about 12.5% globulins, 3.6% albumin and 7.7% casein.

A significant change occurs in the total serum protein content and various protein fractions following the ingestion of colostrums by newborn calves (Tables 4.2

and 4.3). The serum albumin content falls down rapidly and globulins increase (Afzal and Anjum, 1982).

TABLE 4.1: Composition of buffalo colostrums and milk of 7th day

Breed	Day of milking	Total solids	Solids - not fat	Fat	Total protein	Ash.
Murrah	0	31.0	27.0	4.00	23.80	0.90
Egyption	36 h.	-	-	10.29	17.35	-
	7th day	-	-	-	7.38	5.27
Russian	2 h	-	-	10.00	18.80	1.10
	12 h	-	10.00	10.90	10.90	-
	7th day	-	-	-	7.60	7.70
Normal	0	26.60	17.05	9.55	9.59	-
	7th day	18.90	11.29	7.61	5.55	-

TABLE 4.2: Effect of colostrums feeding on serum protein changes in buffalo calves

Serum	Before	Hour	After	Feeding
g/100 ml	feeding	3	12	24
Total serum protein	5.88	-	-	8.47
Albumin	3.45	-	-	2.89
L1-globulin	0.17	0.44	-	-
L2-globulin	0.29	1.08	-	-
Y-globulin	0.64	1.30	2.78	3.16

The average content of manganese, copper, iron, and zinc in first milk is about 125, 357, 1770, and 13013 mg per kg, which fell down to 38, 29, 40, and 61 mg per kg of milk respectively in the fifteenth milking of buffaloes.

TABLE 4.3: Detectable free amino acids in the colostrum of Egyptian buffalo

Amino acids	Hours of milking after calving									
	0	3	15	27	39	63	75	87	99	111
Cystine	+	+					+	+	+	+
Lysine	+	+	+	+		+	+	+	+	+
Histidine						+	+	+	+	+
Arginine						+	+	+	+	+
Arpertic acid	+	+	+	+		+	+	+	+	+
Glycine	+	+	+		+	+	+	+	+	+
Glutamic acid	+	+	+		+	+	+	+	+	+
Alanine	+	+		+		+	+	+	+	+
Proline					+	+	+	+	+	+
Tyrosine					+	+	+	+	+	+
Tryptophane							+	+	+	+
Leucine						+	+	+	+	+

Over feeding should be avoided by restricting the suckling of dam's udder for 8–10 minutes at a time and 2–3 feedings should be allowed daily for 3 successive days. In case of weaning at birth about 800–1200 ml of fresh colostrums of dam should be fed in 2–3 meals to supply about 2.5–3.0 kg colostrums to a calf of normal birth weight of about 30 kg. The bucket, basin or pail used for the milking and feeding of calves should be clean and disinfected by washing in boiling water. In case of a galaction a mixture of 2 eggs and 30–35 ml castor oil should be administered orally and serum of dam should be administered intravenously for 2–3 days to increase the titre of antibody in the body.

Advantages of Hand Feeding of Colostrums

1. Removal of calf immediately after birth significantly reduces the excitement of dam because she does not get chance to lick the calf and develop intenee affinity.
2. Indigestion encountred in suckling is reduced.
3. It is easier to teach pall feeding to calves who have not suckled dams.
4. Incidence of traumatic mastitis caused by bites of calf is reduced.
5. Dam weaned at birth does not produce much problem at milking and let down of milk is easily stimulated by the movement of hand on the teats at the time of milking.
6. The colostrums consumed by calf is recorded and regulated as per the requirement of the calf.

Health Aspect of Colostrum Feeding

The climatic condition of humid-to tropical contries provides favourable environment for the proliferation of round worms. *Neoascaeris vitulorum* are quite common in the colostrums and milk of buffaloes (Mia et al., 1974; Gautam et al., 1976). In addition to the third stage larvae of *Neoascaris vitulorum*, Bruah et al., (1981) have also reported the larvae of *Strongyloides papillpsus*. Therefore, it would be in the interest of calf survivality to deworm the pregnant buffaloes and also the newborn calves. The calves should also be observed carefully for gastric disorders caused by the infection of round-worms in early life.

Systems of Calf Feeding

Two systems of feeding buffalo calves are followed in difrent countries, i.e., suckling of dams and artifical feeding after weaning the calf at birth. Suckling is practiced by private dairy farmers and in swamp buffaloes which is not used for milking. Artificial feeding of buffalo calves on whole milk, and skim milk or milk replace diets are usually followed at the organized dairy farms.

Feeding through Suckling the Dam

This system of calf feeding is common with farmers keeping 1–5 lactating buffaloes partly for domestic consumption of milk and partly as the source of subsidiary income. This is also followed to some extent by the commercial dairies of urban and sub-urban areas. On such farms calves are mostly used for the let down of milk and larger percentage succumb to almost wanton starvation. The situation is somewhat better in rural areas, where female calves of buffalos receive special care to be reared as future daing replacement. Male cavles are neglected creature in Indian subcontinent since anicient time as stated by surapal 'a buffalo that begets a male calf, a bride that gives birth to a daughter and rain that falls in the month of Kartika (October–November) –all these portend aminous times (anonymous, 1964 d).

Same status they had in Egypt (Baelreldin, 1955) and many other countries. The situation is altogether different in the case of swamp buffaloes, which are the main source of power in predominantly paddy growing areas of southeast Asian countries. Almost all calves of swamp buffaloes are reared on dam's suckling for a very long period extending from 6 to 15 months in some exceptional cases. Normally, calves of swamp buffaloes are not separated from their dams even during ploughing the land and pulling the cart. There is no schedule of suckling and it is common seen to observe buffalo calves.

Suckling their dams during the short intervals on work and on the pastures. Although there is no quantification of milk intake by the calves of swamp buffaloes, it is assumed to be about 360–540 kg in calves suckling for a period of one year or more.

In case of dairy buffaloes, young calves are allowed full milk feeding during the first 2–4 weeks of life and then it is gradually restricted to all the let down of milk by 3–4 months of age at which they are able to handle considerable amount of dry feeds and fodders. Succulent green fodder and good quality hays are introduced at 2–3 weeks of age. At this stage calf starter is also offered either in the form of a dry mash or as gruel. Milk intake of such calves varies from 250–300 kg during the lactation period. Ahmed and EI-Sgazy (1975) quantified the intake of whole milk of dawn by suckling either for 45 days (early wearning) or for 123 days (late wearning). Average milk intake was aobut 157.4 and 155.6 kg by early weaned male and female calves respectively. In the case of late weaned calves intake of whole milk was 340 kg the calves were allowed to suckle all the four quarters up to 11 days of age, two quarters during the next 21 days and only one quarter thereaftaer. Feeding of a calf starter containing about 13% protein and 71.5% T D N, green grass and beseam hay started before one week of age. The calves gained at the rate of 0.03 and 0.32 kg up to the age of 125 days, which increased sharply to 0.72 and 0.73 kg daily between 126–363 days, and 0.79 and 0.80 kg from 363 days to finishing at about 400 days body weight in early and late wearned calves respectively. Average T D N intake per kg gain in body weight was 5.15 and 4.95 kg respectively in the corresponding groups, but there was a shaving of about 183.5 kg buffalo milk from early wearing of calves on the complete feeding of calf starter and good quality roughages at 45 days of age.

Artificial Feeding/Pall Feeding/Bucket Feeding of Newborn Calves Wearned at Birth or within One Week of Age

The newborn calves are removed at birth or within one week of birth and reared away from their dams in the calf pens. The calves in early life are either housed individually in metallic cages or kept in groups of 10–20 in calf pens. Normally, calves are feed whole milk at an average rate of 10% of body weight up to 30 days of age followed by about 7% of body weight during the next two weeks and then at 5 percent, which gradually reduces to zero level at about 60 days of age. Milk can be successfully removed from the diets of buffalo calves at 30–45 days of age provided they are fed a balanced and nutritious calf starter. Whole milk requirement ranges from 100 to 200 kg. Average daily gain varies from 200–400 kg depending on the management and climatic factors (Borhami et al., 1967; Khoury et al., 1970; Dave et al., 1971; Sachan and Netke, 1971; Arora et al., 1973; Sohal et al., 1981).

An example of feeding different quantity of buffalo milk for a period of 31 to 126 days including first three days colostrum feeding will provide comparative informations on the permormances of buffalo calves (Table 4.4).

Although better feed gain ratio is obtained on the feeding of larger amount of milk, but there is no appreciable depression in growth on replacement of milk with good quality calf starters (Khourny et al., 1969; Arora et al., 1973, 1976; Table 4.4).

TABLE 4.4: Milk feeding schedule and response of buffalo calves

Age of calf (Days)	Milk feeding schedule per day (kg)			
	1	2	3	4
0–3	2.7	2.7	2.7	2.7
4–14	2.7	2.7	3.6	3.7
15–18	3.6	2.7	3.7	2.7
19–24	3.6	2.7	3.1	2.7
25–31	3.6	1.8	2.7	2.2
32–35	3.6	1.8	1.8	1.8
36–38	4.5	1.8	1.8	1.8
39–45	4.5	1.9	0.9	1.3
46–49	4.5	1.3	-	-
50–55	3.6	1.3	-	-
56–61	3.6	-	-	-
62–84	3.6	-	-	-
85–105	1.8	-	-	-
106–126	1.3	-	-	-
Total milk				
Intake, kg	340	123	120	103
Gain/day, g	380	250	200	270
TDN/kg Gian (kg)	3.3	4.8	5.2	4.4

A standard feeding schedule has been evolved for the feeding of newborn weaned calves from birth to the 3 months of age (Table 4.5). The schedule has been calculated to provide whole milk at the rate approximately 10% of body weight during the first 3 weeks of life, followed by about 1/15th in the next 2 weeks. In the 5th week skim milk feeding started at the rate of 1 kg daily, which was raised to 2.5 kg in the 6th weeks and again reduced to 2, 1.75 and 1.25 kg in the 7, 8 and 9th week respectively. Calf starter and good quality hay were introduced in the diet of calves in the 3rd week of life and they were encouraged to eat ad libitum.

Method of Feeding

Fresh colostrum drawn from the dam is first fed within 1–8 hours of birth and repeated at an interval of 8–12 hours depending on the number of daily meals. Fresh colostrum is fed during the first 3 days of life. From 4th day onward generally milk is fed in 2 meals, that is, morning and evening feeding schedule is followed. Whole milk of buffalo is boiled and then cooled to near body temperature (about 39°C). It is convenient to feed calves through nipples fitted in feeder for individual calf, otherwise calves should be guided to such the middle finger which should be gradually submerged into the milk in a basin or bucket. After 3–4 feedings calves learn to drink milk. The finger should be protected from bityes by thick gloves. Under strick hygienic conditions of feeding the calves of

TABLE 4.5: Feeding schedule of calves from birth to 3 months of age

Age of whole calf (weeks)	Milk (kg)	Skim milk (kg)	Calf-starter (kg)	Hay (kg) equivalent green
1–3 days	2.50 (colostrums)	-	-	-
4–7th days	2.50	-	-	-
2	3.00	-	0.50	0.25
3	3.25	-	0.10	0.35
4	3.00	-	0.30	0.50
5	1.50	2.00	0.40	0.55
6	2.50	0.60	0.60	
7	2.50	0.70	0.75	
8	1.75	0.08	0.80	
9	1.25	1.00	1.00	
10	-	(up to both day only)		
11	-	1.25		1.00
12	-	1.50	1.25	
13	-		1.75	1.75
Total requirement				

healthy hard medication of feeds is not required, but as a preventive measure against scouring an antibiotic feed mix is used either mixed in the milk or in the calf starter.

Feeding of calf starer and hay should be started in the 2nd week. First day a small quantity of calf starter should be rubbed on the tongue and muzzle of calves of develop taste for the feed. Calf starter should be offered in mangers and hay should be kept in hay rack for ad libiturm feeding. A water trough with running water should be available at a suitable place to avoid wetting of shed from the spillage of water during chinking.

In order to save valuable milk for human consumption, milk replacers are used for the feeding of calves. Milk replacer is generally introduced in the second week of life to replace whole milk from the diets of calves. Calculated amount of milk replacer, to supply nutrients almost to supply nutrients almost equivalent to that supplied by milk feeding, is dissolved in warm to make a gruel and fed at the body temperature.

Milk Replacer or Milk Substitute Diets

Buffalo milk is a priced nutritious food in the human dietery. Besides being a very good source of balnced protective protein it is also a rich source of milk fat, which is very much liked as cream, butter, and ghee. In order to spare larger quantity of milk from the feeding of calves, milk replacer or milk substitute diets are used.

Milk substitute or milk replacer diets are special concentrates prepared form palatable and nutritious feeds for the feeding of young calves in place of whole milk. In the preparation of milk replacers efforts are made to simulate the contents and their ratio in accordance with the composition of whole milk. Mostly liquid skim milk or skim milk powder constitute an important ingredients of milk replacer diet. Butter milk and whey can also be used. Milkless replacers are also used but they form mostly poor quality diets. Good mality milk replacers should contain 20–22% crude source (Arora et al., 1973 a,b., 1976, 1978; El-Ashry et al., 1975, El-Serafy et al., 1980; Dass and Arora, 1983). Milk replacers are mostly dry mixtures (Tables 4.6 and 4.7) which are thoroughly

TABLE 4.6: Milk replacers tested in Egypt

Composition and performances	Milk replacer number					
	1	2	3	4	5	6
Skim milk powder, %	40	40	40	55	55	55
Linseed cake, %	15	15	15	-	-	-
Decorticated cotton-seed meal,%	-	-	-	5	5	5
Soyabean flour, %	10	10	10	10	10	10
Corn germ, %	20	20	20	15	15	15
Maiz flouz, %	10	10	10	10	10	10
Dried yeast, %	5	5	5	5	5	
Addition, kg/100 kg						
Linseed oil	-	2.5	-	-	2.5	-
Tallow	-	-	8.0	-	-	8.0
Chemical composition and nutritive value,						
Dry matter, %	92.7	92.3	94.5	92.8	93.0	93.5
Crude protel, %	28.6	27.9	26.5	30.1	29.4	27.9
Ether extract %	6.8	9.0	18.9	8.1	10.6	19.6
D C P, %	24.8	24.2	23.0	26.1	25.4	24.1
T D N, %	78.0	80.3	85.6	79.4	81.6	86.8
M E, Meal/kg	2.85	2.93	3.12	2.90	2.98	3.17
Performance,						
Av. Daily gain, g	343	388	413	387	438	435
Relative gain, %	100	113.1	120.4	112.8	127.7	126.8
Dry matter intake,						
kg/100 kg body wt.	2.29	2.62	2.83	2.27	2.94	2.90
T D N intake per						
kg gain	3.71	3.56	3.56	3.30	3.53	3.54
Relative T D N	100	96.0	96.0	88.9	95.1	95.4
Requirement per unit gain						

TABLE 4.7: Milk replacers tested in India

Composition and performance	Milk replacer number			Whole milk group
	1	2	3	
Wheat flour	8	10	8	
Fish meal	10	12	12	
Skin milk powder	-	13		
Linseed meal	40	40	40	
Coconut oil	14	10	6	
Molasses	6	10	6	
Citric acid	1.5	1.5	1.5	

Contd.

TABLE 4.7: Milk replacers tested in India (*Contd.*)

Composition and performance	Milk replacer number			Whole milk group
	1	*2*	*3*	
Butyric acid	0.66	0.3	0.66	
Mineral mixture	3	3	3	
Linseed oil	-	-	6	
Nutritive value				
D C P, %	17.5	21.2	21.2	
T D N, %	88.0	88.7	91.0	
M E, Meal/kg	3.21	3.21	3.32	
Gain in body weight g/day	368	-	-	453
Total intake (kg)				
Whole milk	149	-	-	333
Milk replacer	31.3	-	-	-

mixed with boiled water in the ratio of 1:4 to 1:6 to prepare a gruel at the time of feeding. Calves are capable to handle adequate amount of milk replacer by two weeks of age and feeding of milk replacer urually starts on 15th day of life. About 200 g dry milk replacer is fed for each litre of whole milk and twice daily feeding schedule is followed.

Any negligence in the maintenance of feeding schedule and hygienic measures may cause gastric disorders leading to abomasal milk impaction in the early life of 3–5 weeks of age (Sharma et al., 1983) and scouring. These conditions may lead to significant calf loss during the rearing period.

▶ CALF STARTER

The requirement of calves increase with the age, which ordinarly becomes difficult to supply through the feeding of liquid diets (milk or milk substitute gruel). Hence, a dry concentrate mixture and good quality hay are offered to calves from the second week of life. These dry feeds are also introduced early life to stimulate the quicker development of functional ruminoreticulum with the earlier establishment of microbial digestion (Naga et al., 1969; Singh et al., 1970).

Since calf starter is fed to supplement the whole milk or milk replacer, it should not be a complex composition. A good quality palatable concentrate mixture containing 13–18% crude protein and 70–72 percent TDN supplemented with adequate minerals and vitamins serve the purpose of calf starter (Table 4.8). Inclusion of high tannin feeds and non-protein introgenous substance are avoided in the calf starter. Maize, wheat, oats, and barley are the good sources of energy feeds and groundnut cake, linseed cake, soyabean cake, cotton seed cake, sunflower seed cake, gram, beans, fish meal and meat meal are the sources of proteins for the preparation of calf staraters. Sorghum, milo and pearl millet may be used to replace part of the energy feeds. In early life stomach capacity of buffalo calf is not fully developed and significant lowering of energy density in calf starter will result in he inadequate intake of available energy consequently leading to poor growth response and reduced. Rolled oats and pearled barley are more suitable substitutes for maize and wheat in the calf starater.

TABLE 4.8: Example of calf starters suitable for different conditions and availability of feed ingredients

Ingredients	Percent composition of calf starter number								
	1	2	3	4	5	6	7	8	9
Crushed maize	35	35	20	50	12	42	30	30	20
Crushed oat/barley	10	10	10	-	10	-	-	-	10
Crushed gram	-	-	-	-	23	-	-	20	15
Crushed beans	30	20	20	-	-	-	-	-	-
Wheat bran	-	-	-	8	10	20	10	6	13
Rice bran	-	-	20	-	-	-	10	-	-
Groundnut cake	-	-	-	30	23	28	-	20	35
Linseed cake Decorticated	15	-	10	-	20	-	40	22	-
Cotton seed cake	-	-	10	-	-	-	-	-	-
Fish meal/skim Milk powder	-	10	-	10	-	8	8	-	-
Mineral mixture	2	2	22	2	2	2	2	2	2
Molasses	8	8	8	-	-	-	-	-	5

N.B. Vitamin premix should contain, Vitamin A activity 20 lakh = I. U., Vitamin D 2.5 lakh I.U. and riboflavin 100 mg per 100 kg mixed feed.

▶ EFFECT OF FREQUENCY OF FEEDING ON PERFORMANCES OF WEANED CALVES

Frequency of milk feeding has some depression effect on growth during the first three month of life when milk or milk replacer is fed only once per day. Increasing the milk feeding frequency to 2 or 3 times daily has no beneficial effect on the performance of calves (Verma and Tomar, 1984). By reducing the number of milk feeding from thrice daily to twice or once daily a significant saving on labourer charges is obtained (Table 4.9). For the raising of replacement stock twice daily feeding in first month followed by once feeding is subsequent months would be quite satisfactory, but for the production of veal calves at 3–4 months of age thrice a day feeding is most suitable.

TABLE 4.9: Effect of frequency of milk or liquid milk replacer feeding on performance of buffalo calves

Observations	Daily frequency of feeding					
	Once		Twice		Thrice	
	Male	Female	Male	Female	Male	Female
Relative time spent on labourer, %	35.0		66.5		100	
Average daily gain (g) in body weight,						
1st month	239	311	340	369	378	359
2nd month	513	411	411	480	602	500
3rd month	583	660	660	689	774	724
4–6th month	379	420	420	435	443	379
Mortality, %	16.67		16.67		9.09	

▶ EFFECT OF ANTIBIOTICS ADDITION ON PERFORMANCE OF WEANED CALVES

Hygienic management and reguiarty of feeding schedule is more important for the production of healthy calves. Several broad spectrum antibiotic premix are available for the feeding in the diets of newborn animals. Antibiotics are generally used for the prevention of gastrointestinal infections and they are more effective in poor hygienic conditions. Variable response of antibiotics feeding may be seen (Table 4.10) and as far as possible their uses should be avoided. Amongst the three antibiotics feed premix used in a study. T M–egg formula gave satisfactory response (Kulkarni et al., 1973). However, overall performances in different treatments were not satisfactory.

TABLE 4.10: Effect of feeding antibiotics premix on performance of calves

| Performance of calves | Treatments | | | |
	Control (no. antibiotics)	TM–egg formula	TM with antigen 77	TM animal formula
Number	14	14	14	14
Death	7	2	5	4
Mortality %	50.0	14.3	35.7	28.6
Mean body weight (kg)				
At birth	35.05	34.51	33.80	34.10
At 6 weeks	39.88	46.05	42.47	38.70
Average daily				
Dain in wt. g	115	275	206	110

A death rate of 50% in non-antibiotic fed animals indicates a very poor hygienic and management conditions, and need the use of effective dose of antibiotic premix.

▶ COMPARATIVE PERFORMANCE ON THE FEEDING OF BUFFALO AND COW MILK IN EARLY LIFE

Buffalo milk contains about 115 kcal energy per 100 ml of whole milk against 67 kcal in cow milk. The growth response of young calves is better on the feeding of buffalo milk than the cow milk (Abou-Hussein and Raafat, 1962). In a veal production study buffalo calves fed buffalo milk gained 1.112 kg daily and consumed 7.116 kg whole milk per day up to 150 kg body weight. Similar calves gained 0.987 kg and consumed about 10.445 kg cow milk. The depression in growth rate was about 11.24% and milk intake was about 65.37% higher for each unit gain in body weight on the feeding of cow's milk. Average gross energy content of buffalo and cow milf fed to calves was about 95 and 65 kcal per 100 ml of milk respectively (Ferrara et al., 1967).

▶ FEEDING OF REPLACEMENT BUFFALO HEIFERS

Heifers of dairy buffaloes are the potential replacement stock, which should be reared at optimum growth rate to ensure timely breeding and production. Plane of nutrition significantly influences the growth and reproductive performances of buffalo heifers (Mudgal, 1979, Gede Puter et al., 1983). Animal gaining at a daily rate of 454 of exhibited significant decrease in age at first service and the age at first conception because they achieved optimum body weight earlier. Age at first calving in different dairy breeds of Indian buffaloes ranges from 41.3 to 55.2 months being lowest in Murrah closely followed by Surti and highest in Marathawada breed. Average body weight at first calving is about 483.4 kg (Bhat, 1979). However, it has been shown in some studies that the age at first mating and first conception can be significantly reduced through the optimum feeding and management practices (Bedeir et al., 1978). On the feeding of protein rich balanced diet age at first service and first conception were 23.9 and 24.4 months in Murrah heifers (Mudgal, 1979), and 25.0 and 27.2 months in the Egyptian buffalo heifers (EI-Shafie et al., 1983). The average body weight ranged from 315 to 346 kg. Therefore, the plane of nutrition during growing period should be adequate to support a daily growth of 400 g in medium and 500 of in large sized buffaloes so that they should attain about 300 and 374 kg mean body weight at about 24 months of age respectively.

The diets of growing heifers should be palatable to ensure about 2.5–2.75 kg dry matter intake per 100 kg body weight in early life up to 6 months of age or 100–150 kg body weight and then 2 kg up to 24 months of age or 300–350 kg body weight. Composite ratios containing 8–10% DCP and 60–65% TDN would be able to meet the requirements of growing heifers reared for replacement. Various factors determine the growth response of heifers and their diets should be not adequate only in protein and energy but also in minerals and vitamins (EI- Harirl et al., 1980).

The following factors should be considered critically at the time of ration formulation for the replacement buffalo heifers:

1. Age of heifers at weaning and ration schedule during the pre-weaning period. Calves feed large amount of milk for longer duration beyond 60 days are less capable to utilize fibrous feeds due to delay in the development of functional ruminoreticulum facilitating microbial digestion of feeds. It is well-developed in calves reared on limited milk feeding supplemented with calf starter and hay feeding.

2. **Age of the heifer:** Early weaned heifers reared on the feeding of limited milk calf starter and hay are capable to eat and utilize good amount of roughages in their rations.

3. **Sources of protein:** Solubility of intact protein feeds considerable influences the requirement of protein. Lower solubility of protein in rumino-reticulum protect if from the microbial degradation and increases their availability through enzymic digestion in the lower tract. Non-protein nitrogenous (NPN) substances should preferable be included after 6 months of age and adequate soluble carbohydrates should be feed for the efficient utilization of NPN compounds.

4. **Sources of energy feed:** They should be palatable, nutrition, and free from contaminants and incrinatig constituents like tannins, saponins, fungal toxins, etc.

5. **Roughages:** Pastures, cultivated fodder and crop residues (straws and stovers) are the common roughages. The last one is available in large quantity in highly populated countries utilizing largest proportion of arable land for the production of food grains. Supplemental feed should be selected to balance the supply of nutrients available from the roughages in the following manner:

   a. With leguminous fodder energy rich feeds like maize, barley, oats, jowar, and bajara should be fed to constitute about 60–70% of total ration up to 100 kg body weight, 50% up to 200 and 15–25 percent thereafter. Supplementation of minerals and vitamins is generally not required.

   b. With cereal fooders like maize oats and pasture grasses like dub, pengola, themeda, panics and timothy a medium concentrate mixture of 8–10% DPC and 65% TDN should be fed at a rate of 1% of body weight in early life reducing the half percent beyond 200 kg body weight.

c. With poor quality roughages like cereal stranos and strovers—strows of wheat, paddy, barley, and ragi, and strovers/kadbies of jowar, pearl millet, and maize and maize are extensively used for the feeding of livestock in developing countries having considerable buffalo population. These fodders are very poor source of protein, minerals and vitamins and they are also low in energy. Large quantity of high protein—higher energy concentrates containing 13–15% DPC and 70–72% TDN are required. About 2–3 kg concentrate mixture is required in the daily diet of growing heifers.

d. A mixture of cereal and leguminous fodder in equal ration is very good source of roughage and ad bibitum feeding of such mixture with half kilogramme concentrate mixture would be adequate to support about 450–550 of daily gain in body weight provided animal inherit the growth potential.

Some examples of growth production rations adequate to support about 40–600 of daily gain in body weight are given for the heifers of different body weights.

EXAMPLE 1: Ration schedule of growing buffalo heifers of 100 kg body weight

Nutrients

	Dry feed kg	DPC g	TDN kg	ME Meal
Requirements	2.5–3.0	212	2.45	9.50
As per NRC (1976)	2.9	240	1.80	6.60
Feeding schedule				
a. With leguminous fodders				
Leguminous fodder	1.25	125	0.85	3.10
Crushed maize/barley	1.50	105	1.13	4.11
Total daily intake	2.75	230	1.98	7.21
b. With green maize/green oats at flowering				
Green fodder	1.5	105	0.98	3.56
Concentrate mixture	1.5	150	1.05	3.83
Total intake	3.0	255	2.03	7.39
c. With wheat strand				
Wheat strand	0.5	-	0.20	0.73
Concentrate mixture	2.5	240	1.50	5.48
Total intake	**2.5**	**240**	**1.70**	**6.21**

EXAMPLE 2: Ration schedule of growing buffalo heifers of 200 kg body weight

Nutrients

	Dry feed kg	DCP g	TDN kg	ME Meal
Requirements	4.5–5.0	268	3.13	11.96
As per NRC	5–6	350	3.40	12.10
Feeding schedule				
a. With leguminous fodder				7.12

Contd.

Nutrients

	Dry feed kg	DCP g	TDN kg	ME Meal
Legume fodder	3.0	300	1.95	4.11
Maize/barley/oats	1.5	105	1.13	11.23
Total intake	4.5	405	3.08	1.46
or				
Wheat/paddy strand	1.0	00	0.40	1.46
Legume fodder	2.5	250	1.63	5.93
Maize/Barley	1.5	1.5	105	1.13
Total intake	5.0	355	3.16	11.50
b. With cereal fodder				
Cereal fodder	3.5	245	2.10	7.67
Concentrate mixture	1.5	120	1.05	3.83
Total intake	5.0	365	3.15	11.49
c. With straws/stovers straw	2.0	-	0.80	2.92
Concentrate mixture	3.0	300	2.10	7.67
Total intake	5.0	300	2.90	10.59
Or when small quantity of greens are available				
Mixed greed fodder	1.0	70	0.55	2.01
Wheat straw	2.0	-	0.80	2.92
Concentrate mixture	2.0	250	1.75	6.39
Total intake	**5.5**	**320**	**3.10**	**11.32**

EXAMPLE 3: Ration schedule of growing buffalo heifers of 300 kg body weight

Nutrients

	Dry feed kg	DCP g	TDN kg	ME Meal
Requirements	5.5–6.5	317	3.72	14.12
As per NRC	6.8	420	3.60	13.00
Feeding schedule				
a. With leguminous fodder				
Leguminous fodder	3.0	300	1.95	7.12
Straw	2.5	-	1.00	3.65
Grains	1.0	70	0.75	2.74
Total intake	6.5	370	3.70	13.51
b. With cereal fodder				
Cereal fodder	5.0	350	3.00	10.95
Concentrate mixture	1.0	100	0.73	0.75
Total intake	6.00	3.73	3.73	13.61
c. With straws and stovers				
Concentrate mixture	2.0	1.46	1.46	5.33
Wheat straw	4.0	1.60	1.60	5.84
Geen fodder	0.5	25	0.25	0.91
Total	**6.5**	**325**	**3,31**	**12.08**

The feeding schedules suggested for heifers of 300 kg body weight may be continues up to conception and also during the first six months of gestation period except than the quantity of half kg concentration mixture should be increased to replace equal weight of straws and stovers.

▶ SUPPLEMENTAL FEEDING OF HEIFERS RAISED ON GRAZING

The quality and quantity of feed required to be supplement the grazing animals depends on the herbage cover, quality of herbage and animal density per unit of land. In hot humid tropical climate grazing requires supplemental feeding of one kilogram concentrate mixture during the rainy season, 1 kg concentrate mixture and ad libitum fodder on return from pastures during the winter season and 2 kg high protein (about 15% DCP) concentrate mixture and roughage in the dry season.

The feeding schedule of buffalo heifers from 3 months of age to the stage of first conception may be followed as per the summarized schedule in Table 4.11 safety to meet the requirement of nutrients due to individual variations in eating capacity and growth potential.

TABLE 4.11: Summary of feeding schedule of buffalo heifers from 3 months of age to first conception

Age (months)	Expected body weight (kg)	Quantity of daily feed (kg)	
		Concentrate mixture	Roughage
3–6	60–110	(i) 1.2–2.0	Green cereal forage ad lib. (5–10)
		(ii) 1–1.5 (cereal grain)	Berseem/Lucame/paddy pea (10–15)
		(iii) 1.5–2.5	Wheat bhusa/paddy straw kadles (0.5–1.0) + Green grass (1–2).
6–12	150–200	(i) 1.5	Cereal fodder ad lib. (20–25).
		(ii) 1.0 (cereal grain)	Berseem/Lucerne/Cowpea (20–30).
		(iii) 2–2.5	Wheat bhusa/paddy straw/Kadbies (2–4) + green grass (1–2).
12 months to age at first conception	200–350	(i) 2.0	Cereal fodder ad lib. @ 10–15 kg/100 kg body weight)
		(ii) 1.0 (cereal grain)	Leguminous fodders @ 12–15 kg/100 kg body weight
		(iii) 1.0 (cereal grain)	Leguminous fodder @ 10kg/100 kg body weight + wheat bhusa @ 1kg/100 kg body weight
		(iv) 2–3	Wheat bhusa/paddy straw Kadbies ad lib (3–6). Green grass (2–3).

NB: The concentrate mixture for feeding with good quality cereal fodders should contain 7–8% DCP, and those for supplementation of straws should have 15–20% DCP. Mineral-vitamin licks should be provided with exclusive feeding of dry roughages.

▶ FEEDING OF PREGNANT BUFFALO HEIFERS DURING THE LAST THIRD OF GESTATION PERIOD

Average gestation period of Indain dairy type buffaloes is 310 (300–315) days, Egyptian buffaloes 317 days, and swamp buffaloes 330 (315–340) days. During the first gestation period pregnant buffalo heifers are still in growing phase. The growth of foetus and increase in the content of concepta are very fast during the last 10 to 12 weeks of gestation period. An average heifer gains about 125–200 kg during the gestation period of which about 50% is gained during the last 10–12 weeks of pregnancy and they should receive additional allowance of good quality feed during this period of active gain in body weight and concepta. The feeding schedule suggested for the growing heifers of 200–350 kg body weight are quite satisfactory for heifers in early pregnancy. The quantity of concentrate should be increased after the sixth month of gestation period. Additional concentrate mixture or grains with leguminous fodders should be fed at a daily rate of 1 kg in seventh, 2 kg in eighth, and 2.5 kg from the ninth months of pregnancy. The latter amount is determined on the basis of the milk production protential of the dam and size or either parent of the animal. Diets are made laxative during the last week of gestation through the replacement of concentrate mixture with wheat bran or a mixture of wheat bran and molasses when dry roughages are fodder sources.

▶ REQUIREMENT OF FEEDS FOR REARING A BUFFALO HEIFER FROM BIRTH TO PUBERTY/FIRST CONCEPTION AND FIRST CALVING STAGE

Great flucuations are generally seen in the market price of feedstuffs and price of rearing a replacement heifer calculated for the present may not hoid good after a few months or year. Since the quantity and quality of feedstuffs required for the rearing of heifer determine the cost of feeding, estimated requirements of different feedstuffs have been given in Table 4.12.

TABLE 4.12: Estimated requirement of different feedstuffs for rearing a buffalo heifer from birth to puberty/first conception and the first calving date

Feedstuff	Requirement
Colostrum	7–10 kg
Whole milk	100–120 kg
Calf starter	60–80 kg
Requirements up to first conception	
Concentrate mixture	
(i) With cereal fodder	100–1200 kg
(ii) With leguminous fodder	600–700 kg
(iii) With straws and stovers	1200–1500 kg
Roughages	
(i) Cereal fodder	20–25 tons
(ii) Leguminous fodder	20–25 tons
(iii) Leguminous fodder	20–25 tons
(iv) Straws and stover	2.5–3 tons
Requirements up to first calving	
Concentrate mixture	
(i) With cereal fodder	1600–1900 kg
(ii) With leguminous fodder	1000–1100 kg
(iii) With straws/stover	200–2500 kg
Roughage	
(i) Cereal fodder	35–40 tons
(ii) Legumious fodder	35–40 tons
(iii) Straws/stover	4.5–5 tons
Mineral mixture (depending upon the quality of fodder)	10–25 kg

The requirement of mineral mixture is low on the feeding of leguminous fodder and highest on the feeding of dry roughages of crop residues. The feeding of rations devoid of green fodders requires the supplementation of vitamin a supplement, because vitamins of B-complex series and vitamin C are synthesized during the fermentation processes in the ruminoreticulum and also for the synthesis of vitatim D adequate solar radiation is available throughout the buffalo raising countries mostly situated in the tropical and subtropical zones.

▶ FEEDING OF ADULT BUFFALOES

Both breeding and working animals are reared by the farmers. For the purpose of feeding adult buffaloes may be classified as follows:

1. Idle adult animals require maintenance ration
2. Dairy animals include:
   a. Dry females
   b. Dry and pregnant females
   c. Lactating females
   d. Lactating and pregnant females
3. Breeding bulls
4. Working buffaloes
   a. Entire or castrated males
   b. Dry females
   c. Dry and pregnant females
   d. Lactating females
   e. Lacating and pregnant females

▶ FEEDING OF IDLE BUFFALOES

Male and female buffaloes not engaged in work and production and the nonpregnant dry females kept under observations before culling require maintenance ration. Free choice grazing for 8–10 hours on natural herbage capable to provide about 1.5 kg dry matter per 100 kg body weight is adeuqte for the maintenance of idle adult buffaloes. On sole feeding of dry roughage like straws and stovers the voluntary intake is about 1.5 kg dry matter per 100 kg body weight and it requires proteinous feeds for balancing. An adult buffalo of about 400 kg body weight should be fed 600–700 g high protein oilcakes like groundnut cake, mustard cake, cottonseed cake or linseed cake or 1 kg concentrate mixture providing 25–27% DCP or leguminous fodder to substitute about one-third dry matter of straw intake.

▶ FEEDING OF DRY FEMALES

Nonpregnant dry buffaloes require a little better deal in feeding and management for efficient breeding. Dry females should be allowed ad libitum feeding of cereal fodders or a mixture of straw and leguminous fodder in the ratio of 1:3 on fresh basis, which will contain about 4–5% DCP and 50–52% TDN on dry matter basis. The voluntary intake will be about 1.75–0.2 kg dry matter per 100 kg body weight. Mineral mixture and vitamin A should be supplemented during the feeding of dry crop residues for longer duration the feeding of dry crop residues for longer duration. When straws and stovers are the sole roughages each dry female should be fed about 2 kg concentrate mixture containing 15–17% DCP and 68–70% TDN along with 3–4 kg mixed green grasses, fodder, tree leaves or edible aquatic plants depending on their availability.

▶ FEEDING OF DRY AND PREGNANT FEMALES DURING THE LAST 3 MONTHS OF GESTATION PERIOD

Active growth of concepta takes place during the last 3 months of pregnancy. In addition to this the animal is required to put some 10–20 kg weight for bearing the sudden stress caused by the flow of nutrients from the body reserves into the milk. Pregnant dry buffaloes are fed additional concentrate mixture over the maintenance requirement at the rate of 1, 2, and 3–5 kg during the 8th, 9th, and 10th month of pregnancy. The amount fed in last month is fixed on the basis of the milk yield in previous lactation. Gradual increase in concentrate allowance before calving makes the animal accustomed the consumption of larger quantity of concentrate mixture and also reduces the scope of gastric disorders occasionally encountered during the sudden feeding of large amounts of concentrates of farm grain mixture.

▶ FEEDING OF LACTATING ANIMALS

Due to high content of protein and energy in milk, the requirement of buffaloes for milk production is higher than the cattle. Average protein content in buffalo milk is 3.6 percent, fat 7.0% and energy 105 kcal per 100 ml of whole milk. Buffalo secretes about 36 g protein, 70 g fat, and 1050 kcal gross energy in each litre of milk produced. To support the milk production without affecting the significant drainage of nutrients from the body tissues, adequate additional feeding is required. The efficiency of DCP utilization for the production of milk protein varies from 60.12 to 79.35% (Kurar and Mudgal, 1980; Sivaiah and Mudgal, 1983). The efficiency of ME utilization for milk production varies from 64.3 to 65.7% (Srivastava, 1970; Kurar and Mudgal, 1980; Sivaiah and Mudgal, 1983). About 1600–1700 kcal ME feeding is required for each kg of whole milk production. Thus, a balanced farm grains or dairy mixture should contain about 8–10% DCP and 70–75% TDN or 2.56–2.74 Meal ME per kg of feed, and it should be fed at the rate of 0.60–0.63 kg per kg milk yield of about 7% fat content, and this allowance for milk production should be in addition to maintain requirement. This is slightly higher than the recommendation 0.5 kg concentrate mixture per kg milk production (Shukla et al. 1972). About 7 kg daily milk yield may be supported by ad libitum feeding of good quality green fodders, a mixture of cereal and leguminous fooders like equal ratio of flowering oats and berseem or Lucern, and green maize at milk stage with cowpea or 1–2 kg wheat straw with ad libitum berseem (60–80 kg). With the feeding of all-roughage ration about 0.5 to 1.0 kg concentrate mixture is fed at each if the two milkings to stimulate the let down of milk (Jackson and Gupta, 1971; Gupta et al., 1983). About 250 g concentrate feeding per kg milk yield is required on ad libitum feeding of cereal fodders palatable to support about 2 kg dry matter intake per 100 kg body weight. From a complete ration of concentrate mixture and maize or oat silage about two-thirds concentrate mixture can be replaced by good quality berseem hay. The replacement value of berseem, hay was 1.25 kg for each kg of concentrate mixture Chauhan and Chopra, 1984). A few examples of dairy mixtures containing 15–17% DCP, 70–75% TDN and 2.56–2.74 meal ME per kg are given considering the variations in the availability of feedstuffs in different agroclimatic conditions (Table 4.13).

Although daily milk yield of larger population of dairy buffaloes is less than 7–8 kg and their production level can be sustained on the feeding of good quality nutritions fodders like leguminous crops and mixed crop of cereal and legume fodders providing about 8–10% DCP, 60–65% TDN and 2.19–2.37 meal ME per kg feed on dry matter basis. However, in most of the tropical countries dry crop residues are the staple roughage in the diets of farm animals, and feeding programs have been mostly developed around wheat *bhusa* and paddy straw supplemented with some concentrate mixture and green fodders. The proportion of green fodder varies from almost zero level in dry hot season to ad libitum feeding in hot-humid season. Some examples of ration calculations with different kinds of feedstuff are as follows:

TABLE 4.13: Composition of concentrate mixture for dairy buffaloes or dairy mixtures

Ingredients	Percent composition						
	1	2	3	4	5	6	7
Crushed maize/barley/oats	50	50	50	40	30	30	50
Sorghum/pearl millet	-	-	-	10	20	-	-
Rice polish	-	-	-	-	-	20	-
Groundnut cake	30	-	15	15	-	-	-
Cottonseed cake	-	30	-	15	-	-	-
Mustard cake	-	-	15	-	20	-	-
Linseed cake	-	-	-	-	10	35	35
Wheat bran	17	17	-	10	-	-	12
Rice bran	-	-	17	7	17	12	-
Mineral mixture	2	2	2	2	2	2	2
Salt	1	1	1	1	1	1	1

EXAMPLE 1: Computation of daily ration for a lactating nonpregnant adult buffalo of 500 kg body weight and yielding 10 kg milk of 7% fat content daily. The break up to daily nutrients requirement for the maintenance and milk production is given below:

Requirements	Dry matter	DPC	TDN	ME	Ca	P
	kg	g	kg	Meal	g	g
Maintenance	7–8	275	3.33	12.95	20	15
Adjustment allowance 10%		28	0.33	1.29	-	-
Total maintenance	7–8	303	3.66	14.24	20	15
Milk production	5–6	630	4.40	15.90	33	26
Total	**12–14**	**933**	**8.06**	**30.14**	**53**	**41**

For the supply of these nutrients different feeding schedules are followed under the different conditions of the feeds and fodders supply. The feeding schedules are decided on the availability of feeds from the farmers field and the local markets, the relative cost of feeds and the voluntary intake of feeds by the lactating buffaloes. There are four possibilities for the determination of a suitable, effective, and economical feeding schedule at an organized farm, viz.,

    i. the feeding of green fodders as the sole ration,

    ii. the feeding of green fodders mixed with wheat *bhusa*, chaffed paddy straw or chaffed kadbies,

   iii. straws or stovers and concentrate mixture, and

   iv. straws or slovers, green fodders and concentrate mixture.

The last system of feeding is more prevalent in many countries of the tropical agro-climatic zone.

Feeding schedules of a buffalo of 500 kg body weight yielding 10 kg milk of 7% fat daily.

Feeds	Quantity kg	DM kg	DCP g	TDN kg	ME Mcal	Ca g	P g
Ration 1							
Green berseem (15 DM, 1.5 DCP, 10 TDN, 0.365 meal ME)	85	12.75	1270	8.5	31.03	255	60
Requirements		12–14	933	8.06	30.14	53	41
Difference			**+337**	**+0.44**	**+0.89**	**+201**	**+19**
Ration 2							
Green Lucerne (20 DM, 2.0 DCP, 13.5 TDN, 0.493 Mcal ME	60	12	1200	8.1	29.58	312	59
Requirements		12–14	933	8.06	30.14	53	41
Difference			**+267**	**+0.04**	**+0.56**	**+259**	**+18**
Ration 3							
Green maize + Cowpea (1:1; DM 20, DCP 1.5, TDN 13.7, ME 0.5 meal)	65	13	975	8.78	32.5	98	20
Requirements		12–14	933	8.06	30.14	53	41
Difference			**+42**	**+0.72**	**+2.36**	**+45**	**−21**

When cereal fodders are fed in large quantity supplementation of phosphorus is required in the diets (ration 3).

Green berseam/Lucerne	50–60	9–10	900	6.5	23.73	150	40
Wheat straw/paddy straw	5–6	4–5	-	2.2	8.00	10	
Total intake		**13–15**	**900**	**8.7**	**31.73**	**160**	**42**
Ration 5							
Concentrate mixture (DM 90, DCP 13, TDN 70, ME 2.56, Ca 1, P 0.7)	7	6.3	910	4.90	17.92	70	49
Straws/Stovers	8	7.2	-	3.20	11.68	16	4
Total intake		**13.5**	**910**	**8.10**	**29.60**	**86**	**53**
Ration 6							
Mixed green grass (DM 25, DCP 1.5, TDN, ME 0.511, Ca 0.5, P. 0.3)	10	2.5	150	1.4	5.11	50	30
Concentrate mixture (DM 90, DCP 1.5, TDN, ME 2.56, Ca 1.5, P 0.3)	5	4.5	700	3.5	12.80	25	15
Straws/Stovers	8	7.2	-	3.2	11.68	16	4
Total intake		**14.2**	**850**	**8.1**	**29.59**	**91**	**49**

Under the grazing conditions feeding schedule is changed and decided on the basis of herbage cover available in the fields for the feeding. Mixed herbage of cereal grasses contain 7–8% DCP and 55–60% TDN or 2–2.2 meal ME per kg dry matter in the hot-humid season; about 4–5% DCP and similar energy during the cold months and 2–4% DCP and 45–50% TDN or 1.64–1.83 meal M E per kg dry matter in the dry hot season. On adequate grazing in hot-humid season, a lactating nonpregnant buffalo of 500 kg body weight consume about 12.5 kg (12–13 kg) dry matter supplying about 938 (840–1040) g DCP, 7.19 (6.6–7.8) kg TDN and 26.3 meal (24–28.5 meal) M E daily. The herbage consumption was adequate to satisfy the appetite and meet the DCP requirement for maintenance and 10 kg daily milk yield but the DCP requirement for maintenance and 10 kg daily milk yield but the availability of energy was marginally short, which is balanced through the feeding of one kg concentrate mixture fed for the let down of milk.

Herbage cover in dry cold season is much less than the hot-humid season and buffaloes consume about 7 kg (6–8 kg) dry matter from 8–10 hours daily grazing. This provides about 315 g (240–400 g) DCP, 4.03 (3.3–4.8) kg TDN and 14.71 (12.05–17–52) meal ME daily. The feed intake was adequate for the maintenance and small quantity of milk production, and needs daily feeding of dairy mixture at the rate of 0.5 kg for each kg milk yield. The situation in hot-dry season is quite unfavourable and buffaloes hardly consume 5 (4–6) kg dry matter from the grazing of almost dried herbage similar in quality to poor quality hay. During such conditions buffaloes should be fed 1–2 kg concentrate mixture for the maintenance in addition to the allowance for milk production.

▶ FEEDING OF PREGNANT LACTATING BUFFALOES

Additional feeding of protein and energy is not required in the early pregnancy and standard rations of lactating animal is considered adequate to take care of the foetal development up to 6–7 months of gestation period. From seventh month the quantity of concentrate mixture is increased at the rate of 1 and 2 kg daily during the eight and ninth month of pregnancy and thereafter the quantity of concentrate mixture is gradually increased to about 75% level of consumption in the previous lactation. Ordinarily pregnant buffalo should start gaining in body weight after 6 month of pregnancy, which should acceierate to about half kg daily gain during the last 60 days when they are dried. During latter half of gestation period buffaloes should receive adequate nutrients to restore the body reserves depleted during the lactation and put additional 20–30 kg to take care of the depletion during the early phase of the next lactation.

In case of dry pregnant buffaloes about 1–2 kg additional concentrate mixture is fed over the maintenance requirement during the eight and ninth month. After this amount of concentrate mixture is increased to about 75% of the requirement of buffalo in the early lactation.

▶ FEEDING OF BREEDING BULLS

Buffalo bulls are used for breeding and semen collection at 3 to 4 years of age in Egypt, Indian subcontinent, and the southeast Asian countries, although meiotic division of the spermatogonial cell lining of the seminiferous tubules has been observed in a one-year-old Indian buffalo bull (Dutt and Bhattacharya, 1952). In Italy and USSR some buffalo bulls are used at an early age of 2 years (May mone, 1942). In reduction of about 25% DCP intake from the diets of buffalo bulls some improvement in semen quality has been observed (Prabhu and Bhaya, 1962 a, b). Partial replacement of protein through urea feeding increased the urea content in the seminal plasma and changed the patern of protein in the seminal fluid (Ahuja and Bhatia, 1974). However, it is not possible with scanty knowledge to suggest deviations from the normal feeding systems being developed on the basis of informations from the normal feeding systems being delevoped on the basis of informations on cattle bulls. Mature breeding bulls in active service should be fed balanced diet to support marginally positive body weight. Over feeding and fat deposition not only makes the bulls unusually heavy and lethargic but also adversely affect the breeding behaviour. When good quality fodders are availale for ad libitum feeding, there is no need of concentrate feeding. Under free living conditions, a common practice in India, buffalo bulls maintain satisfactory vigour and fertility for several years. Such bulls thrive exclusively on the grazing on natural pastures and cultivated crops. Some examples of feeding schedule under different conditions have been given for a mature breeding bull of about 600 kg body weight.

▶ FEEDING SCHEDULES OF BREEDING BULLS

With the large quantity feeding of concentrate mixture and dry crop residues adequate minerals and vitamins should be fed in the absence of any green fodder. (Table 4.14)

TABLE 4.14: Feeding schedules of breeding bulls

	Quantity kg	DM kg	DCP g	TDN kg	ME Meal
Requirements		9–10	360	4.5	16.4
Ration 1					
Cereal fodder					
(5DCP, 55TDN, 2 meals ME)	40	8	400	4.0	14.60
Straw/stovers	1	0.9	-	0.4	1.46
Total intake		8.9	400	4.4	16.06
Ration 2					
Leguminous					
Fodder (10 DCP, 60 TDN, 2.19 meal ME)	25	3.75	375	2.25	8.21
Straws/stover	6	5.40	-	2.40	8.76
Total intake		9.15	375	4.65	16.97
Ration 3					
Concentrate	3	2.7	360	2.10	7.67
Straws/stovers	5	4.5	-	2.00	7.30
Mixed green fodder	5	1.0	40	0.55	2.01
Total intake		8.2	400	4.65	16.98

▶ FEEDING OF WORKING /DRAUGHT BUFFALEOS

Normally males of dairy buffaloes and both sexes of swamp buffaloes are used for working. The main work contribution of buffaloes is in the agricultural operations of paddy cultivation, and a small number is used for haulage of luggage in the industrial towns. Animals involved in agricultural operation are largely engaged in light to medium work like ploughing, thrashing of grains and transportation of agricultural produce. Average working time varies from 3–6 hours a day, whereas those in industrial areas are required to pull heavy cart loads for 6–10 hours daily. The feeding of former group includes 4–6 hours daily grazing supplemented with feeding of paddy straw and a small quantity of concentrate mixture constituted of rice milking bye-products and cakes of mustard, coconut or groundnut, and dal chaunies.

Female swamp buffaloes put to work during pregnancy and lactation also except for the last one or two months of gestation period. In the computation of rations of such animals these conditions of body should be given due consideration for the supply of adequate nutrients to support optimum foetal growth and milk production for nursing the calves.

Some examples of feeding schedules for light (2–3 hours), medium (4–6 hours), and heavy (8–10 hours) works are given for adult buffalo of about 500 kg body weight, although they are put to work in young age of 2–3 years, while they are still growing.

▶ RATION SCHEDULES OF WORKING BUFFALOES

TABLE 4.15: Ration schedles draught and working buffaloes

	Quantity of feeds, kg	DMK g	DCP g	TDN kg	ME meal
Requirements					
(i) Light work		8–9	300	4.95	16.85
(ii) Medium work		9–10	310	5.45	19.25
(iii) Heavy work		10–11	325	5.93	21.65
Daily rations for light work					
Ration 1					
Grazing for 4–6 hours		5.0	200	2.50	9.12
Paddy straw	5	4.5	0	2.00	7.30
Protein supplement	0.5	0.45	100	0.35	1.28
Total intake		**9.95**	**300**	**4.85**	**17.70**
Ration 2					
Concentration mixture	2	1.8	300	1.45	5.11
Straws/stovers	8	7.2	-	3.2	11.68
Total intake	**10**	**9.0**	**300**	**4.6**	**16.79**
Daily rations for medium work					
Ration 1					
Grazing 3–4 hrs.		3.0	120	1.50	5.47
Straw/stovers	5	4.5	-	2.00	7.30
Concentrate mixture	2	1.8	220	1.40	5.11
Total intake		**9.3**	**340**	**4.90**	**17.88**
Ration 2					
Concentration mixture	3	2.7	330	2.1	7.67
Straws/stovers	8	7.2	-	3.2	11.68
Total intake		**9.9**	**330**	**5.3**	**19.35**
Daily rations for heavy work (No grazing)					
Ration 1					
Concentrate mixture	5	4.5	450	3.60	13.14

Contd.

TABLE 4.15: Ration schedles draught and working buffaloes *(Contd.)*

	Quantity of feeds, kg	DMK g	DCP g	TDN kg	ME meal
Straws/stovers	6	5.4	-	2.40	8.76
Total intake		**9.9**	**450**	**6.00**	**21.90**
Ration 2					
Mixed green fodder	25	5.0	250	2.50	9.12
Concentrate mixture	2	1.8	200	1.44	5.26
Straws/stovers	5	4.5	-	2.00	7.30
Total intake		**11.3**	**450**	**5.94**	**21.68**

Pregnant working swamp buffaloes should be fed a concentrate mixture of 10–12% DCP and 67–70% TDN at the rate of 1–2 kg daily during the last 8–10 weeks of gestation period, in addition to normal rations for work. Similarly, lactating buffaloes should be fed at a flat rate of 1.5 kg additional concentrate mixture during the 5–6 months of lactation period, because milk requirement of calves is 2–3 kg daily (Table 4.15). Early weaning should be practiced for restoring the breeding, which delays due to suckling in many cases.

▶ FEEDING OF BUFFALOES FOR MEAT PRODUCTION

Buffalo meat is quite popular in the diets of people in the buffalo breeding countries. In the Indian subcontinent and many countries of southeast and east Asian as well as the island countries of Asia-Pacific region mostly spent buffaloes and sterile females are culled for utilization as meat animal. However, in Europe, Egypt, near east, Russia, Australia, West-Indies, and Latin American countries buffaloes are reared for meat and milk or meat in Australia. In recent years buffalo fattening is becoming a commercial enterprise also in Asian countries due to extensive mechanization of agriculture. Now the male calves are reared for buffveal, yearling and fattened 2–3 years old for buffen or carabeef production.

Buffaloes available for meat production

1. Surplus male calves are reared for veal, yearling and fattened 2–3 years old animals (steer or bulls).
2. Sterile heifers unable to conceive up to 5 years of age.
3. Sterile female buffaloes failed to conceive during different lactation.
4. Spent female buffaloes after 7–8 lactaction.
5. Spent draught buffaloes over 15 years of age.
6. Retired breeding bulls called due to advance age or poor quality seman production.

▶ FEEDING FOR BUFFALO VEAL (BUFF VEAL) PRODUCTION

Good quality buffalo veal (buff veal or cara veal) of white and juicy flesh is obtained from the young buffalo calves reared on high level feeding of diets containing greater proportion of milk or milk replacer. The buff veal calves are finished as young as 4–8 weeks of age to young buff veal calves of about 6 months of age. The diets of baby buff veal calf is whole milk and reconstituted milk while that of young buff veal is milk gradually replaced with high energy-high protein diets of concentrate and mutritious fodder, mostly the legume hay.

Suckling buffalo veals slaughtered at 30–40 days of age consume about 6 kg whole milk of buffalo per kg gain in the body weight. The average milk intake per kg dressed veal is about 8.09 kg (Badreldin, 1955). Whole milk of cow can be fed in place of whole milk of buffalo but due to low energy content and limited stomach capacity buffalo calves fed cow's milk consume less energy which reduces daily gain by about 28% (About-Hussein and Raafat, 1962). The requirement of whole milk of buffalo for each kg gain in body weight is only 6.4 kg intake of later is about 65.6% higher than the milk of buffalo. The depression in growth rate is due to low energy content in cow milk and limited intake capacity of stomach (Ferrara et al., 1968).

On the feeding of reconstituted milk a daily gain of 795 g and about 52.9% efficiency of utilization of milk powder has been found comparable with the cattle veal production (Romita et al., 1976).

For the production of buffalo veal calves of 1 to 4 months of age nutritious diets of 75% milk feeding should be followed up to 4 weeks of age and thereafter it should be gradually reduced to 50 : 50 through the feeding of high energy milk replacer diet by 8–10 weeks of age. In last phase of 4–6 weeks duration feeding of milk may be reduced to 25% of intake or may be stopped completely. Good quality leguminous hay should be fed from 3–4 weeks of age and it may be fed up to 20–25% of daily dry matter intake after 5–6 weeks of age. Incorporation of larger quantity of roughage will dilute the energy content of diet and enhance the development of microbial digestion in the rumino-reticulum of the buffalo calves, which is discouraged in the buffalo veal calves for the better utilization of nutrients similar to that in simple stomached animals. The diets of veal calves shoul be balanced for the adequate supply of essential amino acids, minerals and vitamins. Hence, replacement of milk from the diet shoulb be balanced for proteins through the mixture form the diet should be balanced for proteins through the mixture of vegetable protein and white fish meal or meat meal.

▶ FEEDING OF WEANED BUFFALO CALVES FOR FATTENING

Well-fed calves are available for rearing as 300–500 kg meat animals at 12–30 months of age in Egypt, Italy, Bulgaria, and USSR. In many parts of Indian subcontinent male buffalo calves are mostly the lot of poor animals of 60–100 kg body weight at 8–12 months of age. These are mostly those calves, which were kept for let down of milk and survive the neglected feeding and management. Satisfactory growth response has been observed in such buffalo calves on the feeding of adequate diets containing optimum nutrients (Agrawal, 1974; Pathak and Ranjhan, 1979; Baruah 1982, et al.). There is ample scope for the utilization of this valuable food animals for the production of large quantity of edible meat for consumption at home and also for export in the consumers countries. The situation of calves of Swamp buffalo is far better because in most of the case they suckle the entire milk of dam for a period of 6 months to one year. The body weight of buffalo calves varies from 100–200 kg at weaning before one year of age. Earlier swamp buffaloes were the live tractor for working in belly deep mud of paddy fields of southeast Asian countries, but due to increase in agricultural machanisation, of a good number of animals could be spared for fattening as meat animals (Fisher, 1982). Average weight gain in swamp buffaloes on pasture has been 218 g daily, and could be increased to 0.34–0.65 kg daily on controlled feeding during 2 years period (Voigt, 1977). Grazing is available for longer part of the year in the hot-humid climate of south-east Asian countries, although most of the natural pastures are dominated by grasses with acanty distribution of legumes. Mostly commonly present Kudzu vine is not very palatable to buffaloes and largely distributed *Mimose* spp. are not consumed et al., and they are toxic also. Following three methods of feeding are followed for raising buffaloes for meat production:

1. Intensive system
2. Semi-intensive system
3. Rearing on pastures.

Intensive System of Feeding

The weaned buffalo calves are fed a balanced diet of roughages and concentrates or good quality roughages alone. The system of feeding is selected on the availability of feedstuff and their competitive price and production efficiency. Young buffalo calves are capable to consume dry matter at the rate of 3% of body weight in early life, which gradually decreases with the increase in age to less than 2% of body weight after attaining 400 kg body weight. The feeding schedule of fattening buffalo calves is determined on the basis of body weight and growth potential. Indian buffaloes of 6 months age are capable to deposit 400–800 g body weight daily on the feeding of balanced ration (Sharma and Talapatra, 1962; Agrawal, 1974; Pathak and Ranjhan, 1979; Baruah et al., 1982). A growth rate of more than 0.67 kg daily has been reported in the buffaloes of Trinidad (Faulkner, 1962; Benett, 1964); 0.4–0.8 kg daily in Egyptian and Iraqi buffaloes (Ghonein et al., 1959; El-Ashry et al., 1972; Juma et al., 1972) and almost one kg or even more in many European buffaloes (Proto and Lundi, 1965; Onjanovic et al., 1970; Ferrara et al., 1972). Some examples of ration schedule are given in Table 4.16.

TABLE 4.16: Ration schedule of fattening buffalo for 0.75 kg daily gain

	Feeds kg	DM kg	DCP kg	TDN kg	ME meal
Requirements at 100 kg body weight		3.1	277	3.03	12.45
Ration 1					
Concentrate mixture (DCP 9, TDN 85, ME 3.90)	3	2.70	270	2.55	9.31
Green maize/oats	3	0.45	30	0.30	1.10
Total intake		3.15	300	2.85	10.41
Ration 2					
Containing 8–10% fat					
Concentrate mixture (DCP8, TDN 95, ME 3.47)	3	2.7	240	2.85	10.40
Green fodder	3	0.45	39	0.39	1.10
Total intake		3.15	279	3.15	11.50
Requirement at 200 kg		5–6	333	3.86	14.91
Ration 1					
Concentrate mixture(DCP 9, TDN 70, ME 2.56)	3	2.7	270	2.10	7.66
Green fodder	20	3.0	100	2.00	7.30
Total intake		5.7	370	4.10	14.96
Ration 2					
Berseem/Lucerne	30	4.2	462	2.94	10.73
Maize grain	1	0.9	60	0.84	3.07
Total intake		5.1	522	3.78	13.80

Contd.

TABLE 4.16: Ration schedule of fattening buffalo for 0.75 kg daily gain (*Contd.*)

	Feeds kg	DM kg	DCP kg	TDN kg	ME meal
Requirement at 300 kg		6–7	382	4.45	17.07
Ration 1					
Green Maize/oats	20	4.0	200	2.60	9.49
Concentrate mixture (9 DCP,75 TDN and 2.74 ME)	2.5	2.25	225	1.88	6.84
Total intake		**6.25**	**425**	**4.48**	**16.33**
Ration 2					
Legume fodder	30	4.2	462	2.94	10.73
Maize grain	2.0	1.80	100	1.70	6.61
Total intake		**6.00**	**562**	**4.64**	**16.98**

Residual male buffalo calves available after wearning at 8–12 months of age are poor animals and grow at the rate of 400–550 g daily depending on the density of nutrients in the feeds and the palatability of the feeds (Pathak et al., 1982). Such calves can be finished to 300 kg body weight in about 360–500 days on the feeding of a moderate ration containing 7–8% DCP, 60–65% TDN and 2.19–2.37 meal ME per kg feed on dry matter basis. Fattening of pastures require supplemental feeding during some parts of the year when herbage cover is exhausted (Palo et al., 1971; Carvalho et al., 1982; Robertson et al., 1982).

Feed conversion efficiency of residual male buffalo calves on the feeding of good quality balanced ration has been found to be quite satisfactory, and it ranges from 5 to 9 kg per kg gain in body weight depending on the density of available energy in the feed and its voluntary intake (Agrwal, 1974; Tilakaratne et al., 1926; Pathak, 1979; Pathak *et al*, 1983). Feed requirement per kg gain increases with the increase in age and also the decrease in the available energy content of feeds (Rosa et al., 1980; baruah et al, 1983), but animals of advanced age are capable to utilize higher proportion of fibrous feeds which are otherwise unfit for the human consumption. Good quality red meat of buffalo can be obtained even at 400–500 kg finishing body weight on a moderate energy diet supporting the growth in 35–40 months of age (Charles and Johnson, 1972). From the quality assessment of 1100 buffaloes above 3 years, 1250 buffaloes between 6 months to 3 years, and 1400 calves below 6 years age. Vacarn-Opris and Paul (1981) observed about 70.9, 94.8% of carcasses fall in class I grade in Romania.

▶ FEEDING OF SPENT BUFFALOES FOR MEAT PRODUCTION

Large number of called buffaloes of 3 to 15 years of age are avaible surplus in many countries. These animals usually find their fate in abattoir. The meat available from such animals is mostly fibrous, hard and dark in colour. Since good quanlity meat tenderizing substances is available for the proper cooking, the hardness is not a serious problem. However, there is ample scope of improvement in the meat quality of such poor animals through the feeding of high energy rations for a short period of 8–10 weeks. A very high feed conversion efficiency occurs during the recuperative changes in the body through compensatory growth after a long duration of feeding on submaintained diets.

The feeding resime for such animals should be selected on the basis of their apparent body conditions, viz.:

i. Culled animals with less than 3 visible or exposed ribs may be fed a moderate diet of 6–7% DCP and 55–60% TDN or 2–2.2 meal ME per kg dry feed ad libitum to encourage about 2 kg dry matter intake per 100 kg body weight.

ii. Culled animals with 4–8 visible ribs may be fed at least kg concentrate mixture of high energy grains along with adequate cereal grasses or a mixture of green berseem or Lucerne and wheat *bhusa* or other poor quality fodder in the ratio of 4:1 on as such basis.

iii. Culled animals with exposed joints emaciated conditions should be fed high energy grains enriched with oilcakes to contain about 10–12% DCP and 70–75% TDN or 2.56–2.74 meal ME per kg dry matter and good quality fodders. The proportion of concentrate mixture should be 60–75% in the daily ration.

After these feeding treatments significant improvement will take place and relatively much better carcass would be available for human consumption.

REFERENCES

Abou-Hussein, E.R.M. and Raafat, M.A. 1962. Comparative studies on the feeding of dairy buffalo calves on cow's and buffalo's milk. J.Anim. Prod., U.A.R., 2:27–35.

Afzal, M. and Anjum, A.D. 1982. Serum protein changes in buffalo calves after colostrums feeding. Pakistan Vet. J., 2: 182–183.

Agarwal, V.P. 1974. Studies on growth rate and carcass quality of buffalo calves as influenced by different plans of nutrition. Ph.D. Thesis. Agra University, Agra.

Ahmed, I.A. and Ele-Shazly, K.1975. Early wearing of buffaloes in Egypt.World Anim Rev., 14:26–30

Ahuja, S.P. and Bhatia, I.S. 1974. Effect of prolonged feeding of urea to buffalo bulls on the proteins of blood plasma and seminal plasma. Indian J.Anim. Sci., 44:847–852.

Anonymous 1964. Agriculture in Ancient India. P.106. Indian Council of Agricultural Research, New Delhi, 110001.

Arora, S.P.; Bajpai, L.D. and Dave, B.K. 1973a. Raising crossbred and buffalo calves on milk replacer. Indian J. Anim.Sci., 43:462–466

Arora, S.P.; Abrol, Y.B.; Chatterjee, S.R.; Chopra, R.C. and Tandon, R.N. 1973b. Animo acid composition of buffalo milk proteins for the use in constituting milk replacer. Indian J.Dairy Sci., 28:276–280

Arora, S.P.; Bakshi, M.P.S.; Khirwar, S.S.; Chopra, R.C. and Sarma, P.A. 1976. Effect of feeding milk and milk substitute on the growth of buffalo calves. Indain J.Amim. Prod., 5:52–57

Arora, S.P.; Khirwar, S.S.; Chopra, R.C.; Chhabra, A.; Atreja, P.P and Tomer, O.S. 1979. Economical raising of calves on milk replacer. Indian Vet.J., 56:129–133.

Arumyghan, C, and Narayanan, K.M. 1982. Influence of stage of lactation of the physical and chemical characteristics of buffalo milk fat. Indian J. Anim. Sci., 52:731–735.

Badreldin, A.L. 1955, Dressing out percentage in suckling buffalo veals. Indian J.Vet. Sci. Anim. Husb. 25:61–64

Buruah, P.K.; Singh, R.P. and Bali, M.K. 1981. Relationship between presence of 3rd stage larvae of *Neoascaris vutulorum* and *Strongyloides papillosus* in colostrums/milk of buffaloes and appearance of eggs in the faecal samples of their calves. Indian J.Dairy Sci., 34:76–78

Baruah, K.K.; Ranjhan, S.K. and Pathak, N.N. 1982. Effect of various levels of protein and energy feeding on growth. Digestibility of organic nutrients and carcass characteristics of Indian desi male buffalo calves. Pro. 2nd Anim. Sci. Cong., Asian-Australian Assoc. Anim. Prod. Soc.; PJCC, Manila, Philippines, November 10–13.

Baruah, K.K.; Ranjhan, S.K. and Pathak, N.N. 1983. Dietary energy and protein affecting growth, feed conversion and carcass characteristics of entire Indian desi male buffalo (*Bubalus bubalis*) calves. Proc. 5th world Conf. Anim. Production., Tokyo, Japan, August 13–18.

Bedeir, L.H.; Youssef, M.S.S.;Omara, S.F. and Abdel Halim, H. 1978. The effect of introducing silage in summer rations on the performance of female buffalo claves. Agric. Res. Rev., U.A.R., 56:79–93.

Bhat, P.N. 1979. Genetic Parameters of milk production and scope of increasing milk production in buffaloes vis-a-vis cattle. Buffalo reproduction and artificial insemination, p. 129–141. FAO Animal Production and Health paper 13, Rome.

Borhami, B.E.A.; El Shazly. K.; Abou-Akkada, A.R. and Ahmad, I.A. 1967. Effect of early establishment of ciliate protozoa in the rumen on microbial activity and growth of early weaned buffalo calves. J. Dairu Sci., 50:1654–1662.

Carvalho, L.O.D. De.M.; Nascimento, C.N.B. Do.; Casta, N.A. Da. and Lourenco Junior, J.De.B. 1982. Fattening of Mediterranean race buffaloes on a Brachiaria humidicola pasture on non-flooded land. Circular Temica, Centre de Pesrquisa Agropecuaria do Tropico Umido, No. 25. p.p. 20 (Fide Nutr. Abst. Rev. 1984 3; 54:431; abstr, 3224).

Charles, D.D. and Johnson, E.R. 1972. Carcass composition of the water buffalo (*Bubalus bubalis*). Australian J.Agric. Res., 23:905–911.

Chauhan, T.R. and Chopra, A.K. 1984. Effect of replacement of concentrate mixture by berseem hay in silage based rations on milk production in buffalos. Indian J.Anim. Sci., 54:742–746.

Da-Silva, R.G. 1969. Preliminary study on the nematode parasites of the buffalo in parastate. Pesuisa agropec.bras. Ser. Vet., 4:155–160.

Dass, R.S. and Arora, S.P. 1983. Studies on growth of buffalo calves fed on milk, milk replacer. Indain Vet. Med. J., 7:148–152.

Dave, B.K.; Chabra, S.S.; Ranjhan, S.K. and Upadhayay, R.S. 1971. Effect of limited milk intake on the growth rate of newly born calves up to six months of age. Indain J. Anim. Prod., 2:22–27.

Dutt, N.K. and Bhattacharya, P.1952. Chromosomes of the Indian water buffalo. Nature, London, 170:1129–1130.

El. Ashry, M.A.; El-Serafy, A.M. and shehata, 0.1975. A note on the performance of buffalo calves fed different milk replacers. Indian J.Anim. Sci., 45:234236.

El. Hariri, M.N.; Awad, H.H. and El-Fadaly, M.A. 1980. Increasing the fertility of buffalo heifers by vitamineral and iodinated casein. J.Egyption Vet. Med. Assoc., 40:80–96.

(fide Anim. Breed.Abst., 51:444, Abstr. 3560).

El. Naggar, A.A.; El Shazly, K.and Ahmed, I.A. 1972. Effect of early weaning on the performance of male buffalo and cattle calves. Anim.Prod., 14:171–176.

El- Serafty, A.M.; El-Ashry, M.A.; Zaky A.A. and Khattab, H.M. 1980. Milk repalcer diets for buffalo calves. 1. Effect of level of tallow and skim milk on preweaning performance and digestibilities of diets. Indian J. Amin. Sci.; 50:1039–1042.

El-Shafie, M.M.; Borady, A.M.A.; Mourad, H.M. and Khattab, R.M. 1983. Physiological and seasonal factors affecting reproductive performance of Egyptian buffalo heifers. Egyptian J. Anim. Prod., 23:1–14.

Faulkner, D.E. 1962. Report on livestock development in Trinidad and Tobago. 81 pps. Min. Natural Resources and Agriculture.

Ferrara, B.; Franciscis, G.de.; Minieri, L.and interieri, f.1967. Feeding of buffalo's calves. Atti Soc.ital. Sci. Vet., 21:441–455. (fide dairy Sci. Abst., 30:486, Abstr. 3115).

Ferrara, B.; Zicareleil, Lela, T.Di. and Minieri, L.1972. The performances of young buffaloes slaughtered at approximately 400 kg. Acta Med. Vet., 18(1/2):1–17. (Fide Anim. Breed. Abst. 1973; - 41293, Abstr. 2484).

Fischer, H. 1982. New findings on the gestation, calving and pregnancy of swamp buffalo (*Bubalus bubalis*). Animal Research Development., 16:90–84.

Ganovski,- KH. 1979. Changes in the composition of cow and buffalo colostrums and its significance in the nutrition of newborn calf.

Veterinarnomedisinski. Nauki., 16:3–6 (fide Nutr. Abst. Rev. B, 50:575, Abstr., 5706).

Gautam, O.P.; Malik, P.D. and Singh, D.K. 1976. *Neoascoris vitulorum* larvae in the colostrums/milk of buffaloes. Current Sci., 45:350

Geda Put; Fletcher, J.C. and Riding, G.A. 1983. An effect of nutrition on ovarian activity in Indonesian swamp buffalo cow. Report of Project for Anim. Res. Develop., Balai Penelitian Ternak, Ciawi, Bogor, Indonesia. (fide Anim. Breed. Abst., 52:926; Abstr., 7152).

Ghionna de Maria, C.1978. Change in the trace element content of colostrums in Friesian cows and buffaloes during the first week of lactation. Annali dell Instituto. sperimentale per la zootecnia, 11:165–177 (fide Nutr. Abst. Rev. B, 51:17, Abstr. 76)

Ghoneim, A.; Taha, El Katib, M. and El-Maghrabi, M.1959, study of growth in Egyptian cows and buffaloes up to 1.5 years old.

Gupta, P.C.; Kirpal Singh; Lodhi, G.P.; Gupta, L.R. and sharda, D.P. 1983. Effect of feeding Lucerne and berseem on the milk yield, efficiency of utilization of nutrients and cost of production in Murrah buffaloes. Indian J. Anim. Sci., 53:1181–1185

Jackson, M.G. and Gupta, D.C. 1971. The value of concentrate supplementation of berseem forage for milk production in buffaloes. Indian J. Anim. Sci. 41:86–91

Juma, K.H.; Farhan, S.M.A. and Faraj, M.1972. Feedlot performace of native cow and buffalo calves in Iraq. Indian J. Anim. Sci., 42:406–411.

Khoury, F.K.; Ahmed, I.A. and El-Shazly, K.1967. Early weaning in cow and water buffalo calves. 1. Growth rate, efficiency of feed utilization and cost of unit gain. J. Dairy Sci.; 50:1661–1666.

Kulkarni, P.E.; Sapr, V.A. and Kadu, M.S. 1973. Observations on the effect of feeding various blendings of oxytetracycline on the growth rates of young calves. Indian vet. J., 50: 797–801

Kurar, C.K. and Mudgal, V.D. 1980 Protein requirement of Murrah buffaloes in the early stage of lactation. Indain J. Dairy Sci., 33:443–449.

Maymone, B. 1942. Buffalo breeding in Italy. Z.Tierz. Zuchtbiol., 52:1–44 (fide Anim.Breed. Abst., 10:217.)

Mai,S.; Dewan, M.L.; Uddin, M. and Chowdhury, M.U.A. 1975. The route of infection of buffalo calves by Toxocara (*Neoascaris vitulorum*). Tropical Anim.Hlth.Prod., 7:153–156.

Mudgal, V.D. 1979. Effect of levels of nutrition on reproduction in riverine buffaloes, pp. 247–257. Proc. Buffalo reprod. Artificial Insem. FAO Anim. Prod. Hlth. Paper, 13, Rome

Naga, M.A.; Abou Akkada, A.R. and El-Shazly, K.1969. Establishment of rumen ciliate protozoa in cow and water buffalo calves under late and early weaning systems. J. Dairy Sci., 52: 110–112

Nofal, A.A.; Naghmoush, M.R. and Dawood, A.E. 1974. Free amino acids in Egyption buffaloes colostrums. Alexandria J. Agric. Res., 22:349–347

Ognjanovic, A.; Polikhronov, D. and Joksimovic, J.1970. The possibility of improving the yield and quality of buffalo meat by crossing. Document, 16th European Meeting of Meat Research workers, Sofia, Bulgeria.

Palo,L.P.; Castillo,L.S.; Roas, D.B.; Osunto, G.;Flores, L.P.; Garpacio, A.L.;Panizales,N.; Arganosa, V.G.;Calub, A.D. and Adriano, M.1971. High moisture corn as a supplement to rice straw molasses silages fed to cattle and carabaos with or without diethyl-stilboestrol implantation. Philipins J. Anim. Sci., 8:29–35

Pathak, N.N. 1978. Fattening of residual yearling male buffalo calves on ad lib.feeding of urea-molasses liquid diet. All India Sym. On Protein and NPN ulitilization in ruminants (UNDP/ICAR)., p.10 Sec.I., NDRI, Karnal.

Pathak, N.N and Ranjhan, S.K. 1979. Effect of for maldehyde treated groundnut cake supplementation of urea-molasses liquid feeding on the growth response of residual male buffalo calves. All India Sym. on Protein and NPN utilization in ruminants (UNDP/ICAR). p.13, Sec.II., NDRI, Karnal.

Pathak, N.N., Baruah, K.K. and Ranjhan, S.K. 1982. Nutrient utilization and carcass characteristics of male buffalo calves on different plane of nutrition. Proc. 2nd Anim. Sci. Cong. of Asian-Australian Assoc. Anim. Prod. Soc., PICC. Manila, November 10–13.

Prabhu, S.S. and Bhaya, K.D. 1962a. Semen and reaction time of buffalo bulls kept on different levels of protein 1. Indian J. Vet. Sci., 32:97–105.

Prabhu, S.S. and Bhaya, K.D. 1962b. Semen and reaction time of buffalo bulls kept on three levels of protien.2. Indain J.Vet. Sci., 32:249–259.

Proto, V. and Lundi, F. 1965. Meat production tests with young buffalo bulls. Produz.anim., 4:237–242 (Fide Anim. Breed. Abst., 1966; 34; 176, Abstr. 1048).

Raafat, M.A.; Abou-Hussein, E.S.; Abou Raya, A.K. and El-Shibiny, A.1974. Some nutritional studies on colostrums and milk of cows and buffaloes. Egyption J. Anim. Prod. 14:137–148.

Rathee, C.S. and Yadava I.S.; 1971. Effect of different protein levels on the performance of Murrah calves. Haryana Agric. Uni.J.Res., 1:136–140.

Robertson, J.A.; Ford, B.D. and Morris, C.A. 1982. Live weight changes and carcasss measurements in buffalo (*Bubalus bubalis*) and Brahman Northern territory shorthorn (*Bos indicusx Bos Taurus*) steers up to 4 years of age grazing on improved pastures. Australian J.Agric. Res., 33:755–762.

Romita, A.; Borghese, A. and Maria, C.De. 1976. Comparison of bovine and buffalo calves reared to 20 weeks of age. 1. growth, index of conversion, carcass yield and characteristics.

Annali dell Instituto Sperimentale per la Zootecnia, 9:79–92.

Rosa, A.; Creta, V.; Dzic, G. and Fecloru, R. 1981. Fattening performance of young buffaloes reared semi-intensively Lucrari Stilntifice ale Inst. *De Cercetari pentru Cresterea Taurinelor-Corbeanca*, 7:31–42. (fide Nutr. Abst. Rev., B1982; 52; 651, Abstr., 5185.)

Sachan, D.S. and Netke, S.P. 1971. Raising buffalo calves with limited quantity of milk. Indain J. Anim. Prod., 2(3): 6–15.

Sharma, M.C.; Pathak, N.N.; Hung N.N.; Vuc, N.V. and Thuong, N.V. 1983, Abomasal milk impaction-an emerging disease of buffalo calves. Indian J. Vet. Med., 3:117–119.

Shukla, K.S.; Ranjhan, S.K. and Netke, S.P. 1972. Effciency of utilization of energy and nitrogen for milk secretion by buffaloes fed various levels of concentrates. J. Dairy Res., 39:421–427.

Singh, N.; Pant, H.C. and Roy, A. 1970. Early weaning of buffalo calves. I. concentration of bacteria and protozoa in the rumen. Indain Vet. J., 47:660–667.

Sivaiah, K. and Mudgal, V.D. 1983. Effect of feeding different levels of protein and energy on feed utilization and milk production in buffaloes (*Bubalus bubalis*). Indain J. Dairy Sci. 36:85–92.

Sohal, T.S.; Arora, S.P. and Oberoi, P.S. 1981. Milk replacer feeding to growing calves in rural areas. Indian J. Dairy Sci., 34:229–230.

Soliman, F.A. and Soliman, M.K. 1974. The carotenoid and vitamin A content of buffalo and cow milk. Egytion J. Vet. Sci., 11:33–43 (fide Dairy Sci. Abst. 1979; 41:304, Abstr. 2679).

Srivastava., J.P.1970. Studies on the utilization of dietary energy for maintenance and milk production in buffaloes. Ph.D. thesis. Agra University, Agra.

Tilakaratne, N.; Matsukawa, T.; Buvanendran, V and Thangarajah, P., 1976. Growth, feed conversion and carcass characteristics of cattle and buffaloes fed grass and concentrates. Ceylon Vet. J., 24:9–12.

Vacaru-Opris, I. and Paul, T. 1981. Some meat production characters of buffaloes (*Bos bubalis*).

Lucrari Stiintifice, Inst. Agron. "N Balcescu," C (Med. Vet.). 24:13–16 (fide Anim Breed. Abst., 52:307, Abstr., 2358).

Verma, G.S. and Tomer, O.S. 1984. Effect of frequency of feeding on growth rate and health of Murrah buffalo calves. Indian J.Anim. Sci., 54: 486–488.

5

Management of Buffaloes

Buffalo management is a science as well as art of rearing for animal welfare and human utilities. Riverine buffaloes considered as the native of India is well-known worldwide for their nutritious milk and capabilities of thriving in harsh agriclimatic conditions of the tropical countries besides the adaptation capacity on translocation in different agroclimatic conditions. The species is well-recognized as a multipurpose animal for milk, meat, draught power, valuable hides for leather, leather industry, and organic by-products (dung and urine) for manure. The dairy buffaloes aquired important place long back in the livestock production of many Asian, European, and some of the African countries and still spreading in many countries of Africa and Latin America. The other type of equally important buffaloes are the swamp buffaloes of wet regions of Asia and Asia-Pacific island countries. The swamp buffalo is a valuable animal of paddy growing areas for its ability to work in the knee deep water and mud, and thriving on the inferior quality herbages with some supplemental feeding. Since buffalo holding is highly variable ranging from a single lactating, dry or growing to lots of few hundreds, the management (Macgregor, 1935). On the other side translocation of Indian dairy buffaloes imported from Philippines in India around 1917 AD drastically fell from average 8 litres daily yield to only 2.17 litres in about two decades breeding in a different managemental condition in which buffaloes are more important for draught (Sumulong, 1937). However, during subsequent years the milk production potential of Indian Murrah has been exploited by following desired management and through crossbreeding with Philippine swamp different grades of crossbreeds have been evolved for multipurpose, i.e. milk, draught, meat, valuable hides and organic manure. Crossbreeding of Combodian swamp buffaloes with Philippines swamp buffaloes has improved the traction strength (San Augstin, 1938).

Due to inherent affinity of water and marshy land the buffaloes spent longer time for grazing on marsh lands near the rivers, lakes, ponds and canal, etc. for frequent wallowing. The wallowing in stagnant waters often leads to infestation of different parasites. The pathological changes and clinical manifestations of most parasites remain unnoticed for quite long period. Most of the farmers do not find the causes of fall in milk yield and growth, and suffer significant economic loss from subclinical parasitism (Blood and Henderson, 1971). A tentative estimated economic loss due to subclinical parasitism in Indian dairy buffaloes has been estimated about 25% (Ranjhan and Pathak, 1979). Therapeutic control of gastrointestinal parasitism in Murrah buffaloes increased growth rate by 5.6% and milk yield by 12.3% reared in the southern province of Vietnam (Sharma et al., 1984).

Different climatic factors like ambient temperature, humidity, intensity, and duration of rainfall, wind velocity, and various methods of management practices like shelter, shower bath, air coolig and wallowing for the amelioration of climatic stress on the health, production and reproduction of buffaloes have been found very useful for remunerative buffalo production (Misra et al., 1963; Roy et al., 1964; Soni et al., 1980; Bahga et al., 1985). Exposer to direct sunshine during hot and humid-hot climatic environment for longer duration in the tropical countries produce stress in buffaloes which is expressed by significant rise in respiration rate and body (rectal) temperature. Excessive exposure causes severe effects manifested by restlessness, salivation, dehydration, cessation of rumination and pleothermy (Minett, 1947; Asker et al., 1952; Mullick, 1960; Sadhu, 1969). The reaction may be reverted by providing protection, plenty of cold drinking water and cooling (Badreldin and Ghany, 1952; Mullick, 1960; Radadia et al., 1980 a,b). Significant fall in feed intake and nutrients utilization of buffaloes occurs in hot-humid climate (Raghavan et al., 1951). This is due to disturbance in abomasal secretion in buffaloes which decreases significantly on rise of rectal temperature to 104 to 109°F (40–42.7°C) and the decrease may cause the complete disappearance of hydrochloric acid and loss of digestive activities. The secretary activity of abomasums is restored on providing cool environment through the provision of cold drinking water, cold water bath or wallowing and shade facilities (Aliev, 1961). A natural instinct for wallowing is noncontroversial and buffaloes move to water sources on rising air temperature above 85°F or 30°C (Minett, 1955). The farmers of humid hot tropical countries of the buffalo tract are fully aware with the susceptibility of buffaloes for hot climatic environment. Even in traditional system of management the buffaloes are provided protection from the very hot and extreme cold weathers. In door housing and regular bathing or wallowing ae provided during the hot climate. In the winter season buffaloes are housed indoor during the night and cloudy weather, and some times also covered with a rug which is called 'jhul' or 'chatti' (Promilla, 1983).

The weaning of calves has been found to spare substantial amount of milk for human consumption, reduce the dry period and regularize calving (Singh, 1935). But, in most of the Indian dairy breeds weaning at birth is not successful in true sense and extensive use of oxytocin hormone for let down is common despite ban in many contries including India. Regular culling of poor performers has significant impact on the improvement of production and reproduction (Alim, 1953; Asker et al.; 1955; Afify et al., 1970). The persent day management practices at the organized buffalo farms are that of dairy cattle farm with some minor modifications in the Indian subcontinent.

▶ FACTORS AFFECTING BUFFALO MANAGEMENT

Like the management of any other farm animal the buffalo management is also an art of using science for the benefits of mankind. Some important factors of good management are listed as follows:

1. Pleasant and gentle manners and tactful behaviour of farm maneger.
2. Optimum living conditions for farm workers.
3. Adequate facilities for scientific breeding. Feeding, housing, milking, and health care of farm animals.
4. Easy approach to metalled road and connection with towns and markets, etc.
5. Sufficient arable land and other facilities for fodder cultivation.
6. Assured supply of good running water for drinking, washing, wallowing, and other farm operations.

7. Storage facilities for concentrates, supplements, fodder, and other items.
8. Workshop for maintenance of farm equipments and appliances and also for minor fabrication, etc.
9. Sources of financing institutions like banks and cooperative societies.
10. Maintenance of records for calculation of economic status of farm.

▶ DEFINITION OF COMMON TERMINOLOGIES USED IN BUFFALO MANAGEMENT

Buffalo	=	All animals belonging to buffalo (*Bubalus* spp.) irrespective of age, sex and type.
Buffalo calf	=	The young ones of buffalo irrespective of sex.
Buffalo bull (male) calf	=	Male buffalo calf below one year of age.
Buffalo heifer (female) calf	=	Female buffalo calf below one year of age .
Yearling male buffaloes	=	Growing male buffalo of more than 1 but below 2 years.
Replacement buffalo heifer	=	Buffalo heifer from 1 year to onset of puberty.
Buffalo bull or stud	=	An adult male buffalo used for breeding/semen collection.
Buffalo cow or she buffalo	=	The female buffalo after first calving.
Open buffalo heifer	=	A buffalo heifer which has not yet conceived after puberty.
Entire buffalo	=	An intact adult male buffalo.
Buffalo bullock	=	Working male buffaloes.
Castrated buffalo	=	A male buffalo which has been castrated.
Down calver	=	Pregnant buffalo which has been castrated.
Calf at foot	=	Female buffalo approaching calving in few days.
Buffalo steer	=	A castrated male buffalo over 1 year of age reared for fattening.
Buller buffalo or Nymphominiac buffalo	=	An adult she buffalo always in heat.
Free martin buffalo	=	Heifer calf, of a twin birth of different sex, with abnormal external genitalia and strerile.
Intersexual	=	Buffalo with ill-formed sex organs of both sexes.
crossbreed buffalo	=	Progeny in inter breeding different breeds or types.
Polled	=	Natural hornless buffalo. Extremely rare incidence.
Dehornin or Debudding	=	Destruction of horn buds with in 3–5 days of birth.
Store buffalo	=	Young buffaloes reared at a slow rate for fattening on later date.
Veal buffalo calf	=	Young buffalo calves grown on high energy feeding, usually whole milk for finishing at 15 weeks of age.
Single suckling	=	Buffalo cow nursing her own single calf.
Double suckling	=	A buffalo cow nursing two calves, one from the other buffalo.
Multiple suckling	=	A Buffalo cow allowing suckling by more than 3 calves.
Baby buffalo	=	Reared on high plane of nutrition for finishing at 12–15 months age.
Young buffalo	=	Buffaloes fattened for slaughter at 15–24 months of age.
Spent buffaloes	=	Buffalo females unable to breed further and retired male buffaloes (both working and breeding).

▶ THE POINTS OF BUFFALO BODY

Knowledge of different external body parts of buffalo (Fig. 5.1) is essential for the owners and the staff of veterinary hospitals for communications regarding the exchange of informaions regarding the health and ailments. The body of buffalo is described in four groups of external body parts (Fig. 5.1).

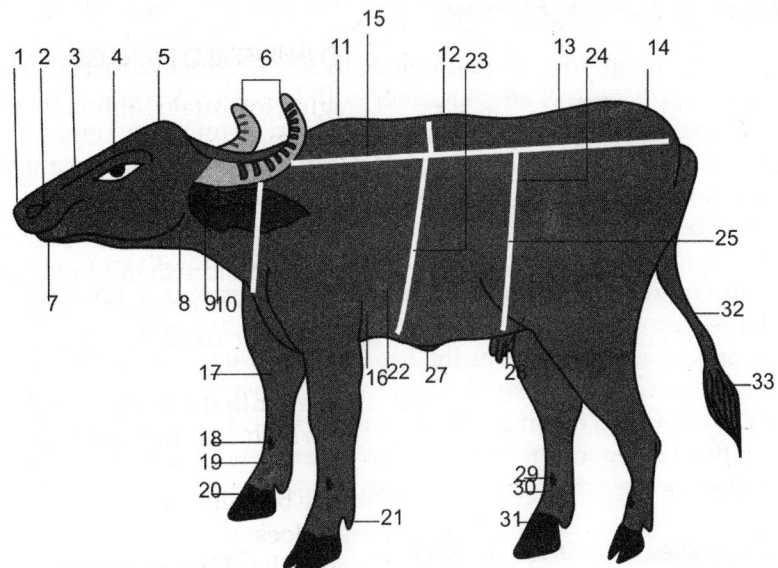

Fig. 5.1: The points of buffalo body

1. Muffle, 2. Nostril, 3. Nose bridge, 4. Eye, 5. Poll, 6. Horn, 7. Lower jaw, 8. Jowl, 9. Ear, 10. Neck, 11. Weather, 12. Back, 13. Rump, 14. Croup, 15. Shoulder, 16, Arm, 17. Fore arm, 18. Knee joint, 19. Cannon, 20. Hooves, 21. Dew claw, 22. Elbow joint, 23. Thorax, 24. Paralumbar fossa, 25. Abdomen, 26. Ahiop joint, 27. Thigh, 28. Stifle joint, 29. Hind cannon, 30. Pastern, 31. Coronat, 32. Tail, 33. Switch of the tail

A. **Parts of head:** The head includes a pair each of lips, nostrils, jaws, eyes, ears, and horns, and also the muzzle, nose bridge, forehead, poli, chin, cheeks and jowl.

B. **Parts of neck:** These are crest, throat, windpipe, jugular groove, dewlap and brisket.

C. **Parts of trunk:** The trunk includes withers, crops, back, chine, loin, rump or croup, buttocks, belly or barrel, chest, chest floor, naval, flank or paralumbar fossa, groin, dock or tail head or root of the tail, tail and switch of the tail.

Sometimes the anterior half is refered as fore quarters and the posterior half as hind quarters.

D. **Fore limb(s):** This starts from the point of shoulder and descends in sequence as shoulder, point of shoulder, arm, armpit or axilla, elbow, forearm, knee joint or knee, shank, fetlock, pastern, dew claw, coronet, hooves, and sole.

E. **Hind limb(s):** This includes thigh, stifle, tendon achillis or hamstring, hock joint, hind shank, fetlock, pastern, dew claw, coronet, hooves, and sole.

F. **Sex specific parts in female buffloes:** The external sex organs are external genitalia or vulva, milk well, milk vein, udder of four quarters each opening independently through teats.

G. **Sex specific parts of male buffalo:** These are sheath, prepuce and scrotum enveloping the testcles.

H. **Parts of eye:** The external parts of eyes require routine inspection and cleaning are the eyelids, eyelashes, inner canthus, outer canthus, and pupil.

I. **External muous membranes:** The external mucus membranes requiring routine examination and cleaning are buccal mucosa, nostrils, eyelids, ears, anus, vulva in females and prepuce in male buffaloes.

▶ REQUIREMENTS OF PHYSICAL FACILITIES

Greater proportion of buffaloes are maintained by small holder farmers in home tract of buffaloes. The main purpose of keeping river buffaloes is milk production and swamp buffaloes for draught purpose. Three types of buffalo farming are common in most of the countries. These are small holder rural farmers keeping 1 to 20 lactating buffaloes and their progeny under different systems of management. However, grazing of 4 hours to 10 hours daily or herding round the clock on scrub lands of highly variable herbage cover. Most of the these owners do not rear dry buffaloes and calves and they are given to another group for rearing on barter basis. The second group is mostly landless farm families with meager resources and unable to purchase buffaloes. Such families raise dry buffaloes growing buffalo heifer for 1 to 3 years or until breeding. These farmers do not pay for the animals but bear all other inputs. Most of the buffaloes are raised on grazing on scrub lands and feeding of grasses collected from road sides, orchards, canal bunds, etc. the third categories that of exclusive commercial farmers maintaining only lactating buffaloes in the urban and periurban areas.

A1. Physical Facilities with Small Holders

Buffalo keeping is a living system in most of the Asian contries and buffaloes are also kept in the limited space of house with a courtyard or some open spaces. The females are let loose in the morning immediately after milking to return back only in the evening for milking. Small amount of dry fodder, some kitchen left over and grain miling by products and small amount of oilseed cake is fed. The requirement for the management of buffaloes is limited.

1. **Housing:** The animals are mostly accommodated in cold night with the family members. No shelter is available during other season. Few farmers may afford an animals shed to tiles, iron sheets, asbestos or thatch materials.
2. **Feeding troughs:** These may be made of clay, wood or bricks, etc. At some places baskets made of bamboo or cazurina are also used.
3. Utensil available in the home are also used for the buffaloes like a bucket is used for watering, washing, milking, and milk supply to consumers.
4. **Storage of dry fodder:** Paddy straw is stored in open on bamboo machan, branches of tree or a high ground.
5. **Disposal of dung:** It is daily made into dung cake. Part of dung cake is used for cooking food and partly sold for supporting daily requirements.

A2. Physical Requirements of Small Holder Swamp Buffaloes

Hardly there is any specific requirements for the swamp buffaloes exclusively reared for draught purposes. Both sexes are used for phoughing, puddling, and pulling cart loads. These buffaloes spent long-time on feeding on marsly land and aquatic plants, wallowing in mud holes and resting in night. However, milking swamp buffaloes require similar facilities mentioned for the dairy buffaloes.

B. Physical Facilities for the Dairy Farms of Private Owners

Large number of commercial dairy farms are engaged in milk production and marketing in the urban and periurban areas of cities, towns and industrial areas for daily supply of local consumers fond of fresh milk in the Indian subcontinent. Hardly any such dairy farmer maintain optimum hygienic conditions and provides optimum comfort. The buffaloes on such farms are exclusively lactating with few calves to stimulate let down of milk in some difficult animals. Intensive system is followed by 70–80% owners (the term farmer appears unethical for such stalls) and buffaloes are mostly maintained under stress.

1. **Animal sheds:** The buffaloes are housed in half-walled sheds of bricks work or put on pillars. Roof is generally made of corrugated iron sheet or asbestos sheet or thatch. A few owners are construct concrete sheds. In very hot season and in very cold season large curtains of jute or bamboo are used for protection.

2. **Water sources:** These may be tap water, tube well, hand pump, lake, stream, canal or river. Natural sources of perennial water supply are preferred due to ample availability without any charges.

3. **Ropes, chains and pegs:** These are required for tethering the buffaloes and also securing the hind legs at the time of milking.

4. **Troughs, buckets, pails and milk cans:** These are require for carrying water for cleaning, washing, milking, and milk collection, etc. Measures of 200 ml, half litre and 1 litre are used for the sale of fluid milk. Bulk saling is rare.

5. **Feeds and fodder stores:** A small shed is available for storing concentrates for a week or a fornight. Wheat straw is mostly stored in a thatch structure called bonga, khopor coop. Some farmers stack in open. Seasonal green fodder are purchased daily or contract is given to fodder grower for daily supply.

6. **Transports:** Most of the dairy owners maintain a horse cart for the daily disposal of dung and farm wastes, and transportation of feeds from markets.

7. **Disposal of dung and farm wastes:** These are disposed in compost pits away from inhabitation or transferred to families engaged in the preparation dung cakes.

C. Physical Facilities for an Organized Dairy Farm

The requirement of physical facilities at a dairy farm depends on the size of herd, types of animals used for milk production, agroclimatic conditions, markets for milk disposal and mode of milk sale.

1. Land for the construction of different kinds of buildings and cultivation of at least green fodder for round the year supply.

2. **Buildings:** At an organized buffalo dairy farm the following different types of houses and sheds are required:

   a. Office building for the farm manager and office staff

   b. Multipurpose dormitory for changing, washing, and lunch, etc. for the farm workers

   c. Animal sheds of different size for housing lactating, pregnant, and dry buffaloes; newborn young calves, growing cavles, yearlings, buffalo bulls, draught animals, and calving pen, etc.

   d. Veterinary hospital and semen processing laboratory for AI, and a sick animal ward for housing 1% animals.

e. Milking barn with attached milk recording room and milk processing and disposal rooms.

f. Godowns for storage of farm appliances, concentrate feeds, feed supplements and agricultural inputs like fertilizers, etc. but not the toxic substances.

g. Fodder storage barn for storing straws, hay and kadbi during the harvesting season when prices are quite low.

h. Housing colony for the farm staff.

i. Tube wells for assured water supply at the buffalo farm and housing colony.

j. Shed fitted with chaff cutters for fodder chaffing.

k. **Compost pits:** The size and number will depend on the herd size and the frequency of turn over of manure from pits to arable land or other disposal.

3. **Sweet water resources:** Natural sources of running water like rivers, streams, and canal or large lakes are considered easily accessible, less expensive and liked by the buffaloes for wallowing. The water supply must be assured for any livestock farm and the requirement of buffaloes is much higher than the other fam animals.

▶ DAIRY FARM EQUIPMENT AND APPLIANCES

Some of the common dairy farm equipments are buckets, baskets, belcha, balances, hauze pipes, ropes, chains, neck collars, halters, milk pail, milk can, refrigerator, hot air oven, sterilizers, milk chilling plant, deep freeze spade, rakes, plough, mowe, tractor, trollies, feed compounding mills (grinder, mixer), etc.

▶ RECORDS TO BE MAINTAINED AT A DAIRY FARM

For the preparation of annual balance sheet of input-output ratio and economic viability it is very important to maintain the proper records of all inputs and return (output) from the farm. These records provide the informations about the skill used and the lacunae requiring attention for improvement through necessary changes in the management during the following year. The farm records provide basis for the estimation of the requirements of replacement stock, feeds, fodder, various appliances, and other necessary inputs. The records of a livestock farm may be categorized into two broad categories, i.e. animal records and the business records. Required at an organized buffalo dairy farm has been listed as follows:

1. Daily livestock inventory register
2. History of animal and pedigree record
3. Breeding record
4. Calving record
5. Calf registed
6. Daily milking record
7. Daily feeding register
8. Stock register for feeds and other consumables
9. Lactation register
10. Herd health register
11. Fodder crop production register
12. Milk and milk products sale register

Proforma: Daily livestock inventory register for the year..............

Date	Female buffaloes		Replace-ment	Buffalo calves		Male buffaloes		Loss or gain		Balance	Remarks
			heifers								
	In milk	Dry		Male	Female	Bulls	Draught	Added	Dead		
1	2	3	4	5	6	7	8	9	10	11	12

Proforma: Animal history and pedigree cord

Brand No....................................... Species and type.................................

Name of animal (if any)............................. Date of birth/purchase...........................

Description of animal:

Date of receipt............................. Source................................

Sire number and breed............................. Dam number and breed........................

Dam' milk yield (kg/L)   1st lact.............. 2nd lact.............. 3rd lact....................

Dam; lactation length (days) 1st lact.............. 2nd lact.............. 3rd lact...................

Dam's dry days   1st lact.............. 2nd lact.............. 3rd lact....................

Paternal grand dam number and breed..

Average milk yield per lactation (kg/L)...

Average lactation length (days)...

Maternal sire number and breed...

Maternal grand dam's number and breed...

Average milk yield per lactation (kg/L) ....

Average lactation length (days)...

Growth performance of heifer calf, weekly up to 13 weeks and monthly up to 30 months or puberty

Reproduction/breeding record;

S.No.	Date of service			Bull number	Calving date	Record sex	Bwt.	Gestation days
	1st	2nd	3rd					
1.								
2.								
3.								
4.								
5.								
6.								
7.								
8.								
9.								
10.								

Lactation Record

Milk yield in 305 days	Peak milk yield (kg)	Date of peak yield	Lactation days	Dry days	Service period	Calving interval	Remark

Health Record

1. Vacccination date	FMD	HS			BQ	Any other
2. Deworming date	1st	2nd	3rd	4th		others
3. Date of sparying against ectoparasites	1st	2nd	3rd	4th		others

Date   Signature of farm manager

Proforma: Breeding record

Brand number of buffalo in heat................Date and time of detection................

Insemination number	Date of insemination	Sire number and breed	Date of pregnancy diagnosis	Remarks
1.				
2.				
3.				
4.				

Proforma: Calving register

S.No.	Date of birth	Number of			Sex of calf	Body size of calf		
		Calf	Dam	Sire		Weight (kg)	Length (cm)	Girth (cm)
1	2	3	4	5	6	7	8	9
1.								
2.								
3.								

Proforma: Calf register

S.No.	Date of birth	Identification number	Sex of calf	Date of deworming	Date of vaccination			Disposal
					FMD	HS	BQ	
1	2	3	4	5	6	7	8	9
1.								
2.								
3.								
4.								

Proforma: Growth record of buffalo calves

Brand no. of calf   Date of birth   Sex   Dam No.   Sire no.

Date	Body weight (kg)	Length (cm)	Girth (cm)	Pounch (cm)	Height (cm)
1	2	3	4	5	6
1.					
2.					
3.					
4.					
5.					
6.					
7.					
8.					

Recorded weekly up to 13th week and then monthly up to puberty.

Proforma: Daily milk yield recording register

Farm   Year   Month

S.No.	Buffalo No.	Calving date		Date of month (1 to 31)					Total (kg/L)
		1		2		3............31			
		M	E	M	E	M		E	
1.									
2.									
3.									
4.									
5.									
6.									
7.									
8.									

Maintained for each buffalo up to last milking

Proforma: Daily Feeding Register

Year 2009   Month   January

Year	Type of buffaloes	Total number	Concentrate mixture (kg)	Dry fodder (kg)	Green fodder (kg)	Remarks
1	2	3	4	5	6	7
1.	Lactating	80	400	400	1000	
2.	Dry pregnant	50	150	250	500	
3.	Bulls	6	18	48	120	
4.	Bullocks	10	30	70	100	
5.	Heifers	20	60	60	200	

(It is maintained daily for every month as per schedule followed at the farm)

Proforma: Stock register for feeds and supplements

Name of feed: Crushed barley

Date	Opening balance (qtl)	Received (qtl)	Total (qtl)	Issued (qtl)	Balance (qtl)	Signature
1	2	3	4	5	6	7
01–01–09	500	Nil	500	150	350	
02–01–09	350	500	850	150	700	
03–01–09	700	Nil	700	200	500	
04–01–09	500	Nil	500	200	300	
05–01–09	300	700	1000	200	800	

Similarly recored up to last date of every month.

NB: This record is maintained for each ingredients on separate pages.

Proforma: Health cord of buffalo for veterinary hospital

Brand number	Date of birth	Sex
Dates of vaccinations		FMD HS BQ
Date of sickness		

Changes in behaviour

Cordinal signs: Rectal temperature   Pulse rate

Respiration

Colour and volume of urine

Consistency of dung

General appearance

Clinicopathological tests

Blood examination

Fecal examination

Urine examination

Skin scrapings

Diagnosis

Line of treatment

Prognosis

Signature of veterinary doctor

Proforma: Fodder crops production input register

Inputs	Fodder of Kharif (humid-hot) and Zayad (hot) seasons				
	Maize	Sorghum	Bajra	Cow pea	Guar
Dates of ploughing					
First					
Second					
Third					
Date of manuring					
Date of sowing					
					Contd.

| Inputs | Fodder of Kharif (humid-hot) and Zayad (hot) seasons | | | | |
	Maize	Sorghum	Bajra	Cow pea	Guar
Dates of irrigations					
First					
Second					
Third					
Fourth					
Fifth					
Date of fertilizer use					
Urea					
DAP					
Murate of potash					
Dates of harvesting					
First cut					
Second cut					
Third cut					
Fourth cut					
Green fodder (Quintals)					
First cut					
Second cut					
Third cut					
Fourth cut					
Total yield					
Remarks, if any					

NB: The selection of fodder crops will depend on the prevalent agroclimatic conditions, availability of resources and qualitative and quantitative need of the farm. A farmer with limited land and cereal crop residue (straws) as staple roughage will prefer to cultivate proteinous fodder (legumes).

Proforma: Record of sale of milk and milk products

| Date | Fluid milk | | Cream | | Butter | | Skim milk | | Ghee | | Total | Initial |
	Qty.	Rs.	Qty.	Rs.	Qty.	Rs.	Qty.	Rs.	Qty.	Rs.	Rs.	
January												
01	500	5000	20	1200	10	800	used		nil		7000	
02	700	7000	10	600	nil	nil	used		nil		7600	
Up to 31												
Total												
February												
01												
02												
Up to December												
Total												
Grand Total												

Similarly recorded daily for the complete year.

▶ HANDLING AND RESTRAINT OF BUFFALOES

The handling is routine activity at the buffalo farm and it is a daily activity with small holders where buffaloes require daily tethering. By and large the domesticated buffaloes are docile. Sometimes a few animals, specially the breeding buffalo bulls may become furious and unruly. It is a common seen on pastures and water sources that the herds of buffaloes are driven and controlled by a young child of 14–15 years or a woman or a senior person of the family. The different appliances and methods of handling buffaloes are as follows:

1. **Ropes and halter:** Ropes and halters (mohair) of sunhemp, patson, cotton, moonj, coconut coir, reed and synthetic fiber are used for the tethering and handling of the buffaloes. Some economically sound farmers also use the decorated halters of leather specially at animal show. A 1.5 m long rope of about 6–8 cm circumference. A long rope of about 10 m is required for costing and securing the animal for showing and clinical management. Neck collar and halters are used for driving the animals in cart and plough, etc.

2. **Bull holder:** It is a metallic rod fitted with a clip like tongue for holding the nasal septum tightly. This is used for controlling unruly bulls during driving out for the collection of semen or covering a buffalo in heat.

3. **Nose ring, nose string and nose peg:** The nose ring is used for handling and controlling the buffalo bulls. A nose ring is inserted by pearching the cartilage of nasal septum at about one year of age when the cartilage is still soft and pliable. The nose string is fixed with the help of a sterilized suja by pearcing the nasal septum in the working buffaloes. The rope string is placed running behind the ears and tied at the level of poll. Fixing of nose string in working male buffaloes is a common practice in the Indian subcontinent. In the southeast Asian and Asia-Pacific regions fixing of a metallic, wooden or bamboo peg is used for the handling and control of buffaloes.

4. **Uses of muzzle:** Use of muzzle in buffaloes is rare and applied only during the thrashing of paddy harvest for extracting grains. Muzzle is made by the farmers or local artisans with rope string, cane, bamboo, leather or metallic (alumunium or copper) wire. It is mostly used for preventing the licking of medicines applied on wounds and abscesses and also protecting the tearing or removal of bandage from dressing. Use of small muzules for calves in more common in loose housing for preventing naval sucking and chewing the ear or switch of the tail. The muzzle is made sufficiently voluminous to allow mastication.

5. **Use of tranquilizers on narcotics:** These drugs are used for sedation in the wild and feral buffaloes for catching and unruly domestic buffaloes for the clinical interventions. These drugs are also used for the long distance transportation in ship, rain wagon, and aeroplanes. A mixture of 50–60 mg piperidine derivative 'Fentanyl' together with 300 mg the butyrophenone neuroleptic drug 'Azaporone' has been used successesfully as a single shot for tranquilizing wild African buffalo (*Syncerus caffer*) of about 900 kg body weight (Plenaar, 1969). About half dose of the drug mixture may be sufficient for controlling the domestic buffaloes of 400–600 kg body weight. For producing sedation in the Egyptian domestic buffaloes a proprietary narcotic 'Rompun' or 'Bay Va 1470' has been used in dose of 3 ml intramuscular injection for a buffalo of about 400 kg body weight. It produces sedation in 7–10 minutes and maintains for 5 hours approximately (Khamis and Saleh, 1970).

Intramuscular injection of 'Xylazine' (2-(2–6 dimethyly-phenyl amino)–4-H–5,6 dihydro 1,3 thiazine hydrochloride) at a dose rate of 0.5 to 1.7 mg per kg body weight has been found to produce satisfactory tranquilization in domestic Indian buffaloes (Kumar et al., 1976). In case of overdosing of this drug, exhibited by profuse salivation the administration of atropine is quite effective. Chloral hydras and other common analgesics may be used for controlling the animals for clinical examinations and surgical manipulations.

6. **Neck cradle:** This is used for preventing the licking of medicines applied on the body, tearing of the bandage and self suckling in lactating buffaloes.

7. **Cattle crush or travis:** It is made of wooden slabs or poles, bamboo poles and galvanized iron pipes. Several designs of travices have been developed for different uses.

8. **Side rod:** It is an indigenous device developed by the livestock owners for the prevention of self-sucking and licking of externally applied medicines, etc. It is normally a bamboo stick or pole of 100 to 125 cm with rounded ends. A hole is made on either side foe fixing a neck collar and larger girth rope for placing the side rod on the animal.

9. **Mouth gag:** It is metallic age or a flat piece of smooth plank of 25 cm length and fixed with a 50–60 cm long rope for securing the gag at place to keep the mouth open. It contains a round hole of about 2–3 cm diameter in the center for passing a stomach tube or brobang either for the collection of rumen contents, evacuation of rumen opr administration of large amount of fluid (drug or liquid feed).

▶ CASTING OF BUFFALOES

The common methods of casting cattle, i.e. Reuff's and alternative are also used for the casting of buffaloes. Sometimes these methods do not work in few obstinate buffaloes and a local method is used.

1. **Reuff's method of casting buffaloes:** For this purpose a strong rope of about 9–10 m (30 feet) length is required. A running noose is prepared at one end of rope in such a way that its sliding is restricted by a knot for preventing fatal choking by asphaxia. The noose is tight fixed along the base of hours and free end of rope is used to make two half hitches, first around the chest just behind the shoulders and second around the belly in front of hook bone running along the stifle. The operation is normally started from the left side of the buffalo. One person is required to hold the animal firmly and two persons are required for fastening of the rope. The front and rear loops are kept reasonable tight and the joining portion of rope is placed straight about 10–20 cm below the dorsal line. After this the free end of rope is pulled strongly while holding the head tilts face over the neck by holding inter dental place by second hand. A second person is required to pull the tail through groin on the flank and hold tightly. The legs are tied by persons. Therefore, minimum 4 person are required for the casting of a buffalo. The knot used should be easy to open free without any obstruction. The animal falls on the side of the parallel rope along the dorsal line.

2. **Alternative method of casting:** In this method a central noose wide enough to place around the neck is made. It should not be running. Two free parts of rope are passes from the ventral aspect of neck through the fore limbs and passes alternate over the back and then taken out through the groin behind the animals. At the same time

free ends of rope are pulled with full force. After falling the operations described for Reuff's method are repeated.

3. **Indigenous or farmer's method of casting buffaloes:** In this method 2 ropes of 5 m (15–16 feet) each are required. Each rope is used for fastening the fore and hind limbs just above the dew claw separately. After this free end of front rope is passed behind through the rear limbs and rear rope through the forelimb above the knot. Now, the head is held and tilted by one person and the rope ends are strongly.

▶ ESTIMATION OF AGE AND BODY WEIGHT OF BUFFALOES IN FIELD CONDITION

It is often required to estimate the age and body weight of the buffaloes for the assessment of their productive life and production capacity. Age is estimated with the help of the eruption pattern of milk teeth and permanent teeth or the number of rings and grooves on the horns. Since growth of horns is dependent on nutritional status, it has little use in the calf rearing systems of riverine buffaloes the Indian subcontinent.

Common Terms of Denture

1. **Dentition:** The eruption of temporary and permanent teeth.
2. **Alveolus:** The cavity of origin of a tooth on the jaw.
3. **Lingual or inner surface of tooth:** The surface of tooth facing the tongue.
4. **Buccal surface of tooth:** The surface opposing the inner wall of lips.
5. **Incisors:** The front row of teeth. Only lower 4 pairs are present in buffaloes. Any shortage in incisors is considered in auspicious and significantly reduces the value of buffalo. These are initially deciduous and replaced by permanent teeth at different age and the replacement pattern is used for the estimation of age.
6. **Canine teeth:** These are next to incisors and absent in buffaloes.
7. **Premolar teeth:** Also known as anterior cheek teeth. These are 3 pairs on each jaw initially deciduous and replaced by permanent teeth at different age.
8. **Molar teeth:** These are 3 pairs of cheek teeth and initially erupt permanent.
9. **Eruption or cutting of teeth:** The processs of emerging teeth through the gum is known as **eruption** or **cutting of teeth**. The crown of tooth is visible.
10. **Milk teeth:** These are also known as **deciduous** or **temporary teeth**. In buffaloes incisors and premolars are deciduous.
11. **Permanent teeth:** The teeth replacing the milk teeth are called **permanent teeth**. These replace deciduous incisors and premolars at different age. Age of buffaloes is estimated from the eruption of temporary and permanent incisors.
12. **Dental pad:** The place of incisor teeth on the upper jaw is made of a hard band which is called **dental pad** in buffaloes and other ruminants.
13. **Parts of tooth:** A tooth of buffalo contains three parts. The upper visible part is **crown**, the middle part at the level of gum is called **neck** and lowest portion embedded in the socket is called **root**.
14. **Dental table:** The upper wearing surface of the teeth is called **table**.
15. **Dental formula:** The method of presentation of the teeth in sequence starting from the incisor to end at the molars on both jaws is called **dental formula**. Two dental formulae, one for depicting milk teeth and second for depicting permanent teeth are used. The symbols for depicting incisor, canine, premolar and molar teeth are I, C, P and M respectively. The teeth on the upper jaw are numerators and that on the lower jaw are denominator.

▶ DENTITION FOR THE ASSESSMENT OF AGE

Estimation of approximate age of cattle and buffaloes with the sequence of eruption of milk (deciduous) incisor teeth and their replacement by permanent incisors is quite popular among the livestock owners. Although eruption of teeth is influenced by several factors like breed, level of feeding and environment, indeed it is useful for the estimation of age of buffaloes in the absence of recorded age.

Dental Formula of Buffalo

Like other bovines buffaloes also do not possess canine teeth. The dental formulae of deciduous and permanent teeth of buffaloes are as follows:

Milk (deciduous) teeth = I 0/4 C 0/0 P 3/3 M 0/0 = 20
Permanent teeth = I 0/4 C 0/0 P 3/3 M 3/3 = 32

The minimum, maximum, and average age of eruption of milk or deciduous and permanent teeth (Saini et al., 1984) are presented in Table 5.1.

TABLE 5.1: Eruption pattern of milk teeth in buffalo calves

Incisors (pair)	Age of teeth eruption (days)		
	Minimum	Maximum	Average
Central/First	0	9	1.77 ± 0.14
Second	0	30	11.19 ± 1.29
Third	6	119	40.80 ± 2.51
Fourth	46	159	118.82 ± 3.79

From the eruption pattern of temporary or milk teeth approximate age of young buffalo calves may be assessed as 0–3 days, 1–2 weeks, 5–6 weeks, and about 4 months on the complete visible eruption of the first (central), second, third and fourth pair of incisor teeth respectively in optimum management. So far, there is no such method for the assessment of age of growing buffalo calves of 4 to 30 months of age. It depends on the physical appearance of the calf and information given by the owner. The teeth eruption pattern is hereditary but it is also significantly influence by the system of feeding. For the normal eruption of temporary teeth the calves should be either fed adequate milk or milk replacer with comparable content and quality of minerals that present in the dam's milk.

TABLE 5.2: Replacement pattern of milk incisors with permanent incisors

Incisor teeth (pair)	Murrah type buffaloes (age)			Swamp buffaloes (age in month)
	Minimum	Maximum	Average	
First (Central)	908 (30.0)	1217 (40.5)	1045 + 11 (34.8)	30–36
Second	1043 (34.8)	1556 (50.2)	1282 + 20 (42.2)	36–48
Third	1205 (40.0)	2060 (68.7)	1570 + 19 (51.9)	48–60
Fourth	1463 (48.8)	2063 (68.8)	1814 + 85 (59.6)	60–72

The replacement of deciduous incisor teeth by permanent teeth provides more accurate estimates of age between 30 to 72 months of age (Rollingon, 1974, Saini et al., 1982). The pattern of replacement of temporary incisors with permanent incisors is shown in Table 5.2. The size of permanent teeth increases till the buffalo becomes full mouth at 6 to 9 years of age in different breeds and in different agroclimatic conditions. In the estimation of age buffaloes from the eruption of deciduous and permanent incisors the general condition and sexual maturity should also be considered for more accuracy. In some buffaloes only 3 pairs of incisor teeth are erupted. Reasons for such deviation is not fully known.

▶ ASSESSMENT OF AGE FROM THE RINGS AND GROOVES ON THE HORNS

Large variations occur in the shape, size, and volume of the horns and influenced mainly by breed and sex. The differential growth in the thickness of buffalo horns before and after calving is said to be responsible for the formation of horn rings although they are present on the horns of infertile buffaloes and the male buffaloes. There is great difference in the intercalving period of buffaloes of different countries, the average being approximately 18 months in Egyptian buffaloes (Mourad, 1978), 13.5 months in Italian (Salerno, 1960) Iraquis buffaloes (El-Wishy, 1979), and 14–18 months in the buffaloes of India (Bhat, 1979) and Paksitan (Wahid, 1979). In case of swamp buffaloes average intercalving period has been reported 18.5 months in China (Wang Pei Chein, 1979), 14 months in Mayanmar, 14.5 months in Philippines, 16.5 months in Thialand (Chantalakhana, 1979), and 17.5 months in Malayasian swamp buffaloes (Jainudeen, 1977). The average age at first calving is about 42 months in riverine dairy buffaloes, 48 months in swamp buffaloes and 36 months in European dairy buffaloes. Therefore, approximate age of different buffaloes may be estimated as follows:

  i. Age of riverine buffaloes = Number of horn rings × 16 + 42 months
  ii. Age of swamp buffalo = Number of horn rings × 16 + 48 months
  iii. Age of European buffaloes = Number of horn rings × 14 + 36 months

Since there is wide variation between the types and countries, this method of age assessment has little application. For making it more useful informations for each breed or related breeds are required.

▶ ASSESSMENT OF BODY WEIGHT OF BUFFALOES

Heavy balances for weighing the large animals like buffaloes are not avialble in the remote areas, ranges, and pastures. The estimation of body weight of buffaloes is often required to have some idea about the production potential and also for the assessment of carcass yield. Significant correlations between body weight and different body measurements of buffaloes have been developed (Mullick, 1959, Bhandari et al., 1951, Jawarkar and Johar, 1975; Manik et al., 1981; Verma and Hussein, 1985). The different prediction equations presented as follows may be used for the estimation of body weight of buffaloes in absence of weighing bridege.

Estimation of the body weight of adult buffaloes,

  i. $Y = 25.156\ X - 960.232$, where Y is body weight and X is heart girth in inches at wither (Mullick, 1950).
  ii. Separate equations for the dry nonpregnant, dry pregnant, and lactating pregnant buffaloes (Bhandari et al., 1951),
    a. Dry nonpregnant adult buffaloes
       $Y = 26.35\ X_1 + 21.50\ X_2 - 2123.73$

  b. Dry pregnant buffaloes
    $Y = 20.25 \, X_1 + 25.90 \, X_2 - 1934.48$
  c. Lactating pregnant buffaloes
    $Y = 27.14 \, X_1 + 24.55 \, X_2 - 2387.60$
  where, Y is body weight in lb and X_1 and X_2 are heart girth and body length (from pin bone to point of shoulder) in inches respectively.
iii. With the use of single measurement on body in cm (Manik et al., 1981),
  a. $Y = 5.22 \, X_1 - 527.75$, where X_1 is heart girth
  b. $Y = 5.33 \, X_2 - 286.92$, where X_2 is body length,
  c. $Y = 3.89 \, X_1 + 2.09 \, X_2 + 1.41 \, X_3 - 766.13$
iv. Estimation of body weight of buffalo calves (Verma and Hussein, 1985),
  a. Male buffalo calves,
    $Y = 1.6235 \, X - 88.4957$
  b. Female buffalo calves,
    $Y = 1.6490 \, X - 87.3357$
  where, Y is body weight in kg and X is heart girth in cm.

▶ TRANSPORTATION OF BUFFALOES

Transportation of dairy buffaloes is more common in the Indian subcontinent and too in the terminal stage of gestation or the first month of calving. The distance to be traveled may ranges from few kilometres walk to more than one thousand kilometres on rail. Sometimes transportation by air and ship is also carried. Larger number of dairy buffaloes are reared up to last month of pregnancy to first month of calving and then purchased for translocation to towns, cities, and highly populated industrial areas with the main purpose of supplying fresh fluid milk. The main destination of milch buffaloes are the Delhi, Mumbai, Kolkata, Ahmedabad, Kanpur, Lucknow and almost all towns of Punjab, Uttar Pradesh, Madhya Pradesh, Gujarat and Maharashtra in India, Karachi, Lahore, Faisalabad, and other cities of Pakistan. The various modes of transport are walk on the foot, motor vehicles, railway wagons, boat, steamer, ship and airplane.

1. **Movement onfoot:** Short distance travel to local markets, dairy farmers and abattoirs are covered onfoot. The distance covered onfoot is mostly up to 10 km but it may be up to 15–20 km or even more in some remote areas. It is often difficult for the young calves to travel such distance and the calves are carried in a large sixe shallow basket on the carrier of bicycle, on a rikshaw, tonga or bullock cart along with the dam onfoot following the calf. The culled buffaloes for slaughter are moved in groups of 3 to 5 tied together by neck are driven to destination. Movement of buffaloes is preferred during late hours for avoiding the problems of motor vehicles and their horns.

2. **Transport on tractor driven trollies, minitruck and truck:** The choice of vehicle depends on the distance to be covered and number of animals to be transported. These are mostly used for transportation up to 200 km. However, in some cases trucks are used for transportation up to 500–600 km. In long distance travel the buffaloes are offered drinking water at an interval of 8–10 hours but no feed during a one day travel. Use of a mild tranquilizer may be required for the transportation of breeding bulls. At the animal markets of the buffalo breeding tract plateforms are made for the easy loading of buffaloes on the trucks.

3. **Transportation by rail:** Transportation by rail is more common from the buffalo breeding tract of northwest states to metropolitan cities of Mumbai and Kolkata. The buffalo carrying capacity in a wagon of meter gauge is 6 adults and progeny and in broad gauge 8 adults and their progeny along with 2 attendants, essential utensils, first aid medicines and limited amounts of food, feed and fodder. The distance normally covered daily may be 400–500 km and journey break is preferably at place of water supply and markets for foods and feeds.

4. **River transportation:** It is carried for crossing a river for avoiding long travel by road. Large size boats are used for the ferry of buffaloes. The duration of journey may be 1–2 hours only for 1–3 km navigation. Steamers are also used but mostly for the transportation of buffaloes between the islands of Asia-Pacific countries. In such cases use of mild tranquilizers may be required.

5. **Transportation in ship:** Large consignments of fattened buffaloes are transported to slaughter houses of Hong Kong, Singapore and other countries of the pacific region from Australia and other countries.

6. **Air transport:** Special designed aeroplane are required for the transportation of buffaloes for covering very long distance of more than 2000 km when other transports are not available and traveling by road through different countries will require long quarantine periods. Some examples of air lifting of buffaloes are that of swamp buffaloes from Australia to New Guinea and 502 adult and mostly pregnant Murrah buffaloes with few breeding bulls from India to Ho Chi Minh City in S R Vietnam.

   Some precautions required for long distance transportation of buffaloes.

1. The buffaloes should not be driven tired. About 30 km on foot journey is considered optimum for a day.

2. Journey during hot season should be avoided, if not essential. Otherwise, it should be performed in cool hours of night.

3. Sufficient feeds and fodder should be carried along with essential utensils, ropes and pegs, etc.

4. There should be complete information of markets, water sources, shelter places, and veterinary clinics in the route.

5. First aid box of human and animal medicines should be carried.

6. Camping should be preffered at market places for the easy disposal of milk and purchase of essential foods and feeds.

7. The camp should be also near a Police Station or Sarpanch of the village should be informed and requested for necessary safety.

▶ ROUTINE MANAGEMENT PRACTICES

The various activities carried daily, weekly, fornightly, monthly or seasonally at the organized buffalo farms and some of them also used by other buffalo farmers are presented briefly.

▶ IDENTIFICATION OF BUFFALOES

In small holding system the buffaloes are mostly given a short name for calling. The names generally depict the body colour, horn type, eye colour, behaviour or other common names used in the area. Some of the names in India are bhuri, maini, chanda, kabari, bala, etc. At the organized farms the common methods of identification are the branding, ingraving on horn, tattooing, ear tag, and ear notching. The use of ear notching is gradually disappearing because most of the farm manegers do not want to disfigure the natural look of ears of buffaloes.

1. **Ear tag:** Light metallic and plastic ear tags engraved and painted brightly with large size numbers alone or in combustion capital letter are fixed on the dorsal surface of ears so that they may be easily read from a long distance without disturbing the animals in the herd.

2. **Necklace with number:** Use of necklace or collars made of colored beeds and colored ropes or leather strips tagging a number locket are quite common in many countries. The small holders generally use a specific design or some ornamental article for identification.

3. **Branding:** Two common methods of branding the buffaloes are hot method using red hot numbers of iron and cold method using branding fluid. The hip is considered suitable site for branding but shoulders are also used. Branding operation is carried out under the supervision of a veterinary surgeon or a trained stockman.

4. **Tattooing:** It has become more popular in recent years because it does not live any apparent mark on the body and sites used are either anterior surface of the ear or under surface of tail near the root of tail.

5. **Ear notching:** This is a very old system in which different sites of left and right ear has been assigned a number for depicting date, month, and year of birth in young calf. This system disfigures the ears and now it is obsolete.

▶ DESCRIPTION OF BUFFALO

For the preparation of animal history cord, soundness certificate and marketing the description of buffaloes is required which is generally presented in the following order:

1. Date
2. Name of buffalo, if any
3. Identification number, if marked
4. Color of the buffalo
5. **Sex of the buffalo:** Female/entire male/castrated/hermaphrodite/rig. The adult female buffalo is described according to physiological status, viz. dry, early lactation, mid lactation, late lactation or the month of calving, and also with or without calf on foot. Stage or months or pregnancy or date of insemination. The buffalo heifers of more than 2 year of age are described as nonpregnant, maiden or open and pregnant or in calf buffalo heifer.
6. **Age:** Date of birth is given for the farm bred buffaloes. For other buffaloes age is estimated on the basis of dentition and eruption of permanent teeth. The rings or grooves on the horns.
7. Special distinguishing characteristics like:
   a. Shape and size of face with markings like star or blaze, etc.
   b. Color and appearance of muzzle, viz. wet and glossy or dull dry.
   c. *Horns*: Shape, size, length, color, coils, rings and extension, etc.
   d. Tail includes length and color of switch.
   e. Chervron on neck-number, position, and color intensity.

f. Udder and teats-shape, size color, and also supranumerary teat or short number of teats along with clinicopathological status.
g. *Whirls on the body*: Size, location, and number.
h. *Color of extremities*: This is a trait of Nili-Ravi breed.
i. Abnornalities like walled eye in other than Nili-Ravi breed, broken rib(s), broken horn, short number of incisors, etc.

▶ GROOMING

Unlike cattle and horses daily grooming of buffaloes is not required because wallowing and bathing serves the purpose. However, cleaning of eyes, nostrils and external genitalia will be helpful in maintaining good health. This may be done at the time of washing the buffaloes. The lactating buffaloes should be washed properly before milking for the production of clean milk. A dandy brush or long straw may be used for cleaning the body during bathing under the shower, running tap or wallowing. Regular grooming of indoor housed buffalo bulls is a routine exercise.

Application of mustard oil or linseed oil at an interval of a month or two is quite popular in the riverine buffaloes of the Indian subcontinent.

▶ CLIPPING

Healthy buffaloes have scanty hairs on the body which becomes somewhat dense during the winter season. Therefore, at the end of winter season almost all buffaloes are clipped close to remove the breeding and hiding places of lice, ticks and mites, etc.

▶ SPRAYING OF INSECTICIDES

The humid-hot tropical climate is favorable for the multiplication of different kinds of ectoparasites, which should be controlled to reduce the menace to buffaloes and controlling the tick-borne infectious diseases. Most of the insecticides used for the protection of crops are also effective against the ectoparsites of buffaloes. Spraying should be kept under secured storage separate from the feeds, fodder, water, and other things in routine use. A muzzle should be applied during the treatment and should be removed only after washing the buffaloes insecticide free.

▶ WASHING THE BUFFALOES

Buffaloes possess inherent instinct of wallowing for several hours even during the winter season. Dairy type riverine buffaloes prefer free wallowing for several hours in clean water and the swamp buffaloes like lying in the mud holes and plastering the body with wet mud at frequent interval. All buffaloes enjoy rain water during the hot season. Amelioration of heat stress through the provison of cold water bath, shower, splashing of cold water, wallowing and cooling of sheds provided comfortable environment and improved feed intake and productivity of buffaloes (Sinha and Minett, 1947; Misra et al., 1963; Singh et al., 1976; Gangwar, 1984).

▶ BEDDING

Bedding is not important for the adult buffaloes of tropical region but use of a light bedding on the pucca floor of brick works or concrete helps in cleaning by soaking the urine. The buffaloes housed on earthen floor do not require bedding and wet soil due to urine is replaced by dry soil or ash. The young buffalo calves should be provided bedding of long straw, wood savings or dry sawdust during the cold months of winter season.

▶ CLOTHING

In hot season buffaloes do not need any clothing but in very cold season a rug may be required for the young calves. The application of rug on the buffaloes is more a psychological reaction of the owner and not the requirement of buffaloes. In the month of May to August the buffaloes grazed and herded in open on the; bugiyals (natural grassland on the high hills of Himalayan region at 6000 to 7000 m above the mean sea level). Only the young calves are housed inside the tents. Since most of the farmers are not aware with this fact, they take care of buffaloes too when they themselves fill cold.

▶ EXERCISE

The female buffaloes spending 6–10 hours on grazing and wallowing do not require further exercise, and grazing of female dairy buffaloes and all swamp buffaloes is quite common in almost all tropical countries. Similarly, loose housed females and replacement heifers at the farms also do not require additional exercise. Actually, regular exercise is only required for the confined buffalo bulls at the farms and artificial insemination centers. These bulls are either driven on walk for an hour or placed in a bull exerciser for half an hour daily.

▶ DISBUDDING OF HOURS OR DISHORNING

The destruction of growing ability of the horn buds in early life to make the buffaloes polled by the application of chemical method or red hot iron is known as **disbudding** or dishorning. This is not common in buffaloes and used only on some organized farms. **Dishorning** may be practiced in buffalo calves for fattening on range land to avoid injury due to fighting and also to divert the nutrients for body growth. The following two methods are used for disbudding the horns.

   i. **Disbudding by caustic cauterization:** The hair around the horn bud is close clipped or saved, washed, dried, painted with antiseptic lotion and a ring of Vaseline or white greese is made around the horn buds to prevent the flow of caustic containing fluid into the eyes. After this a stick of caustic soda (sodium hydroxide) or caustic potash (potassium hydroxide) is rubbed wet on the surgace of horn buds until blood oozes out. Now, the wound is wiped dry with sterilized gauze cloth and antiseptic dressing is applied for few days to prevent contamination and earlier healing.

   ii. **Hot iron method:** In this method a fire heated or electric heated iron rod with flat end is applied for dishorning. After making necessary preparations as described for caustic dishorning. The red hot iron rod is applied firm on the horn buds to live behind a burnt horn surface.

The calves should be secured properly during the operation of dishorning and corneal nerves are blocked with the injection of local anesthetics for avoiding pain. The oozing fluid should be wiped off carefully. A negligence may damage the eyes by caustic solution. The wounds are dressed aseptically for few days required for healing.

▶ DEHORNING

Amputation of emerged horns on clinical basis or otherwise is called **dehorning**. The horns are charactheristic trait of some breeds and normally dehorning is not practiced unless it becomes essential in clinical cases and also for protection from the charging of unruly buffaloes. The area around the base of horn is saved, washed with soap and water, dried and disinfected by painting an antiseptic lotion. The corneal nerves are blocked with the injection of a local anesthetic. The animal is secured in the recumbent position and horns are cut close to skull with the help of a saw to live a smooth surface. Bleeding is checked and wounds are dressed with antiseptic drug on alternate day until complete healing requiring 3–5 dressings. Parentral administration of antibiotics is required in the case of injured horns. The stum of cancerous horns may be sealed with the application of red hot iron. Dehorning should be avoided in young buffaloes otherwise stubs may grow. As far as possible dehorning should also be avoided during the humid and very cold climatic conditions.

▶ TRIMMING OF HOOVES

The buffaloes housed indoor for very long duration sometimes develop long hooves. The elongated hooves disturb the gait of buffaloes and may be break off accidentally to cause lameness. The excess growing hooves are cut-off with the help of a hoof trimming knife and the cut surface is rounded smooth with the help of a wrasp. The job is done by a trained farrier.

▶ SHOEING OF THE DRAUGHT BUFFALOES

The working buffaloes do not find any difficulty in ploughing and puddling the wet paddy fields but it is painful to drive a cart load on the metalled roads and ploughing dry and hard field with unshod feed. Shoeing is necessary for the buffaloes engaged in haulage of materials on the metalled roads and in the rocky areas. One draught buffalo requires eight shallow semilumar shoes to be shod at a time. For the fixing of one shoe 3–4 first head nails are required. Monthly shoeing may be required in the buffaloes put on heavy works everyday. The shoes used for draught buffaloes are normally made of iron plates and shoeing is done by a local farrier. In some paddy growing countries of southeast Asia shoes made of long aquatic grasses like reed or unserviceable tyres of motor vehicles are used. Unshod animals should not be put for working on hard ground for long otherwise they will become lame due to extensive wear and tear of the hooves and sole. Any negligence may expose the sole for infection and that will require long treatment and rest.

▶ CASTRATION OF MALE BUFFALOES

The castration of male buffaloes is uncommon in most of the countries, but in some European and west Asian countries male calves are castrated at young age of 6–9 months for fattening. The working males are castrated only on turning unruly and making the management and handling difficult. Retired buffalo bulls are castrated at about 7–8 years of age for draught purpose. The cart loading pooling capacity of castrated buffalo bulls is much higher than the common draught buffaloes. Burdizo castrator is used for the castration.

▶ **PREPARATION OF TEASER BUFFALO BULLS**

The teaser buffalo bulls are prepared surgically either by deflecting the sheat at one side from the plane for protecting the intromission of penis during mounting on oestrous buffalo. The other surgical method is the vasectomy or the ligation of vas deferens.

▶ **REMOVAL OF SUPRANUMERARY TEATS**

Occurrence of supranumerary teats is quite common in some breeds of dairy buffaloes, e.g. Murrah, Nili Ravi, and their grades with local buffaloes. These supranumerary teats are mostly on functional and these are unwanted appendes spoiling the shape of udder. These teats are extirpated aseptically at very young age and wound is painted with tincture benzoin co. or tincture iodine for few days to facilitate healing. Humid climate is avoided for the removal of supranumerary teats to avoid complications of healing.

▶ **DOCKING OF TAIL**

The docking of tail is not a common practice and highly undesirable in the homelands of buffaloes. However, in some cases tail of dairy buffaloes are docked near the root for preventing inconvenience to milkers due to frequent movements of the tail for removing the fly menace. Sometimes it is also used for the idenitification of buffaloes in the mixed herd of grazing swamp buffaloes. In this case the size of tail stum is highly variable and indicates ownership. Docking of tail is an important surgical intervention and used for checking the spread of infection at the terminal end of tail due to crushing by other animal, chewing of switch of the tail in loose housed calves or chewing of the switch by the buffalo for relief from itching produced by infestation of ticks, lice, mange mites or fungal infection, which may develop into gangrenous wound. In clinical cases docking of tail also include a small healthy part as a precautionary measure for stopping the recurrence of inflammation. The docking is done under the effect of local anaesthesia eith with the help of a red hot docking iron applied at the junction of coccigeal vertebrae to be removed or by flap method in which a linger flap of tail skin is sutured for closing the open end of dock. Aseptic procedure and regular dressing assures good healing in short time.

▶ **MILKING OF LACTATING BUFFALOES**

The buffaloes are either hand milked or machine milked. Machine milking is used only at some organized farms in a few countries. Stripping and full hand milking are the common procedure of milking the buffaloes. In most of the buffaloes full hand milking is facilitated by large size voluminous teats and stripping is used only in the buffaloes with very small teats. Wet hand milking, and fisting or knuckling should not be permitted because these are predisposing factors for the injury of teat canal often causing mastitis.

▶ **LET DOWN OF MILK**

In buffaloes weaning at birth has been less successful due to problem of let down of milk without suckling. In case of weaning despite statutory ban oxytocin or crude pituary extract injections are extensively used for let down of milk. In India there are at least tow wonderful breeds of dairy buffaloes, the Pandharpuri of Maharashtra and Tarai breed of Uttar Pradesh due to their characteristic milking behaviour. Let down of milk has been made possible 3 to 5 times at a short interval for door to door supply of fresh drawn milk. Calf mortality in early life is high in dairy buffaloes and straw stuffed dummy calf made of the skin of deceased calf is used for stimulating the let down of milk. The straw stuffed dummy calf is called 'mahua' or 'putla' in different parts of India. In many parts of the Indian sub continent the owners have evolved methods for stimulating let down of milk without suckling. The let down is stimulated by mild massage with warm water and intermittent light stripping. At the same time buffalo is offered a small quantity of concentrate mixture at milking.

▶ DISPOSAL OF BUFFALO DUNG AND FARM WASTE

The dung, soiled feeds and other organic wastes are collected together and disposed at an isolated place in a compost pit far away from the dairy farm and human habitations. Some amount of dung diluted with water is used for the charging of biogas plant, if operational. In many countries substantial amount of dung by small holders is used for making dung cakes required as fuel for cooking and warming the house in winter season. Although use of dung of manure is more advantageous but dung cake making will continue until fuel gas is not available at a low price with in the reach of economically weaker farm families.

▶ TRADITIONAL HOUSING AND MANAGEMENT IN MOST OF THE ASIAN COUNTRIES

The traditional housing and management of riverine and swamp buffaloes in their home tract are quite simple ad have been evolved on the basis of experience for generations and the availability of resources in the area. Longer part of the year in western parts of the tropical region remain dry hot and humid hot. Cold span of about 2–4 months is found north to the line of cancer in the north hemisphere and south to the line of Capricorn in the south hemisphere and also at high altitudes in the hilly region of the tropics. Although both riverine and swamp buffaloes have great affinity for water, the riverine buffaloes like to rest at a dry and clean place in sheds, whereas swamp buffaloes enjoy lying in the mud holes. The difference in behaviour is perhaps due to the agro-climatic conditions in their home tracts in which they are evolved. The buffaloes of coastal and southern parts do not require shelter from protection against cold while that in northern region are housed indoor during night in the winter season and some farmers also cover the buffaloes specially the young calves with a rug or jhool, when ambient minimum temperature may fall below 50°C for a month or two. The dairy buffaloes are also housed indoor during the hot hours in summer and kept cool by splashing cold water 2–3 times daily or given shower bath at the farms. The buffaloes on pastures and other grazing lands in villages either cluster beneath the trees if water sources are not available, otherwise enjoy wallowing for several hours. The sheds of buffaloes may be made of thatch, long grass, bamboo, mud or brick works depeding upon the economic status and the availability of housing materials either free of cost or on very low price. There is no doubt that the life of huts made of long grasses and thatch materials is short but the system is prevalent in many Asian countries due to very low initial cost. Most of the farmers are able to erect such sheds themselves during the lean period. There is no specific measurements and designs for sucj houses and farmers make all possible efforts to provide protection to their buffaloes against the critical climatic conditions. The effect of region is quite apparent on the feeding also. The buffaloes of dry zone are mostly fed wheat straw and stovers of sorghum and pearl millet with little grazing on scrub and fallow lands whereas that in wet areas allowed grazing to meet their greater feed requirements.

Larger number of swamp buffaloes of hot-humid tropics live on pastures, mud holes and the shelte of tree during the hot hours of grazing time in the day. In the night all buffaloes are either tethered (if few) or herded in open place with or without few small huts without side walls. The open paddocks are fenced with bamboos, wooden logs or barbed wire. At certain places the swamp buffaloes are tethered with one of the fore limb which is altered almost daily for preventing brusing and necrosis. These herding places are invariably constructed at a raised ground with sufficient slope for the drainage of urine. These drains discharge in a compost pit, fish pond or paddy field wherever it is possible.

Washing bathing or wallowing is a daily routine before the milking of dairy buffaloes. Young buffalo calves in Indian villages are allowed adequate suckling during the first 4 to 8 weeks and most of the farmers allow full suckling of one quarter by changing the quarter at eash milking. The female calves receive better care than the male calves because they are valuable future replacement buffaloes. Milking of swamp buffaloes is uncommon in most of the countries or they are milked only once daily. However, in the Brahmaputra valley larger number of swamp buffaloes are milked twice daily because of their evolution for higher milk production (Tamuli, 1986, Singh, 1088). In some of the region the calves always remain on pasture with dams and frequent suckling even through the inter limb space is quite common in swamp buffalos during grazing, ploughing or pulling a cart. The calves of swamp buffaloes are weaned at 9 to 15 months due to ceasure of lactation. This is followed by redbreeding within 4–8 weeks in most of the buffaloes (Pathak, 1975).

The buffaloes in so called backyard system with small holders are provided adequate shelter and open space for rest, whereas at commercial dairy buffalo stalls of the Indian sub continent in the urban and peri urban areas are kept crowded in small encloser with slant roof of coorugated asbestos or galvanized iron sheets or thatch and rarely of concrete on a single wall along the manger and only pillars at the rear end. Long curtains of bamboo or gunny bags are used for providing protection from cold breeze of winter in night and hot wave during summer months. A thick layer of straw or long hay is also spread on the roof specially that made of asbestos and iron sheets.

There is large variation in feeding of buffaloes starting from exclusive grazing on natural herbage cover of uplands, diara (seasonal river islands) and marshy low lying areas to intensive stall feeding prevalent at the commercial dairy buffalo stalls. Some types of swamp buffaloes inhabiting along the coastal areas have great tolerance for the saline water and dive long distance in lakes and streams for grazing on the submerged aquatic herbages. In certain areas grazing is supplemented with the feeding of paddt straw on the stack itself. Chaffing of paddy straw had started in recent years in many areas due to recurring scarcity of fodder. Chaffing reduces the wastage and improves utilization. The quantity and quality of supplemental concentrates are highly variable and these are mostly milling by products of cereal grains, pulses and oild seeds. The later is the main source of dietary protein in straw based diets. The common oil cakes supplemented in the diets of buffaloes are that of groundnut, nustard, linseed, sesame, safflower, sun flower and soyabeans. Feeding of water soaked boiled cotton seed is quite popular in the diets of lactating buffaloes of the cotton growing areas. It is believed by the farmers that feeding of cotton seed increases the yield of milk fat and recovery is higher on churning for the separation of cream and butter. Special care is taken by the farmers for the feeding of lactating and working buffaloes. In certain part of the Indian sub continent feeding of water soaked chaffed straw or stovers (kadbies) mixed with concentrates and a handful common salt is quite prevalent. This system of feeding of water soaked mixed feedstuffs is called 'sani' in some parts of India.

▶ VICES OF DOMESTIC BUFFALOES

The unwanted and bad habits of domestic animals are called vices and require correction. Some common vices of domestic buffaloes are listed as follows:

1. **Self sucking:** It is a vice of lactating buffalo that develops taste for the milk and becomes habitual of sucking her own udder. The actual cause of this vice is not definite but it is assumed that initially lactating buffalo start self sucking for releasing the pressure of udder engorgement causing discomfort to animal. The self sucking is prevented by fixing a nose plate that prevents the holding of teats. Self sucking is a very rare vice in domestic buffaloes.

2. **Milk sucking of other buffaloes:** This problem is also very rare in buffaloes and after identification such buffaloes should be removed from the loose housing and tethered away individually. The animal is also not allowed grazing in the herd.

3. **Naval sucking:** This is a common vice in young calves and a serious problem in loose housed early weaned calves. Frequent naval sucking often causes injury and infection resulting in the development of naval ill. For the control of naval ill a non irritant antiseptic lotion or ointment of offensive odour like neem seed oil is painted 2–3 times daily. In few cases separation and isolation of naval sucking calf may be essential.

4. **Licking of soil and wall of the shed:** Aged calves and mature buffaloes deprived of salt and mineral supplements frequently develop the habit of licking soil and walls of the shed. Few may also start sipping of urine to make up the deficiency. The vice is normally corrected after the incorporation of composite mineral mixture in the diets and also by providing free access to mineral licks.

5. **Furious nature:** It is sporadic in diary type buffaloes and may be observed in few working entire males and some of the breeding buffalo bulls. These animals frvelop the habit of hitting other animals and also humans. Such unruly animals become controllable after the insertion of a nose ring or string. Castration of such unruly male buffaloes has been found quite effective. If correction of vice is not effective the beast should be disposed with declaration of vice. Most of the furious buffaloes terminate their life in abattoirs. In case of pedigreed buffalo bull of a very high heritability appropriate arrangements should be made for controlling during handling.

▶ PRECAUTIONS TO BE TAKEN FROM THE UNUSUAL BEHAVIOUR OF BUFFALOES

Few buffaloes often exhibit unusual behaviour with the strangers and rarely seen objectives. Considerable loss is incurred during the capture of feral buffaloes in the northern Australia due to use of motor driven vehiclea and helicopters in place of horses. The feral buffaloes not exposed to the horns and sounds of mechanical vehicles frequently meet with the serious accidents. In order to orevent such accidents the buffaloes should be driven during the late hours when movements of vehicles is minimum.

Bright and dark colour clothes particularly bright white, red and black and also the open umbrella have been found to offened even the domesticated dairy buffaloes of very remote areas. Therefore, use of bright clothes and umbrella etc should be avoided during visiting these areas.

▶ CARE OF BUFFALO AND CALF AT CALVING

The pregnant buffalo is moved to a clean, dry and disinfected calving pen about 10–15 days before the expected calving. The claving pen is a loose house single accommodation provided with manger for feeding and a water trough. The calving pen is fitted with doors which open in a half walled paddock. The buffalo is offered feed and water inside the house. The doors are kept open during the day time for allowing free movement, but closed in night. Moreover a sincere attendant is posted during the night for keeping an eye on the animal. The animal attendant should be experienced for handling the buffalo during claving and understanding the problems of calving for timely information to veterinary personnels. During these days amount of concentrates is reduced by half and nutritional requirements are compensated by increase the quantity of succulent green fodder. In absence of green fodder greater proportion (almost 50%) of concentrates mixture is replaced with wheat bran or a mixture of wheat bran (60–70%) and molasses (30–40%) for facilitating the easy evacuation of bowel due to laxative property of wheat bran and molasses. This facilitates easier parturition in relatively much short time.

Generally no problem of parturition is encountered during calving on range in dry season. Approximately 48 hours before ensuing calving a clear depression on either side of sacrum is seen which is due to extensive relaxation of the sacro-sciatic ligament. A few hours before the calving vulva tuns engorged, swollen and pinkish, and strings of transparent mucous secretion may be seen. At this stage buffalo should not be disturbed but should also not be left alone and watched from a distance without drawing the attention of buffalo in labour. Normally the process parturition is complete in less than 2 hours from the appearance of water bag and animal does not require any assistance. If delay in expulsion of calf is more than 4–5 hours, a veterinary doctor should be called for necessary clinical or surgical intervention for facilitating smooth delivery and relieving the agony of buffalo in labour.

The naval cord generally breaks from the jerk caused by sudden rise of buffalo just with the expulsion of calf in recumbent delivery and due to weight of calf in standing delivery, and there is little bleeding. An intact naval cord should be cut immediately with a sharp sterilized blade, knife or scissors after ligating towards the naval end at a distance of 5–6 cm. Tincture iodine or tincture benzoin or any other antiseptic lotion or ointment is painted for disinfection and sealing the cut end. The calf should be removed immediately from the site of the dam before licking, if weaning is followed at birth otherwise she should be allowed to clean and dry the calf by licking. The licking stimulates peripheral blood circulation and respiration. Some times first calvers are found reluctant to lick the calf. In such buffaloes licking is encouraged by sprinkling a little salt on the body of calf or it should be cleaned dry with a piece of clean and dry cloth. First of all the layer of mucous is cleaned dry with a piece of clean and dry cloth. First of all the layer of mucous is cleaned from the nostrils, mouth and face followed by the whole body through mild rubbing. In very rare cases artificial breathing may be required and mouth to mouth blowing has been found very effective for restoring breathing. After cleaning the calf rises on its feet in about an hour and moves towards the dam for nursing, In this process the calf is guided and assisted by the dam for reaching the udder and suckling. This is a natural instinct and in very rare case human assistance is required. The udder and teats of the dam should be immediately cleaned with warm water or lightly chlorinated water, if available. The calf must consume colostrums within 3–4 hours of birth either by suckling the dam or with the help of a feeding bottle in case of weaning at birth. The intake of colostrums at first suckling should be 800–10000 g. a delay beyond 4 hours in colostrums feeding reduces the rate of absorption of immunoglobulins and decrease is significant after about 8–10 hours of calving. The total daily intake of colostrums may range from 2.0 to 4.5 kg depending upon the birth weight which ranges from 20 kg in some small breed like Jerangi to up to 45 kg in mature Jaffarabadi buffaloes. The colostrums may be fed in 2–3 meals but first feeding must be within 3 hours of birth. In cold weather of winter season both calf and dam should be provided dry and soft bedding of straw, grass hay or wood savings. They should be protected from heat waves and housed in well ventilated cool sheds. In the villages in northern parts of India young calves are mostly retained tethered indoor and dams are let loose for grazing and wallowing as per need and choice. The calves and buffaloes are also tethered beneath tree sheds of banyan tree, peepal tree or pakar tree and in archards of mangoe and guava.

▶ HOUSING AND MANAGEMENT OF CALVES

The young buffalo calves are housed in calf shed partitioned in pens for providing indivisual accommondation for 20–30 animals. The pen size shoul be 1.2 m × 1.5 m with a manger for feeding calf starter. Hay and other fodder are offered in paddock. The calves may also be housed in a group of 20–30 but in group housing incidence of naval sucking is quite high. In group housing about 1 m² covered and 2 m² paddock area are sufficient up to 3 months of age. The average length, width, depth and height of the inner wall of manger for each calf may be about 50 cm, 40 cm, 30 cm, and 35 cm respectively. This manger can also be used for the feeding of chaffed fodder during rains and extremely hot or cold climates. Water trough of about 1m width, 3m length and 0.5 m depth is stalled along the outer wall of the paddock and fitted with a tap for regular supply of fresh drinking water. The sheds should be half walled fitted with strong hooks along the upper beam for hanging thick curtains during very hot and very cold climate. Daily schedule of inspection, cleaning, grooming, feeding and watering should be strictly followed to keep the calves in good health and satisfactory growth performance.

▶ PACKAGE OF PRACTICE FOR REDUCING CALF LOSS IN EARLY LIFE

Buffalo calf mortality is very high in the buffalo production systems prevalent in the hot-humid tropical climate of Asian countries. The causes are mostly calf scour, ascariasis, gastroenteristis and pneumoenteritis. These are due to gross negligence in care, unhygienic rearing conditions, infections, worm infestation, ectoparasites and various degree of poor feeding and under feeding etc. At the commercial buffalo dairy stalls it is a prevalent practice to eliminate the calves by a highly inhumane practice of intentional under feeding to the extent of starvation. In rural areas also situation is not very good but starvation is not practiced. A simple management schedule may be highly useful for saving the life of neonatal calves (Table 5.3).

TABLE 5.3: Package of practice for the protection of young buffalo calves

Age of calf (weeks)	Milk feeding (kg/day)	Medication schedule	For prevention of (infection)
1	3 kg (Clostrum for first 3 days @ 10%)	(i) Sealing of naval cord with Tr. Iodine/Tr. Benzoin	Naval ill
		(ii) Antibiotic/probiotic	Calf scour
2–3	@ 10% of bwt.	(i) Anthelmintic	Round worms
		(ii) Vitamin supplement	(Ascariasis)
12–15	@ 5% of bwt.	(i) Anthelmintic	Roundworms (Ascariasis)
		(ii) Acricide sprey	Ticks and lice, etc.

Note: At about 12 weeks of age milk is drastically reduced and suckling is allowed just for let down. Main diet is calf starter and good fodder.

Surgical intervention for disbudding of horns and the extirpation of suranumerary teats in female calves are preferably carried in early life. Complete record of history and health coverage should be maintained. Under optimum feeding and management the buffalo calves attain 50 to 65 kg body weight in different breeds at 3 months of age. However, buffalo calves reared on high level of energy feeding may attain more than 90 kg body weight at 3 month of age and more than 150 kg at 6 month of age in different breeds.

▶ **HOUSING AND MANAGEMENT OF REPLACEMENT BUFFALO HEIFERS**

The heifers of dairy type buffaloes are the future valuable dairy animals and receive special care for rearing because buffalo heifers fetch much higher price even after weaning at 10–12 months of age. At medium and large farms only selected heifers of standard breeds are reared for replacement. At weaning about 20–25% more buffalo heifers are retained for rearing for rearing as replacement and at a later stage at puerty or calving a second from the male calves at about 6 months of age and raised in a byre with open wall shed over the manger and spacious paddock with provision of continuous running or scheduled (2 or 3 times daily) drinking water supply along the side wall and having link with drain. Optimum floor area requirement in covered shed is about 2m² and paddock space 4 m² for rearing up to puberty. Average width, depth and height from the ground of common manger may be about 70 cm. 40 cm and 50 cm respectively, and each heifer should be provided about 75 cm length on the manger for comfortable feeding of concentrates ad fodder from 6 months to puberty at 18 to 24 months of age. The inner surface of manger should be reasonably rounded U-shaped for facilitating easy cleaning. Such surface does not provide places for deposition of feeds foor the growth of decaying microorganisms and multiplication of pathogens particularly the fungi during the wet season. The floor of paddock may be bricks paved, half part bricks paved or complete soil ground. The second option is more comfortable in all climates. All soil paddock is good but creates problem of cleaning during the wet season. Heifers frequently make mud holes in the absence of wallowing facility due to which it becomes difficult to keep the animals clean. Buffalo heifers may be well maintained on a relatively lesser flooe space (53 cm) without any significant effect on growth performance (Verma and Tripathi, 1980). However, this space will be insufficient for the adult dry and pregnant buffaloes, whereas the dimension suggested earlier will be multi purpose for housing growing buffalo heifer, dry buffaloes and also pregnant buffaloes up to mid gestation period thereby providing better utilization of space and saving of manpower and materials. The heifers or mixed buffaloes may be fed a common balanced diet to support about 400–500 g daily gain in the body weight of heifers to attain about 300–350 kg body weight at about 18 months of age. The female buffaloes should be provided cool environment by water slashing, shower bath or wallowing etc for efficient breeding.

▶ HOUSING AND MANAGEMENT OF DRY, PREGNANT, AND MILCH BUFFALOES

The housing and management described for the replacement buffalo heifers are equally applicable for the dry and pregnant buffaloes except that the number of dry buffaloes are only 20 to 30% of total buffaloes in the paddock. The shed for lactating buffaloes should be nearer to milking barn joined with a passage or should be designed for feeding and milking at the same place. Arrangement for wallowing or a shower bath before milking is considered advantageous for let down of milk.

Milking barn: It is a well ventilated, fly proof, dried damp free and clean shed fitted with stanchion for holding the buffaloes at a place during milking. Hygienic condition in milking barn is maintained by regular disinfection. However, care is taken to avoid the use of harmful and off odour chemicals because milk is a high absorber f odours form the vicinity. In routine practice concentrates mixture is fed at the time of morning and evening milking. A double row tail to tail arrangement has been found convenient for a milking barn. A manger width of about 60 cm and standing floor 1.75 m terminating in a 20 cm wide U shaped shallow drain on either side. The manger should be fitted with stanchion at a distance f 1.2 m for securing individual buffalo at the time of milking. The moderately convex central passage continuous with shallow drain on either side shall be about 1.5 m wide for the free movement of trollies and milkers. The milking barn should preferably be connected through a continuous closed wall passage with the recording and milk collection room. A light solution of potassium permanganate and clean dry towel shall be placed by the side along a wash basin near the entrance of milking barn for rinsing the hands by milkers before milking. First few streams of milk shall be stripped on strip cup for routine milk inspection for any abnormal change in the milk. Any change in the physical appearance of milk is referred for further investigation in the clinical laboratory.

▶ HOUSING AND MANAGEMENT OF BUFFALO BULLS

Buffalo bull sheds are preferably constructed at the distal end of the farm near to veterinary clinic and artifical insemination laboratory. Breeding bulls should be housed in individual pens separated by strong metallic bars or galvanized iron pipes so that they can see each other but should not come in close contact. Average size of bull pens may be 3 m × 4 m covered area extended in a paddock of about 100 m². Each pen is provided with a manger of 100 cm × 70 cm × 40 cm and a water trough of 100 cm × 70 cm × 50 cm size along the side in the paddock with running water supply. The covered area should open in the paddock. Half walled shed covered with slanted roof is quite comfortable. Provision of a shade tree or spread of a creeper on the roof is added advantage for protection against heat of the summer season. Cooling arrangements are also made with the help of water sprinkled thatch curtains and fans for keeping the temperature below 35°C and alos by providing wallowing for several hours in relatively cold running water of a river or stream. In many villages of India large size ponds connected with canal are made for the wallowing of buffaloes.

▶ **HOUSING AND MANAGEMENT OF WORKING BUFFALOES**

Working buffaloes may be entire or castrated male. Both sexes of swamp buffaloes are used for draught purpose but females are preferably used for lighter works of ploughing, puddling or thrashing. These buffaloes are kept in group in an encloser or thethered individually in a common shed for draught animals. No special arrangements are made at the farms because normally not more than 5 pairs are maintained for routine local works on the buffalo farm and fodder farm.

▶ **MANAGEMENT OF CALVING PEN**

A medium size shed partitioned in pens of about 3 m × 5 m rectangled should continue with a paddock of about 3 m × 5 m size. Although calving pen many also be half walled but open space must be made inaccessible for dogs, cats, mongoose and large lizards by fixing windows of iron bars. The pen shall also have a door which will be kept closed to houdse the dam and calf indoor in early life. Calving pens should be well ventilated and free from dampness.

▶ **ISOLATION WARD**

The isolation ward is constructed far away from the animal houses and other buildings. It would be advantageous to construct in restricted area with adequate provision of detachment from the appliances and attendants of healthy buffaloes.

▶ **LAYOUT PLAN FOR DAIRY FARM**

For the establishment of a dairy buffalo farm the following factors should be considered thoroughly:
1. Land for farm buildings and fodder cultivation.
2. Distance from main road and availability of approach road.
3. Distance from market, milk collection center or dairu plant.
4. Markets for the purchase of feeds, dairy appliances and veterinary products etc.
5. Availability of skilled and common man power for dairy farm operations and fodder cultivation.
6. Location of Veterinary hospital and artificial insemination center.
7. Nearness of buffalo markets for the purchase of producing buffaloes and disposal of surplus calves at weaning and culled buffaloes.
8. Perennial source of non polluted water supply.
9. Topography and pattern of seasonal changes.

A lay out plan of 100 lactating buffaloes and their followers has been outlined as follows:
1. **Selection and purchase of buffaloes:** This depends on the objective of dairy farming. If, it is only for milk production and commercial marketing, then graded buffaloes of prevalent dairy breed of the area are generally more remunerative. The only criteria for the selection is the milk yield and lactation length. It would be better to purchase second parity buffaloes in first month of calving after verifying the performance record of previous lactation. Such buffaloes may be kept economically for 3–4 lactations. The farmers with objective of milk production and maintenance of pure breeds for commercial farming with objective of milk production and

maintenance of pure breeds for commercial farming should identify the most popular breed of the area and should purchase the best available buffaloes falling under the breed standard. Such farmers may select buffaloes of even third and fourth lactation if performance is outstanding period, viz, a Murrah buffalo yielding 2500 kg milk in third lactation against the average 2000 kg may be purchased in fourth lactation also, and if follower is female calf then some premier may also be paid.

For starting a dairy farm 100 good lactating buffaloes in first month of calving and second or third lactation are purchased in a staggered manner so that supply of milk could be maintained round the year. Therefore, if would be better to start with 25 lactating buffaloes with a provision of adding 25 freshly calved buffaloes every quarter until the number of lactating buffaloes is 100. Disposal of a poor performer should not be delayed. In addition to 100 lactating buffaloes and their followers there will be need of a teaser male and pair of working bovine.

2. **Infrastructure, dairy equipments and appliances of buffalo farm:**

Following is the tentative list of office, animal sheds, feed godown, store, equipments and appliances generally required at a dairy farm of 100 lactating buffaloes:

2.1 Two large size half walled shed with provision for feeding and milking and an attached paddock with a drinking water tank along a border. Each shed should house 50 buffaloes.

2.2 One shed of 50 capacity for housing recently dried and 20–30 pregnant buffaloes in different stages of pregnancy.

2.3 Calving pens for at least 5 buffaloes.

2.4 Bull shed of 10 pens for housing a teaser, 2 good bulls and 1 or 2 pairs of draught animals.

2.5 One calf pen for housing 30 calves up to 3–4 month of age.

2.6 One shed for housing 50 growing cavles up to weaning at 10–12 months.

2.7 One shed for housing 30 selected weaned heifers for the replacement of less productive and surplus uneconomical buffaloes.

2.8 Godowns, one each for storing comounded feeds and feed ingredients and another for the storage of dairy farm equipments and appliance.

2.9 A large size barn for storing hay, straws and stovers.

2.10 A fodder chaffing shed attached with workshop and open sheds for tractor, trollies and carts etc.

2.11 A office building with milk collection, processing, packaging and disposal and also an attached change cum lunch shelter with separate toilets and bath rooms for the ladies and gents.

2.12 Milk utencils like milking pails, milk collection cans, buckets, washing tubs, balance for milk recording and large size scanner or sieve for filtering milk.

2.13 Two medium size tractors and 3–4 trollies.

2.14 Compost pits for dumping 20–25 tonnes dung and wastes daily with a provision of frequent disposal at 1 to 3 month interval

2.15 Farm land: Approximately 20–25 hectare satisfactory land for the erection of farm houses and cultivation of fodder for the buffaloes.

2.16 Surces of good quality fodder seeds and fertilizers, etc.

2.17 Markets for the purchase of feed ingredients and fodder, if not cultivated at the from.

▶ FODDER REQUIREMENT AND CULTIVATION CALENDAR

For successful dairy farming assured supply of adequate quantity of nutritious and palatable fodder is one of the most important factors.

A. **Selection of fodder crops:** High yielding nutritious fodder of good feeding value should be preferred for cultivation. Selection should be made to supply bulky cereal fodder and proteinous leguminous fodder in 1:1 to 2:1 ratio. Such selections help in reducing the cost of concentrates and improving the production, condition and reproduction of the buffaloes. Besides being nutritious the fodder should also mature late. Fodder should be shown in split plots at an interval of 2 to 4 weeks for the maintenance of quality. There should be also provision for the cultivation of surplus fodder during favourable season for conservation as hay or silage for the lean period. Some fodder suitable for cultivation in tropical and sub temperate zones are listed in Table 5.4.

TABLE 5.4: Some fodder crops for dairy farms

S.No.	Common nane	Botanical name	Season of sowing	Green fodder yield (quintals/hectare)
1.	Mauze or corn	Zea mays	Year round	300–500/crop
2.	Sorghum/jowar	Sorghum vulgare	Rains, Summer	300–500
3.	Sudan grass	Sorghum sudanense/is	Do	300–450
4.	Pearl millet/bajra	Pennusetum typhoides	Do	250–500
5.	Teosinte		Do	400–500
6.	Cow pea/lobia	Vigna sinensis	Do	300–350
7.	Cluster bean/guar		Do	300–350
8.	Moong	Phaseolus aureus	Do	200–250
9.	Oats	Avena sativa	Winter	350–500
10.	Barley	Hordeum valgare	Do	350–500
11.	Berseem	Trifolium alexandrinum	Do	600–800
12.	Lucerne/alfalfa		Annual	700–900
13	Mustard/rape/cabbage	Brassica spp.	Winter	300–350

B. **Estimated requirement of fodder:** At a buffalo dairy farm of 100 breedable females the strength of animals may very from 120 to 125 equivalent of adult animals provided male calves and surplus heifers are regularily disposed at 3–4 months of age. About 60 buffaloes are expected to be in different stages of lactation producing about 400 to 500 litres milk daily, if herd average is about 2000 litres milk in 395 days. The average body weight of Murrah and Nili Ravi breeds may be expected 500 kg The dry matter requiremen of 125 adult equivalent may be about 17.2 quintals daily and will include about 5.7 quintals concentrate mixture and 11.5 quintals good quality fodder. Daily requirement of green fodder will be 55 to 60 quintals. Therefore, annual estimated requirements may be,

   i. Compounded concentrates mixture about 230 tonnes,
   ii. Green fodder of 20% dry matter about 2200 tonnes. Asuming 2 crops per year and 50 tonnes green fodder yield per hectare, the requirement of arable land with assured irrigation may be about 25 hectares giving margin for 10% crop failure.

C. **Fodder cultivation calendar:** Most of the cereal fodder are preferably harvested from 10–20% flowering oe emergence of buds or head to dough stage of maturity with 15 to 25% dry matter. The cow pea, peas and cluster beans are harvested from budding to immature pod formation. The multicut leguminous crops are ready for harvesting after 45 to 60 days followed by every 6 weeks. It may be more advantageous to place two-third land under cereal crops and one-third under legumes. However, acrage under leguminous fodder crops may be increased if farming also includes cereal grain cultivation providing straws and stovers as low grade and low protein dry fodder. A tentative fodder cultivation schedule has been presented as follows for the climates and soils like Indo-Gangatic plains of India:

  i. **Oats:** Mid October to end to November in split plots at 2 weeks interval.
 ii. **Berseem:** October to mid November. It may be sown either as monocrop or mixed with oats or barley. In monocropping also small amount of Chinese cabbage, kale or mustrud is mixed for higher yield of first cut.
iii. Maize, teosinte sorghum or bajra alone or in different combinations are sown from March to November in split plots at 2–4 weeks interval.
 iv. Cowpea, cluster bean, moong bean are sown during April to August in split plots. Some small farmers often mix these with maize, sorghum, and bajra, etc.

▶ **FIRST AID FACILITY**

Some medicines, appliances and other items required for handling emergency cases should be always available at the medium and large buffalo farms and in the office of Gram Panchayat for the use of common livestock owners of the village. A first aid box should contain at least the following items with the arrangement for quick replacement. The community facility should be available at no profit no loss basis. There should be also provision for providing facilities on credit because many times some of the livestock owners lack cash in hand for immediate payment.

List of items in a first aid box

1. Few strong and smooth ropes of different thickness ranging from 0.3 cm to 2 cm diameter and 1 m to 10 m length.
2. Gauze cloth and bandage cloth 10 m each or more.
3. Sterilized absorbent cotton wool bundles of 100 g to 500 g
4. Disposable syringes and needles of different size.

REFERENCES

Afifi, Y A, Shahin, M A and Shirbij, A 1970. Agric. Res. Rev., Cairo, 48; 1–12

Aliev, A A 1961. Fiziol., USSR, 47; 1156–62

Alim, K A 1953. Nature, London, 171; 755

Asker, A A, Ghany, M A and Ragab, M T 1952. Indian J. Dairy Sci.; 5; 171–182

Asker, A A Ragab, M T and Ragab, M T 1955. Indian J.Dairy Sci., 8; 39–64

Badreldin, A L and Ghany, M A 1952. Nature, London, 170; 145–458

Bahga, C S, Gangwar, P C, Mehta, S N and Dhingra, D P. 1985. Indian J. Dairy Sci., 38; 36–40

Bhandari, M L, Puttuswamy, G, Narayan, D and Rangaswamy, M C 1951. Indian J Dairy Sci., 4; 106–111

Bhat, P N 1979. FAO Production and Health Paper 13; 129–142

Blood, D C and Henderson, J A 1971. Venterinary Medicine, 3rd ed., London

Chantalakhana, Charan, 1979. FAO Production and Health Paper 13; 173–181

Chaudhary, R A and Ahmed, W 1979. FAO Production and Health Paper 13; 173–181

El-Wishy, 1971. Z. Tierzucht Zucht Biol., 86; 81–88

Gangwar, P C 1984. Indian Dairyman, 36; 451–453

Jainudeen, M R 1977. Proc. Jt. Conf. On Reprod. In Malayasian Swamp buffalo, Min. of Agric., Malayasia, pp. 162–169

Jakhmola, R C, Kamra, D N, Singh, R, Pathak, N N 1984. Agric. Waste, 10; 229–237

Jawarkar, K V and Johar, K S 1975. Indian J. Dairy Sci., 28; 54–59

Khamis, M Y and Saleh, M S 1970. Vet. Med. Nachr., 4; 274–284

Kumar, A, Pandiya, S C, Peshin, P K and Singh, H P 1976. Ceylon Vet. J., 24; 22–25

Manik, R S, Jadhav, K E and Iqbal Nath 1981. Indian J Dairy Sci., 34; 448–450

Macgukin, C E 1935

Saini, A, Gill, R S and Gill, S S 1982. Indian J. Dairy Sci., 35; 257–262

Salerno, A 1960, Atti soc. Ital. Sci. Vet., 14; 259–261

San Augustin, g 1938. Philippines J. Anim. Ind., 5; 261–270

Sharma, M C, Pathak, N N and Hung, N N 1984. Indian J. Vet. Med., 4; 97–100

Singh, K, Joshi, B C and Bhattacharya, N K 1976. Indian J. Dairy Sci., 29; 110–113

Singh, S D 1935. Agriculture and Livestock, India; 499–502

Sinha, K C and Minett, F C 1947. J. Anim. Sci., 6; 258–264

Srivastava, P L and Promila, 1983. Indian J. Anim. Sci. 53; 771–772

Soni, P L, Gangwar, P C, Bahga, C S, Srivastava, R K and Dhingra, D P 1980. The Indian J. Nutr. Dietet., 17; 220–227

Sumulong, M D 1937. Philippines J. Anim. Ind., 4; 253–264

Verma, A K and Tripathi, V N 1980. Haryana Agric. Uni. J. Res., 10; 594–603

Verma, D N and Hussein, K Q 1985. Indian Vet. Med. J., 9; 112–114

Wang Pei-Chien, 1979, FAO Production and Health Paper 13, 152–154

6

Reproductive System of Water Buffalo: Female Reproductive System

The reproduction system of buffalo extends from the ovaries located in the abdominal cavity to the vulva opening below the anus and produces the female gamete, ovum. The entire channel is distinguished in different compartments for specialized functions. It provides suitable environment for the fertilization of the ovum, formation of the zygote and development of the embryo (foetus) by supplying necessary nutrients from the day of conception to the termination of pregnancy lasting 305 to 330 days in different types and breed of buffaloes. In addition to carrying the foetus, the female buffaloes also provide post-natal nourishment to their calves in the early life through the feeding of the normal lacteal secretion, the milk. The reproductive organs of a female buffalo include a pair of ovaries, a pair of oviducts or fallopian tubes, a pair of uterine cornua (horns), the body of uterus, cervix, vagina and the external genitalia called vulva. The parts of the reproductive tract extending form the ovaries to the cervix are held in position by the broad ligament (Fig. 6.1). The genitalia of buffalo is muscular and smooth and the uterine cornua are tortuous. The shape and size of different reproductive organs are influenced by the age, parity, breed and nutritional status (Polding and Lall, 1954, Damodaran, 1958, Luktuke and Rao, 1962, Bhalla *et al*, 1964, Sane *et al*, 1964, 1965, Toellherem 1980, Torres *et al*, 1980). The various reproductive organs are smaller in maiden buffalo heifers than the parous buffalo cows (Table 6.1).

▶ PRE-NATAL DEVELOPMENT

In the embryonic stage the reproductive system develops from the two germinal ridges on the dorsal side of the abdominal cavity. The gonads are formed by the 2 invasions of the germinal rudges by a group of large granulated yolk sac cells. The first invasion is abortive but the second forms the sex cord which spreads upwards into the primordial germ cells. The ovary is formed from the cortex of the gonads. Many oogonia are formed in the 3 month old foetus and their number decrease gradually and they are rarely present in 6 month old fetuses. The maturation of oogonia to oocytes begins during the third month and prenatal period and the zygotene and pachytene stages of the meiotic pro-phase represent the most stable phases of the maturation division (El-Ghannam and El-Naggar, 1975). In the early prenatal life of the sexually undifferentiated embryo, both ducts i.e., Wolffian and Mullerian are present and the Mullerian duct forms the gonaductal system. Whereas Wolffian duct undergoes disuse areophy. The Mullerian ducts join posteriorly to form the uterus, cervix and anterior part of the vagina. The coiling of oviduct and the formation of fimbriae takes place in the terminal phase of the

TABLE 6.1: Average measurements (cm) and weight (g) of genital organs different types of female buffaloes

Genital Organs		Nulli-parous	Multi-parous	Murrah	Surti	Jaffarabadi	Egyptian	Swamp
Genitalia wt.	Wt.	234	508	578	-	-	-	-
Rt. ovary	L	2.28	2.53	2.91	2.08	3.12	2.63	2.44
	W	1.52	1.32	1.39	1.20	1.49	0.27	1.79
	T	1.20	1.64	1.17	1.22	1.19	0.59	1.34
	Wt.	2.56	3.97	3.81	2.24	4.01	-	3.71
Lt. ovary	L	2.38	2.60	2.97	2.25	3.13	2.63	2.42
	W	1.58	1.34	1.37	1.23	1.44	0.28	1.72
	T	1.23	1.55	1.13	1.20	1.15	0.60	1.27
	Wt.	2.73	3.93	3.66	2.50	3.87	-	3.56
Rt. oviduct	L	19.17	22.30	22.56	18.82	24.41	24.30	
	W	0.52	0.32	-	-	-	-	
Lt. oviduct	L	20.07	21.80	22.38	19.80	24.49	24.08	
	W	0.50	0.32					
Rt. horn	L	26.43	36.20	39.18	25.21	51.38	34.80	26.19
	W	2.82	2.45	2.18	2.50	2.87	5.88	2.65
Lt. horn	L	26.97	36.30	38.76	24.92	50.27	25.61	
	W	2.84	2.32	2.62	2.42	2.73	-	
Corpus-uteri	L	0.74	0.94	1.38	1.74	1.49	2.73	2.15
	W	3.22	2.79	-	2.86	-	7.82	2.87
Cervix	L	6.34	5.90	7.82	5.54	8.09	7.69	
	W	2.86	3.56	2.79	2.65	5.07	3.46	
Vagina	L	22.10	21.26			23.92		
	W	6.26	6.44			5.34	0.46	0.46
Vulva	L	10.54	12.48			5.75		
	W	9.54	12.46			2.66		

feotal growth. The vestibule is formed by urogenital sinus and the fold of skin bordering the sinus forms the labiae of the vulva.

▶ NEONATAL DEVELOPMENT

The different organs of the reproductive tract are fully formed and distinct at birth (Tiwari, 1972). The morphology at 3–4 days of age included the following:

1. **Ovaries:** The ovaries divided into cortex or zona parenchyma and the medulla or zona vasculasa. The connective tissue stroma of the cortex is compact on the surface to form the tunicainea covered by the germinal epithelium of a single layer of the cuboidal cells. The tunicainea is formed of the dorsal collagenous fibres and a few cells. It lacks in vascularity and the average thisckness is about 37.5 u. the cortical stroma is rich in fusiform cells containing elongated nuclei. They are arranged parallel to the surface of the ovary or follicles and the blood vessels enclosed by them.

The stroma has characteristic swirly appearance. It prossesses numerous ovarian follicles in different stages of development. Just before the tunica albuginea the small primary (pyramidal) follicles are distributed and blood vessels are present below the layer of follicles. Average diameter of the developing ovum is about 18.28 µ and that of the primary follicle is 40.6 µ. The nucleus is placed accentrally and contains distinct nucleolus but poor chromatin.

The medullary substance contains cells of the cortical stroma, several blood vessels, nerve fibres and smooth muscle fibres. A net like arrangement of the medullary tubules lined by cuboidal to columnar cells representing the vestiges of rete overii are present in the medulla.

2. **Oviducts:** The wall of the oviducts is formed of the mucosa, muscularis and serosa layers. The mucosa forms the primary and secondary longitudinal folds lined by tall columnar epithelium, part of which is psuedostratified. Only part of the cells lining the mucosa are ciliated. The core of the mucosal fold is highly vascular. The lamina propria is made of the connective tissue having cells and vessels but devoid of the glands. The tunica muscularis is formed by the inner circular layer and the outer longitudinal layer of the isolated muscle fibre bundles. The stratum vasuclaris separates the two layers of the tunica muscularis. The outer covering is formed of the tunica serosa.

3. **Uterus:** The wall of uterus is composed of the tunica mucosa lining the luminal surface, the tunica muscularis giving the strength and the tunica serosa a protective outer layer. The mucosa of endometrium is longitudinally folded and contains nonglandular portions known as caruncles. In the uterine cornua the epithelial lining is psuedostratified and occasionally ciliated. The epithelium possesses simple tubular glandular crypts of varying depth lined by the columnar cells embedded into the lamina propria. Fully formed glands are absent. The structure of the lamina propria is fibrillar and contains abundance of blood vessels. The tunica muscularis of myometrium is made of a thick inner layer of circular muscle fibres and a thinner layer of the longitudinal muscle fibres. The two layers are separated by the stratum vascularis containing numerous vessels and nerves. The lamina propria of the corpus uteri has a few developed uterine glands. The outer covering is formed of tunica serosa called perimetrium.

4. **Cervix:** The structure of the cervix is similar to the uterus but it is highly folded and devoid of the glandular crypts.

5. **Vagina:** The wall of the vagina is made of the tunica mucosa, the tunica muscularis and the tunica adventitia. The mucos of cranial (neck) region is folded and lined by the columnar epithelium. The tunica propria is highly vascular. The tunica muscularis is formed of the thicker inner circular and the thinner outer longitudinal muscle layers. The outer covering is made of the tunica adventitia.

6. **Vulva:** The cutaneous mucosa of the vulva is covered by the stratified squamous epithelium. The basal layer of the epithelium is folded. A layer of blood vessels extends below the epithelium in the core of papillae. The submucosa is formed of collagenous tissue and the smooth muscle is the continuation of the vaginal musculature.

▶ GENITAL ORGANS OF THE ADULT FEMALE

Broad Ligament

The ovaries, oviducts, uterus and cervix are held by the broad ligament in position. The broad ligament is composed of the double serous folds and in between the folds flat sheets of smooth muscle fibres, blood vessels, nerves and connective tissue are present. The smooth muscle bundles spread parallel to the cervix, corpus uteri and the uterine cornua in diverging fashion, and they are absent in the posterior region attached to the proximal extremity of the vagina. The ligament is thinner and soft in the non-gravid, and thicker and slightly rigid in the gravid animals. The ligament is differentiated 3 parts, themeso-ovarian, the mesosalpinx and the mesometrium, and provided support to the ovarian, the mesosalpinx and the mesometrium, and provided support to the ovaries, oviducts and layer of the myometrium are continuous with the respective components of the broad ligament. A few lymphoid nodes are found in the mesoovarian region of the broad ligament in Surti buffaloes. The average number of smooth muscle cell nuclei is 8676 per mm^2 in the non gravid and 11160 per mm^2 in the gravid animals. The average length and breadth of the nucleus is 10.5u and 3.0 µ in the non-pregnant, 16.5 µ and 1.5 µ in the pregnant buffaloes respectively. The significant increase in the number of nuclei associated with the increase in their length and decrease in breadth indicate hyperplasia and hypertrophy during the pregnancy (Bagi and Vyas, 1983). Somewhat thicker and rigid broad ligament in Jaffarabadi buffaloes (Sane et al., 1964) and muscular feel in the Egyptian buffaloes (Largerlof, 1959) have been reported.

Ovary

A pair of ovaries are found one on either side of the median line and situated deep in the pelvic cavity near the border of the abdominal cavity. The ovary is held in position by the mesoovarian part of the broad ligament. The ovary is irregularly oval or almond shaped and varies in size with the stage of the oestrus cycle and the breed of the buffalo. In young heifers the ovaries remain quiescent and becomes functional with the onset of puberty. The main tissue of ovary is cortex, which is surrounded by the outer layer of the germinal epithelium formed of a simple squamous layer showing sporadic stratification. The subepithelial tunica aluginea is a dense layer of thick and thin collagenous fibres, scattered reticular fibres and a few elastic fibres (Prasad et al., 1979). The primary follicle is spherical in shape and develops individually in the ovarian cortes embedding beneath in the tunica albuginea. It is composed of a thin layer of the epithelial cell enclosing a spherical ovum. The follicular corona cells are cuboidal and some times may be flattened or columnar. The latter type of cells are usually found in the follicles having larger ova, whereas the flattened cells are more common in the small sized zones. The primary follicles are 34–48 µ in diameter containing an ovum of 21–28 µ diameter. The oogonium contains a large prominent nucleus. The diameter of the secondary follicles is 43–60 µ and that of ovum is 24–38 µ in the Egyptian buffaloes and 114–133 µ in the Indian buffaloes. The average diameter of the tertiary or Graafian follicles is up to 21.5 mm across the long axis (El-Sheikh and Abdellhadi, 1970 and Prasad et al., 1979). The follicles are filled with the follicular fluid and the average quantity fo the follicular fluid is 1.32 + 0.32, 0.87 + 0.37 and 0.61 + 0.30 g in the follicles during the follicular phase, luteal phase and subactive condition respectively, and corresponding density of the gonadotropic cell in the adenohypophysis is about 12.92, 16.04 and 7.25%. Large sized follicles are not found in the anoestrus ovaries (Namboothripod and Luktuke, 1978). On laproscopic examination the Graafian follicles appear walled, translucent bulge on the ovarian surface on the day of oestrus (Jainudeen et al. 1983). The follicles remain in various stages of atrasia on the day of parturition and thereafter develop gradually with corresponding regression of the corpus luteum of the pregnancy. A few follicles may mature by 30 days post partum and many by the end of 60 days. The frequency of ovulation significantly differs between the ovaries, and in one observation about 80% of the total ovulation has been recorded in the right ovary (Agrawal et al., 1979).

The ovaries perform two main functions:

    i. They are the primary organs of reproduction and produce female gamet (ovum) and

   ii. the endocrine function.

The ovaries synthesize and secret hormones required of the oestrus cycle, fertilization, implantation of the zygote, development of the foetus and the foetal membranes and the development of the mammary glands.

Oviducts or Fallopian Tubes

A pair of tubes, one on either side extend from the vicinity of ovaries to the proximal end of the uterine cornua. Each oviduct is a tortuous tube suspended in the mesosalpinx

TABLE 6.2: Average measurements (cm) of oviducts at different post-partum intervals in adult Indian buffalo

Stages of oviduct	At parturition	Post-partum interval (days)				
		7	15	30	45	60 (Oestrus)
Gravide side						
Weight (g)	2.50	1.80	1.75	2.00	1.30	1.50
	+0.23	+0.06	0.02	0.08	0.22	0.25
L with fimbriae	21.0	24.5	22.0	23.0	22.5	19.5
	+2.00	+0.75	+0.92	+0.50	+1.12	+0.95
L of fimbria	2.5	3.7	3.2	3.0	3.5	2.5
	+0.25	+0.47	+0.13	+0.20	+0.45	+0.14
Br of fimbria	4.5	3.8	4.3	4.2	4.8	4.6
	+0.05	+0.31	+0.10	+0.30	+0.40	+0.23
Breadth of oviduct						
At fimbriated end	0.45	0.35	0.35	0.30	0.40	0.39
In middle	0.18	0.15	0.13	0.16	0.13	0.14
At Uterotubal joint	0.33	0.35	0.25	0.28	0.35	0.38
Non gravid side						
Weight (g)	2.30	1.80	1.84	1.95	1.42	1.35
	+0.15	+0.07	+0.03	+0.06	+0.25	+0.22
L with fimbriae	21.0	23.5	21.5	22.7	21.0	19.5
	1.80	+0.85	+0.25	+1.12	+0.20	+1.34
L of fimbria	2.5	3.0	2.6	3.5	3.0	0.25
	+0.25	+0.02	+0.31	+0.25	+0.50	+0.30
Br. of fimbria	5.5	5.0	3.8	4.6	6.2	5.6
	+0.90	+0.45	+0.35	+0.40	+0.25	+0.26
Br. of oviduct						
At fimbriated end	0.40	0.33	0.40	0.35	0.40	0.41
In middle	0.15	0.15	0.18	0.18	0.13	0.15
At Uterotubal joint	0.32	0.30	0.35	0.30	0.32	0.34

Note: L = length, Br = breadth.

part of the lateral layer of the broad ligament. The length, breadth and degree of convolution differ between the types, breeds and status of the individuals of the same breed. The oviduct may be differentiated into the fimbriae, the infundibulum, the ampula and the isthmus connecting with the uterine horn. Pronounced fimbriae are present only in the infundibular part that attaches with the mesoovarium (Girish Chandra, 1979). The fimbriae are finger like projections lining the open margin of the infundibulum. Significant variation are finger like projection lining the open margin of the infundibulum. Significant variation occurs in the size of the fimbriae at different intervals from parturition in adult riverine buffaloes (Raizada et al., 1978). The average weight of both oviducts is maximum on the day of parturition (Table 6.2). The funnel shaped opening of the infundibulum is located in a pouch like structure of the peritoneal and the supraperitonial fasciae called ovarian bursa. The infundibulum continues as a wide tube known as ampulla which tapers posteriorly as isthmus forming more than half of the fallopian tube joining distally with the uterine horn of the respective side. A diverticulum generally extending from the ampulla and isthmus towards the uterine or ovarian end has been observed in about 3% females (Chandra and Bhardwaj, 1981).

The tunica mucosa is formed of the thin longitudinal folds decreasing in height and intensity towards the uterine end. The epithelial lining is generally pseudostratified and columnar. The mucosal folds in the ampulla are prominent and virtually fill the lumen during the oestrus. The height of the epithelium ranges between 24 and 55 µ in the middle region and 18 to 39 µ at the uterine end. Some cell are ciliated and others are non-ciliated columnar cells are larger than the ciliated cells towards the uterine end. Appreciable difference is not seen in the height of the cells (6–12 µ) in the mid region and the tubulo-uterine junction. The tunica muscularis is formed of an inner layer of the circular muscle fibres, 39–90 µ thick in the mid region and 190–325 µ thick at the junction of oviducts with the uterine horns. This is surrounded by a thin longitudinal muscle layer, 22–50 µ and 39–75 µ thick longitudinal muscle at the corresponding site (El-Sheikh and Abddelhadi, 1970,a). The height of the cilia of the surface epithelium decline progressively from 0 to 15th day post partum, remain almost unchanged between day 16 and 30, and then increase to reach normal height on day 60 post partum when the animals are in oestrus. The average height of the surface epithelium is about 31.5, 18.9, 18.2, 18.0, 21.9 and 36.5 µ on the gravid side oviduct; and 23.1, 18.3 15.7, 16.0, 16.8, 21.3 and 30.1 µ on the non-gravid side oviduct; on day 0, 7, 15, 30, 45 (non-cycling), 45 (cycling) and 60 (oestrus) post partum, respectively. A few goblet cells are found on the day of parturition and the day of oestrus, and it may be related with the release of secretion during these periods. The cell contents of the tunica propria are minimum on the day of parturition, increases during the next 6–7 weeks and then decreases during the oestrus. The tunica muscularis is formed of a thick inner layer of he circular muscle fibres and thin outer layer of the longitudinal muscle fibres. This layer is generally thicker at the isthmus and gradually reduced in thickness towards the fimbriae (Pandey and Roy, 1968, Raizada et al., 1978).

Uterus

The uterus of buffalo is distinguished into 3 parts, the 2 uterine cornua (hours), the body (corpus uteri) and the cervix (neck). This type of uterus is known as uterus bipartitus. It is a muscular and irregular tubular structure supported by the mesometrium portion of the broad ligament attached with the walls of the pelvis and abdomen. The size of the uterus increases in the subsequent pregnancies. The weight of the uterine horn of gravid side is almost double than the non gravid side on the day of parturition, which regresses rapidly up to day 30 post partum or the normal involution period (Table 6.3). The weight of corpus uteri horn caruncles also decreases (Agarwal et al., 1978). The gravid horn takes a little longer for complete involution than the non-gravid horn.

The wall of the uterus is made of four layers of tissues, i.e., the endometrium, the stratum compactum, the myometrium and the outer layer of peritoneum or serosa

TABLE 6.3: Mean weight (g) and measurements (cm) of the uterus at different Post partum interval in the river buffaloes

Parts of uterus	Day of calving	Post partum interval (days)				
		7	15	30	45	60
1	2	3	4	5	6	7
A. Average weight						
Corpus uteri	283 + 60	302 + 10	55 + 8.5	32 + 3.5	30 + 4.2	16 + 1.0
Caruncles of Corp Ut	22 + 1.2					
Gra horn	2800 + 75	1375 + 122	322 + 29	150 + 15	115 + 4	105 + 16
Caruncles of gr. horn.	600 + 46	210 + 17				
Non gravid horn (ngr)	1375	520 + 43	197 + 52	119 + 11	114 + 25	95 + 15
Caruncles of ngh	338 + 15	45 + 2				
B. Average measurements						
L of corpus uteri	9.7 + 1.9	8.2 + 0.8	3.5 + 0.5	2.6 + 0.3	2.3 + 0.4	1.7 + 0.1
Maximum width	15.0 + 2.4	14.5 + 2.2	6.0 + 2.2	4.8 + 0.4	4.2 + 0.7	3.7 + 0.3
Thickness	5.1 + 0.8	3.0 + 0.2	2.7 + 0.2	2.5 + 0.1	2.4 + 0.2	2.1 + 0.1
Fused Uterine cornua, L.	43 + 2.5	27 + 1.0	14 + 3.4	6.6 + 0.8	7.2 + 2.0	5.9 + 0.7
Maximum width	28 + 3.1	25 + 2.5	8.2 + 0.4	6.5 + 0.3	6.3 + 1.1	5.0 + 0.8
Gravid Uterine Horn						
L from bifurcation	63 + 1.0	72 + 1.5	38 + 4.8	23 + 0.6	19 + 3.0	17 + 1.2
L from Corpus uteri	104 + 5.4	93 + 1.1	53 + 3.7	32 + 0.2	23 + 2.3	26 + 2.4
Wth at corneal jnc.	17 + 1.8	12 + 2.1	5 + 0.2	4 + 0.2	3 + 0.1	2.9 + 0.3
Wth in middle	30 +2.3	15 +0.3	6 + 0.3	4 + 0.3	3 + 0.5	2.5 + 0.3
Wth at uterotubal jnc.	9 + 1.4	5 + 1.3	2 + 0.1	2 + 0.2	1.7 + 0.2	1.5 + 0.1
Thk at corneal jnc.	2.5 + 0.2	1.9 + 0.1	2.2 + 0.2	1.9 + 0.1	2.5 + 0.3	2.6 + 0.1
Thk in middle	2.1 + 0.3	1.7 + 0.1	1.8 + 0.1	1.6 + 0.3	1.7 + 0.1	1.4 + 0.1
Thk at uerotubal jnc.	1.8 + 0.2	1.4 + 0.2	0.7 + 0.1	1 + 0.2	0.9 + 0.1	1.0 + 0.1
Non gravid Uerine Horn (cornua)						
L from bifurcation	44 + 2.6	37 + 0.2	31 + 2.5	17 + 1.5	19 + 1.0	16 + 1.4
L from corpus uteri	86 + 3.5	53 + 1.0	43 + 4.1	24 + 2.0	23 + 1.2	22 + 1.9
Wdh at corneal jnc.	13 + 0.3	9 + 0.1	4 + 0.5	3.6 + 0.5	3.1 + 0.5	2.2 + 0.3
Wdh in middle	16 + 0.9	8 + 1.8	4 + 0.6	3.1 + 0.3	3.3 + 0.4	2.5 + 0.3
Wdh at uterotubal jnc.	6.5 + 0.4	5 + 0.4	2.2 + 0.1	1.8 + 0.0	1.7 + 0.2	1.7 + 0.1
Thk at corneal jnc	2.2 + 0.3	2.0 + 0.2	2.2 + 0.2	2.4 + 0.2	2.3 + 0.4	2.1 + 0.1
Thk in middle	1.8 + 0.1	1.4 + 0.1	1.5 + 0.2	1.7 + 0.2	1.5 + 0.1	1.2 + 0.2
Thk at uterotubal jnc	1.2 + 0.1	1.0 + 0.1	0.6 + 0.2	1.0 + 0.3	1.0 + 0.0	1.0 + 0.0

Note: gr = gravid; hrn = horn; jnc = junction; L = length; Thk = thickness

(Table 6.4). A significant increase takes place in the thickness and the volume of these layers during the oestrus and pregnancy. The number of caruncles (cotyledons) ranges from 105 to 172 arranged in 3–5 rows (Girish Chadra, 1979). The uterine caruncles are quite prominent, stalked and easily separable at the time of parturition, and their regression occurs earlier than the caruncles of the uterine horns. The regression of uterine caruncles is almost complete by day 15 and by day 30 post partum the uterine endometrium becomes apparently patent (Agarwal et al., 1978).

The endometrium can be differentiated into 4 areas i.e., a superficial layer of the psuedostratified columnar epithelium of 14–24 μ thickness, the stratum compactum, the stratum spongeosum and the stratum basalis. The thickness of the endometrium is maximum on the day of parturition and decreases thereafter to attain almost normal

TABLE 6.4: Average thickness (u) of the layers of the various uterine tissues at different postpartum interval (days)

Uterine wall layer	Day of partum	Postpartum interval (days)					
		7	15	30	45	60a	60b
1	2	3	4	5	6	7	8
Endometrium							
Corpus uteri	2713	2212	1730	1700	1650	2576	3000
Gra Ut cornua	4984	3054	1854	1850	2288	3033	2988
Ngra Ut cornua	3228	2943	1980	1700	1603	1833	2933
Corpus uteri	272	177	223	-	201	229	307
Gra Ut cornua	681	540	329	-	227	260	303
Ngra Ut cornua	519	490	369	-	273	230	307
Myometrium							
Corpus uteri	5666	7393	6570	6238	5862	4554	7513
Gra Ut cornua	5831	6382	6021	5575	4484	4539	4987
Ngr Ut cornua	6816	6090	4695	4702	4704	4717	4712
Perimetrium							
Corpus uteri	346	323	47	-	-	107	64
Gra Ut cornua	250	220	47	-	-	75	81
Ngr Ut cornua	313	205	34	-	-	58	76
Average height of the surface and glandular epithelium (u)							
Surface Epithelium							
Corpus uteri	15.3	15.6	20.0	-	-	28.8	17.4
Gra Ut cornua	16.6	24.0	29.8	-	34.2	33.1	29.4
Ngra Ut cornua	19.4	28.0	26.3	-	26.8	25.8	24.3
Glandular Epithelium							
Corpus uteri	24.0	19.2	15.7	12.9	15.2	18.7	27.2
Gra Ut cornua	20.5	17.6	19.0	-	-	24.7	27.2
Ngra Ut cornua	20.1	16.3	18.0	-	-	25.6	24.5
Uterine glands (outer diameter)							
Corpus uteri	101.4	77.7	51.0	-	-	70.5	100.8
Gra Ut cornua	118.5	69.3	60.2	70.8	76.8	71.5	83.8
Ngra Ut cornua	104.6	53.8	53.1	58.4	66.0	80.4	75.8

Note: Gra = gravid; Ngra = non gravid; Ut = uterine

thickness between 30–45 days post partum interval and again increases during the dioestrus and oestrus at about 45–60 days post partum in most of the animals. The lamina propria increases in volume at the time of parturition due to heavy oedema. The oedema of stratum spongeosum also occurs during the oestrus due to significant increase in the concentration of the oestrogen. The surface epithelium is generally absent from most of the surface probably due to the pressure of the developing embryo during the gestation period and also due to the phagocytic effect of the attantochorion. The epithelial height again increases during the post partum period to attain normal appearance by day 15 in the corpus uteri, about day 30 in the non gravid uterine horn and about day 45 in the gravid uterine horn, but they are shorter during the oestrus. The height is relatively more on the caruncles than the intercaruncular spaces. Similar changes are observed in the stratum compactum (Agarwal et al., 1978).

The uterine glands ramify in the stratum spongeosum and extend up to the statum basalis. They are coiled and tubular in structure and maximum coiling is observed during the early and mid stages dioestrus and anoestrus. The glands become more straight showing maximum height of the epithelium and minimum diameter of the lumen during the early and mid stages dioestrus and anoestrus. The glands become more straight showing maximum height of the epithelium and minimum diameter of the lumen during the metoestrus. The glandular epithelium is almost similar to the surface epithelium and does not contain ciliated cells. The height of the glandular epithelium is 20–25 µ in the stratum spongeosum and 5–7 µ in the stratum basalis (El- Sheikh and Abdelhadi, 1970a, Girish Chandra, 1979). The superficial glands are larger with distinct lumen while the deep one resembles the solid epithelial cords with undifferentiated lumen. The enlargement of the uterine glands during the pregnancy takes place for the supply of nutrients to the uterine glands during the pregnancy takes place for the supply of nutrients to the foetus through the histotrophic pathway. A few cells of the glandular epithelium are ciliated on the day of parturition but their number increases during the postpartum period reaching about 20% by the end of 45 days. The clear cells present in between the glandular cells on the day of parturition decrease subsequently and by the end of day 45 postpartum they are not seen (Agarwal et al., 1978).

The myometrium can be differentiated in to 3 zones, viz.,

 i. Stratum submucosa formed of the irregular circular, oblique and longitudinally arranged smooth muscle fibres. Its thickness ranges from 920 to 1670 µ,

 ii. Stratum vasculare is composed of loose connective tissue and irregular smooth muscle bundles. The rich vascularization gives it spongy appearance. It is 1130–1180 µ thick in the adult Egyptian buffaloes and

 iii. Stratum submucosa is 1240–2160 µ in thickness and contains longitudinal muscle bundle arranged into large faciculi by the inversion of the connective tissue from the perimetrium (El-Sheikh and Abdeladi, 1970a). The thickness of the myometrium increases many folds due to hyperplasia of the muscle cells.

The perimetrium or tunica serosa is formed of the fibro-elastic tissue containing collagenous fibres. The number and size of the elastic fibres and the thickness of the perimetrium increase during the oestrus period, increase many folds during the gestation period and reaching the maximum at the terminal stage of pregnancy.

The uterus performs many important reproductive functions like transport of the inseminated spermatozoa to the place of fertilization. The transport is assisted by the peristaltic contractions in the wall of the uterus and oviducts. The uterine contractions are controlled by the level of oestrogen and progesterone during the different stages of oestrus. The ovulation changes the trend of contractions and the uterus becomes quiescent before the migration of ovum in its lumen and remains so during the entire gestation period in the pregnant animals. The fertilized zygote is transplanted in one of the uterine horn where it is provided suitable environment for the normal development of foetus during the gestation period. The attachment between the maternal and the foetal components of the placentome begins to develop at the end of the first month of the pregnancy and it is fragile in early pregnancy. Numerous crypts develop on the surface of the maternal cotyledons and they appear congested and spongy. The development continues with the progress of the gestation period and firm attachment develops between the maternal and the foetal cotyledons. The number of maternal caruncles (cotyledons) may vary amongst the types, breeds and also individuals of the same category during different stages of foeta development (Hafez, 1954, Abdel-Raouf and El-Naggar, 1969, Girish Chandra, 1979, Raja Ram and Chandra, 1979). At the termination of the gestation period (300 to 330 days) the uterine contractions of very high intensity start for the expulsion of the foetus and the foetal membranes. After the parturition, rapid involution of the uterus takes place to regain almost normal size of non gravid stage in about 4–6 week. However 8–12 weeks post partum rest is normally suggested before rebreeding the females.

Cervix

The small muscular tube joining the corpus uteri with the vagina is called cervix or neck of the uterus. The luminal mucous membrane lining of the cervix is folded into few thick plica varying from 2 to 5 in different animals (Bhalla et al., 1964, Sane et al., 1964, Torres et al., 1980). The mucous lining of the cervix is formed by a single layer of columnar to cuboidal epithelium. There may be some patches of stratified columnar cells in the middle and terminal parts of the cervix. The cervical plica is formed of a central core of connective tissue, and the stroma of the cervix is composed of loose connective tussue having many smooth muscle fibres (El-Sheikh and Abdellhade, 1970, Girish Chandra, 1979). The cervix plays an active role in the transport of the spermatozoa and during the pregnancy its orifice is plugged by a highly viscid, thick and turbid mucous plug.

Vagina

The vagina is a posterior tubular connection of the reproductive tract extending from the cervix to the vulva. It is a common urinogential passage. The recto-genital pouch of peritoneum holds the vagina in position beneath the terminal part of the rectum. The wall of the vagina is relatively thinner than the wall of the uterus. The mucous membrane of the vagina is thrown into many longitudinal folds, which are relatively higher and flexuous towards the cervical end. The epithelial linning varies from simple columnar to stratified columnar cells. The height of superficial epithelium ranges from 15 μ to 23 μ and that lining the vaginal crypts is about 32 μ. Goblet cella are clearly present. The stroma is composed of the irregular bundles of the smooth muscle fibres and loose connective tissue richly ramified with the blood vessels and nerve fibres. The epithelial layer of stroma is lined by 1 to 9 layers of the stratified polyhedral cells (El-Sheikh and Abdellhadi, 1970a, Girish Chandra, 1979). The vagina is the organ of coitus and semen is deposited in it for transportation to the cervical reservoirs and the uterus. Its wall is highly flexible and extensive dilatztion occurs at the time of parturition.

Vulva or External Genitalia

The external genitalia includes the 2 labiae, the vestibule, the clitoris, the dorsal and vental commissures and the suburethral diverticulum. The vulva is a somewhat inverted cone shaped structure located beneath the anus. Its dorsal commissure is more or less arched while ventral one is tapering. The outer skin is wrinkled due to several folds. The glans clitoris is rudimentary structure and a distict fossa clitoris is absent. On the dorsal surface of the suburethral diverticulum a tubercle presents the V-shaped external urethral opening on the ventral aspect of the vulva. The vestibule or Bartholin's glands are found as 2 to 3 pin head sized glandular masses laterally present in the wall of the suburethral diveritculum (Girish Chandra, 1979).

▶ THE PUBERTY

Puberty is a stage of growth at which secondary sexual characteristics appear in the animals for the first time. It is influenced by the growth of body, functional development of the reproductive organs and endocrine glands involved in various reproductive functions. The sequence of the growth of the reproductive organs may be phased as the development of adenohypophysis (posterior pituitary) gland in the early post natal life., which stimulates the ovarian activities and finally both the glands play active role in the development of the uterus.

Buffaloes are considered late maturing animals attaining puberty at 2–4 years of age in the tropical countries (Dave, 1940, Mcgregor, 1941, Leupold, 1968). This observation is applicable to buffalo rearing in backyard system of management on low level of nutrition prevalent in most of the tropical countries. The age at puberty can be significantly reduced to even less than 1 year on raising the heifers on high plane of nutrition (Mohammed et al., 1980). Feeding of adequate balanced rations support higher growth by providing conditions for genetic expression including the development of the reproductive organs which significantly reduces the age at puberty to less than 2 years (El-Nauty, 1971; Franciscis, 1979, Mudgal, 1979, Polikhronov and Peeva, 1982). For optimum production life, buffaloes should be preferably bred for the first time at 18–24 month of age on attaining about 75% of the mature body weight.

▶ THE OESTRUOUS CYCLE

The specialized rhythmical reproductive changes in pubertal and post pubertal active reproductive life of mammalian females is known as oestrous cycle. The oestrous strats at puberty which is influenced by several factors like inherent character of the breed, the agroclimatic conditions, the nutritional status and the management practices. Poor nutrition and harsh climatic conditions adversely affect the health and reproduction functions (Bassir, 1968). The growth rate and levels of various hormones involved in different reproductive activities are the most important factors which control the oestrous cycle. The follicle stimulating hormone (FSH) of the adenohypophysis stimulates the development of ovarian follicles, and during the development of ovarian follicles the ovaries start the synthesis of another important hormone, oestrogen. The increase in production of oestrogen reaches a periodic peak at which females show the apparent signs of oestrous (heat). They become receptive to the bull and allow coitus. Another hormone of the adenohypophysis known as leutinizing hormone (LH) causes the ovulation and initiates the formation of corpus luteum. The corpus luteum (CL) starts the production of progesterone which inhibits the development and maturation of the other follicles. The progesterone brings significant changes in the uterus for providing suitable environment for development of the zygote. In the absence of conception, the activity of CL is normally ceases in 15–20 days. This is followed by the development of next follicle due to stimulation by the FSH. The oestrous cycle continues at an interval of 20–37 days in different types and breeds of buffaloes during the active breeding season (Kaleff, 1942, Hafez, 1952, Bhattacharya, 1954, Roy et al., 1968, Kemonpatana et al., 1979). The buffaloes have been identified as seasonally polyoestrous. The intensity of oestrous in hot season is either quiescent or there may be complete anoestrous. However, this is not true for the buffaloes raised in the less fluctuating hot-humid climate of the southern region of the Socialist Republic of Vietnam (Verma et al., 1984).

▶ PHASES OF THE OESTRUOUS CYCLE

The oestrous cycle of buffaloes may be divided into 5 phases, viz. proestrous, oestrous, metoestrous, dioestrous and anoestrous.

Proestrous: The short period before the onset of oetrous is known as proestrous. In this period ovaries are more active and FSH stimulates the development of the Graafian follicles which sectete more oestrogen. This phase is also known as the follicular phase or oestrogenic phase. The size of tubular genitalia increases and the endometrium becomes congested due to increased supply and oedemous swelling. Its duration may be 15 hours to 2 days (Wang et al., 1975).

Oestrous: Oestrous or heat is the period when female buffaloes become receptive. It is characterized by the typical breeding behaviour (Janakiraman, 1979). There is strin like transparent glossy discharge from the vagina and marked oedematous swelling of the internal and external genital organs (Riazada et al., 1978). The cervical mucous is highly elastic and it lasts for 12–48 hours in different types of buffaloes (Hafez, 1952, Singh et al., 1984).

Metoestrous: Immediately after the oestrous phase the granuloma cells of the ovulated Graafian follicle produce lutein cells and formation of the corpus luteum starts. There is sharp reduction in the secretion of oestrogen and cervical mucous. The external and internal genital organs shrink to original size.

Dioestrous: In this phase active development of corpus luteum occurs, which secretes significantly higher amount of progesterone. In pregnant animals CL persists during the gestation period for the maintenance of pregnancy. It is also called luteal phase of the oestrous cycle. In the absence of fertilization the dioestrous phase extends from 10–20 days.

Anoestrous: Dry hot climatic conditions suppress reproductive functions in buffaloes, which results in the prolonged anoestrous phase. During this period ovaries are smooth and quiescent. The development of follicles is almost absent and CL is also non-funtional.

Postpartum Oestrous: The first appearance of oestrous signs after the parturition is called postpartum oestrous, and the length of time between the parturition and the appearance of following oestrous is called postpartum oestrous interval. This may range from as little as 10 to even longer than 410 days (Ocampo, 1939, Mcgregor, 1941, Hafez, 1952, El-Dessouky and Rakha, 1964, Rao et al., 1973, Wang Pei Chien, 1979). Ameliorative measures for reducing the heat stress significantly reduce the postpartum oestrous interval and improve fertility (Roy and Pandey, 1971, Mehta et al., 1979).

Gestational Oestrous: This is an abbresion of reproductive physiology. The appearance of signs of oestrous during pregnancy is called gestational oestrous. It occurs generally during the first 3–4 months of gestation period and incidence may be 6–18% (Luktuke et al., 1964, El-Wishy, 1979).

The duration of Oestrous or Oestrous period: Average duration of oestrous in the normal cycling buffaloes is about 24 hours in most of the riverine breeds of the Indian subcontinent, 12–36 hours in the Egyptian, 24–36 hours in the Bulgarian and 36 hours in the swamp and Murrah buffaloes of the Thailand (Hafez, 1952, Chantalakhana, 1979). In some animals the duration of oestrous may vary from a short 3 hours to long 72 hours and is influenced by feeding, management and climatic conditions (Bhattacharya, 1954, Ishaque, 1956, Khanau and Shimizu, 1982).

▶ **THE SIGNS OF OESTRUOUS OR HEAT**

The intensity of heat is generally lower in buffaloes (Hafez, 1952, Luktuke and Rao, 1954) which becomes still weaker during the hot season (Rao et al., 1968, Gill and Gangwar, 1972). The problem of oestrous detection in buffaloes is one of the main constraints of efficient breeding (Rife, 1959, Roy and Pandey, 1971 and Kamonpatana et al., 1979). The incidence of silent or quiescent heat is very high in buffaloes due to which many animals are left unbred. The intensity of oestrous may be classified as normal, medium and weak, and has been recorded in about 18, 17 and 55% cases in a small study of 164 oestrouses (Roy and Pandey, 1971). The incidence of silent heat may be responsible for about 81% occurrence of long cycles in the buffaloes (El-Sheikh and El-Fouly, 1971a).

Diurinal oestrous behavior is quite common in the buffaloes and majority breed in the cool hours of morning, night and evening (Macgregor, 1941, Hafez, 1954, Luktuke and Ahuka, 1961, Gill and Gangwar, 1972, Agarwal and Pandey, 1983) which is contrary to earlier report of nocturnal mating in swamp buffaloes (Macgregor, 1941). The various signs of oestrous observed in different breeds (Table 6.5) showed great variations (Toelitere. 1980b, Vale, 1983, Danell et al., 1984, Ullah and Usmani, 1985).

TABLE 6.5: Signs of oestrous/heat in buffaloes (% activity)

Signs of Oestrous	Nili-Ravi	Surti	Brazil	Swamp
Swollen vulva	96.0	100.0	42.0	31.8
Raised tail	20.0	100.0	42.0	25.3
Frequent urination	-	27.6	54.0	-
Bellowing	8.0	24.1	50.3	29.5
Mounting/Mounted	24.0	20.7	19.3	58.1
Restless	-	10.3	-	13.1
Loss of appetite	4.0	3.4	-	29.7
Mucous discharge	96.0	100.0	60.6	25.3

Seasonal variations in oestrous behaviour of buffaloes are quite common and most of the classical signs of oestrous are either undetectable or absent during the unfavourable breeding seasons, i.e. summer and hot-humid monsoon (Table 6.6). In Surti buffaloes the common signs of oestrous are more pronounced in the winter season. Frequent urination may be one of the important visible sign of oestrous in Surti (Janakiraman, 1979).

TABLE 6.6: Signs of oestrous in Surti buffaloes during different season

Signs of oestrous	Winter	Summer	Monsoon
Bellowing	Present	Absent	Absent
Mucous discharge	Present	Absent	Present
Swollen vulva	Present	Absent	May be in few
Restlessness	Present	Absent	Present
Frequent micturition	Present	Present	Present
Uterine tone	Present	In few cases	Present
Open cervix	Present	Present	Present

The intensity of oestrous may be classified as good or normal, medium and weak on the basis of the external signs of oestrous and rectal palpation of the tubular genitalia for the degree of uterine tone and the condition of the Graafian follicle (Roy and Pandey, 1971). During the oestrous mature Graafian follicle is more than 10 mm in diameter and palpable as turbid area slightly bulging from the surface of the ovary. On examination with laproscope the mature Graafian follicle appears thin walled and translucent bulging area on the surface of the ovary, and on rectal palpation it gives a soft fluctuation feel on the day of oestrous (Jainudeen et al., 1983).

▶ **HEAT DETECTION**

Since there is a great variation in the intensity of oestrous and the incidence of silent heat is high in the buffaloes, a combination of different procedures should be adopted for the detection of oestrous (Pandey et al., 1979).

1. A vasectomised or tearser bull should be paraded in the sheds/herd of breedable buffaloes twice daily, i.e. in the morning before 8 am and in the evening after 5 pm. during the normal breeding season. The frequency of teaser parade may be increased to 3 times a day during the off season when the intensity of oestrous in very low in most of the females. The third period may be at noon but it may be better to parade at equal interval with necessary adjustment of the time.
2. The breedable open buffaloes should be checked frequently for the vaginal discharge. The ventral aspect of tail should be examined for the smearing of the vaginal discharge. The cervical mucous flows as a string from the vulva of females in heat.
3. The cervical mucous should be examined for the crystallization pattern, which is usually fern like in oestrous.
4. The genitalia is examined per rectum for the uterine tone and palpation of the mature Graafian follicle on the ovary.
5. Breeding bulls and females should be provided protection from the solar exposure during the hot season and also from the extreme climatic changes. Some cooling arrangement should be made for the amelioration of the heat stress.
6. Buffaloes showing long oestrous period should be inseminated 2 times or given double service at the interval of 8–12 hours.

▶ **OVULATION**

Ovulation is perhaps a gradual process and normally one ovum is shed out at a time in buffaloes. Incidence of double or triple ovulation is less than 1% (El-Sheikh and

El-Fouly, 1971a). Right ovary has been found to be more functional than the left one as evident from the higher rate of ovulation in the right ovary (Hafez, 1955; Wang et al., 1965; Roy and Pandey, 1971). Ovulation normally occurs after the end of the oestrous period and time of ovulation may vary from 0 to 40 hours from the end of the oestrous (Luktuke and Ahuja, 1961, El-Sheikh and El-Fouly, 1971b, Roy and Pandey, 1971, Jainudeen, 1977, Kanai and Shimizu, 1982). Some reports have shown ovulation after 16 hours of the onset of oestrous (Shalash, 1958; Basirov, 1964; Singh et al., 1984). The incidence of silent ovulation is quite high in buffaloes, which is maximum in the hot season. Most of the short oestrous cycles are non-ovulatory, while largest silent ovulation is associated with the long oestrous cycle (El-Sheikh and El-Fouly, 1971a, b, Borady et al., 1982).

▶ SEASONALITY OF SEXUAL ACTIVITY

The seasonality of breeding is one of the important function limiting the overall production of the buffaloes. This is due to a very high incidence of anoestrum and silent oestrous during the hot season in tropical countries (Dave, 1938; Venkayya and Anantakrishnan, 1957; Singh et al., 1966; Majeed et al., 1974; Agarwal and Purbey, 1983).

▶ FERTILIZATION

The biological union of a viable ovum and spermatozoan is called fertilization. The process of fertilization uncludes (i) the transportation of ovum into the oviductm. (ii) the transportation of spermatozoa into the oviduct, (iii) the penetration of a potent spermatozoan into the ovum and (iv) the formation and fusion of the male and female pronuclei (syngamy). The site of fertilization in buffaloes is normally the upper third of the oviduct or ampullar region (Roy and Pandey, 1971).

After deposition of the semen in the genitalia of female certain changes take place in the spermatozoa which are necessary for the fertilization of ovum. The spermatozoa in semen do not have all the properties of fertilization. During the course of traveling through the cervical mucous following changes take place in the spermatozoa and the process is called capacitation:

  i.   Elevation occurs in ionic strength of the sperm contents.
 ii.   The oxygen intake rate of spermatozoa is increased.
iii.   Adenyl cyclase activity of the sperm is increased.
 iv.   An increase occurs in the potassium: sodium ratio and cyclic adenosine monophospahte.

After capacitation the spermatozoa can achieve fertilization by actively penetrating into the ovum. During penetration, the acrosomal enzyme viz. hyaluronidase, corona penetrating enzyme and acrosin of the spermatozoa play a catalytic role (Mc Roie and Williams, 1974). The penetration of outer layer of the ovum, cumulus oopharus is activated by hyaluronidase, corona radiate by corona penetrating enzyme and zona pellucida by acrosin for final fertilization. Normally one spermatozoan penetrates the zona pellucida and at the time of penetration specific reaction of sperm head with vitellus makes the membrane nonresponsive for the penetration of sperm head with vitellus makes the membrane nonresponsive for the penetration of the other spermatozoa. In some abnormal conditions more than 1 spermatozoa may enter into the ovum, and it is called polyspermy. The occurrence is very rare and results in the failure of the zygote development and extremely rarely in the development of abnormal foetus.

Implantation: After fertilization the zygote is carried down the oviduct and it has a loose outer membrane while entering the uterine cornua. The early cleavage of the zygote may occur in the fallopian tube and at about 8 cell stage it enters into the uterine cornua. The development of vesicle or embryonic membrane occurs with the cell division of the embryo, which lies in close contant with the uterine lining. A firm attachment between the maternal and foetal cotyledons occurs after about 34 days of the gestation period and implantation starts during this period. The elevation of uterine cotyledons starts but foetal cotyledons are not visible on the chorion (Roy and Pandey, 1971).

Development of Embryo: The early embryonic development after the fertilization takes place in the fallopian tube up to 4 cells cleavage in about 3 days after the insemination. It is difficult to determine fertilization in single cell stage due to presence of the large number of fat globules in the vitellus. The 8 and 12 celled zygotes are present in the uterine cornua on fifth day post service. At day 10 of gestation period the embryo is a multicellular honeycomb like morula. At this stage the cells shrink away from the zona pellucida leaving behind a large perivitelline space indicating the blastocyst stage in some of the buffaloes. The early blastocysts are oblong-shaped. Late blastocysts are seen at 15–16 days post service and they are thin white elongated structures. The embryos. Obtained on day 34 post service had vertebral column imprint, formed eyes and limb buds (Table 6.7). The embryonic membranes had an average length of 60 cm occupying the entire gravid horn and also extending partly into the non-gravid horn

TABLE 6.7: Development of ovum and embryo at different post service intervals in early pregnancy

S.No.	Interval from the end of oestrous	Development stage of ovum/embryo	Dimension (Length × Breadth)	Site of recovery
1.	Late oestrous	Single cell	-	Mature Graafian follicle
2.	9 h	Single cell	154 μ 154 μ	Do
3.	10 h	Single cell	133 μ 126 μ	Do
4.	14 h	Single cell	234 μ 233 μ	Do
5.	20 h	Single cell	91 μ 84 μ	Do
6.	Day 3	Single cell	180 μ 132 μ	do
7.	Do	Single cell	172 μ 156 μ	Do
8.	Do	2 cells	160 μ 146 μ	Do
9.	Do	4 cells	-	Do
10.	Day 5	8 cells	98 μ 91 μ	Uterine cornua
11.	Do	12 cells	112 μ 108 μ	Do
12.	Day 10	Blastocyst	436 μ 364 μ	Do
13.	Do	Blastocyst	419 μ 258 μ	Do
14.	Do	Morula	105 μ 91 μ	Do
15.	Do	Morula	161 μ 154 μ	Do
16.	Day 15	Blastocyst	3.28 cm 1.7 mm	Do
17.	Do	Blastocyst	3.80 cm 2.00	Do
18.	Day 34	Embryo	1.70 cm 1.40 cm	Do
19.	Do	Embryo	1.70 cm 1.30 cm	Do
20.	Do	Embryo	1.75 cm 1.25 cm	Do

through the corpus uteri. No physical connection develops between the chorion and the mucosa of the uterus up to this stage but they lie in close opposition (Roy and Pandey, 1971).

The sex of the foetus can be identified at about 6 weeks gestation period. The size of fetuses of the Surti buffaloes at 30 to 228 days gestation period (Table 6.8) shows 3 stages of significant incat about day 45, day 114 and day 148 of pregnancy (Kodagali and Deshpandey, 1969).

TABLE 6.8: Size of foetuses of Surti buffalo at different interval of gestation period

S.No.	Age (days)	Weight (g)	Length of embryo in cm		Sex
			Pin to crown	Pin to shoulder	
1	2	3	4	5	6
1.	20	0.12	-	-	-
2.	35	0.18	-	-	-
3.	40	0.32	1.5	-	-
4.	45	0.89	2.1	-	Male
5.	45	-	2.3	1.5	Female
6.	56	5.2	4.0	2.2	Male
7.	58	5.7	4.0	2.5	Male
8.	62	7.5	5.0	2.6	Male
9.	63	11.2	5.0	2.6	Male
10.	64	13.0	5.2	3.2	Female
11.	66	13.2	5.3	3.3	Male
12.	67	12.9	5.5	3.4	Male
13.	75	25.0	6.1	3.5	Female
14.	76	24.2	6.5	3.6	Female
15.	77	22.0	6.5	4.0	Male
16.	78	25.8	6.5	3.8	Female
17.	90	25.7	6.6	3.9	Male
18.	91	39.3	8.9	5.5	Male
19.	93	39.8	9.1	5.5	Female
20.	93	42.0	9.0	5.8	Female
21.	93	44.0	9.1	5.5	Male
22.	93	40.2	9.5	5.5	Male
23.	93	42.2	9.0	5.9	Male
24.	94	44.1	9.5	5.7	Female
25.	94	46.2	9.7	5.6	Female
26.	95	50.8	10.0	5.8	Female
27.	103	69.8	12.3	7.1	Female
28.	104	69.6	12.3	7.1	Male
29.	106	76.0	12.5	7.2	Female
30.	114	84.4	13.2	7.3	Female
31.	116	139.1	14.0	8.5	Female
32.	120	140.0	15.0	9.0	Female
33.	124	200.0	16.0	10.0	Female

Contd.

TABLE 6.8: Size of fetuses of Surti buffalo at different interval of gestation period *(Contd.)*

S.No.	Age (days)	Weight (g)	Length of embryo in cm		Sex
			Pin to crown	Pin to shoulder	
1	2	3	4	5	6
34.	126	199.0	16.0	10.3	Male
35.	135	273.0	19.0	12.2	Male
36.	135	300.5	19.0	12.0	Male
37.	137	323.5	19.7	13.0	Male
38.	140	422.0	21.5	13.5	Female
39.	148	800.0	23.0	15.0	Male
40.	176	-	32.0	19.5	Female
41.	201	-	37.0	24.7	Male
42.	228	-	49.0	30.3	Male

▶ PREGNANCY

Pregnancy is one of the most important reproductive functions of female. The process of of hosting, nourishing and providing optimum environment in utro for the development of th embryo from the date of conception to the date of parturition is known as pregnancy. In buffaloes the development of foestus takes place in the uterine horn and involvement of the right horn is generally more than the left horn. This is due to higher activity of the right ovary (Reddy, 1960, Faszil, 1970, Reddy and Rai, 1979). Migration of zygote is also observed in some buffaloes (El-Wishy, 1979).

Gestation Period

The time required for carrying the developing foetus from the date conception to the date of parturition is known as gestation period. The development of foestus and thus the gestation period is affected by several factors like type of buffalo, breed, parity, age at calving, season of breeding, sex of the calf and nutritional status of the dam (Table 6.9). Average gestation period usually exceeds 300 days. It is shortest in Murrah,

TABLE 6.9: Effect of various factors on gestation period of buffaloes

S.No.	Factors	Gestation Period (days)	
		Range	Mean
1	2	3	4
1.	**Type/Breed**		
	Murrah	270–339	305
	Nili-Ravi	285–325	306
	Marathawada	-	309
	Surti	299–325	312
	Jaffarabadi/Jafari		316
	Egyptian		316
	Italian	287–337	311
	Bulgarian		315
	Russian		318

Contd.

TABLE 6.9: Effect of various factors on gestation period of buffaloes (*Contd.*)

S.No.	Factors	Gestation Period (days)	
		Range	Mean
1	2	3	4
	Chinese swamp		312
	Indian swamp	290–336	315
	Malayan swamp	320–340	332
	Philippines swamp	291–335	314
	Taiwan swamp		315
	Thialand swamp		330
2.	**Sex of Calf**		
	Murrah:		
	Male		306
	Female		305
	Egyptian:		
	Male		317.5
	Female		315.8
3.	**Parity (Nili-Ravi)**		
	Primiparous		318.5
	Pluriparous		308.7
4.	**Season of calving (Murrah)**		
	Summer	270–332	303.8
	Monsoon	272–339	305.0
	Winter	285–332	305.7
5.	**Month of insemination**		
	January		308.9
	March		315.1
6.	**Effect of sire**		
	Buffalo Bull No.		
	1		310.9
	2		311.7
	3		311.9
	4		311.9
	5		312.4
	6		314.1
7.	**Calving sequence**		
	First		308.1
	Second		309.6
	Third		318.7
	Fourth		309.6
	Fifth		304.5
	Sixth		311.2
	Seventh		313.6
	Eight		308.8

Nili-Ravi and Kundi (Arunachalam et al., 1952, Nambier and Raja, 1962, Wahid, 1975), longer is Surti, Jaffarabadi, Italian, Egyptian, Bulgarian and Russian buffaloes (Dave, 1940, Maymone, 1942, Ahmed and Tantawy, 1956, Kerur and Kodagali, 1969, Polikhronvo et al., 1978) and longest in most of the swamp buffaloes of south-east Asian countries (Jainudeen, 1977, Chantalakhana, 1979).

Formation of Placenta

In the early gestation period the embryo receives nutrients from the uterine milk (Fluid) for few days. During the differentiation of the 3 germinal layers (entoderm, mesoderm and ectoderm) the embryonic membranes are also formed. The amnion is formed by a fold of mesoderm and ectoderm, and the allantois is formed from the hind gut of the embryo. The allantois together with the serosa form the chorion, which is a 4 layered membrane an completely surrounds the embryo, amnion and allantoic cavity. This membrane is extensively ramified by the blood vessels and lies close to the uterine mucosa. This close contact facilitates the exchange of gases and nutrients between the vascular system of the embryo and the blood vessels of the dam through the processes of osmosis and diffusion.

The placenta is formed by a close union between the chorion and the uterine mucosa, which is cotylendonary type. Histologically this type of placenta is known as syndesmo-chorial type and it is characterized by the absence of uterine epithelium over the caruncles. Attachement between the maternal caruncles and the cotyledons of the foetal membrane increases with the advancement of the gestation period being maximum during mid pregnancy. The foetal cotyledons attached with the maternal caruncles (maternal cotyledons) through villi are known as placentomes. The placentomes are differentiated into (i) the placentomes and (ii) the interplacental areas.

The placental membrane is formed of 6 layers comprising 3 each of maternal and foetal origin. The maternal layers are the endothelial lining of the endometrial blood vessels, endometrial connective tissue and endometrial lining of the crypts. The foetal layers include the chorionic villus lining epithelium, chorionic villus connective tissue and chorionic villus core blood vessel endothelium (Yap, 1974).

Placentome

The placentome is usually a mushroom shaped structure having a free convex surface and a short and broad stalk. The stalk of placentome develops from the elevation of the underlying endometrial stratum compactum including parts of the stratum spongiosum beneath (Yap, 1974). The number of placentomes (Table 6.10) and their number is normally more in gravid than the non-gravid uterine horn (Hafez, 1954a, Abdel-Raouf and El-Naggar, 1969, Raja Ram and Girish Chandra, 1979). The shape of placentomes is spherical, bean or kidney shaped or horse shoe shaped during early pregnancy; mushroom shaped and elliptical during mid-pregnancy; and elliptical, beaded and irregular shaped in late pregnancy (Raja Ram and Girish Chandra, 1984). The surface of larger placentomes mostly had a honeycomb like central depression, which becomes prominent after about 17–18 cm crown-rump length (CRL) of the foetus. These depression are formed by the interconnections between the adjoining maternal septae. Large variation has been observed in the size of maternal cotyledons and placentome (Table 6.11), which are generally larger in gravid than the non-gravid uterine horn (Raja Ram and Girish Chandra, 1979).

TABLE 6.10: Number of placentomes in different phases of gestation in buffaloes

CRL (cm)	Number of placentomes		
	Gravid horn	Non-gravid horn	Total
Early pregnancy (CRL < 9 cm)			
1.2	48	44	92
2.0	46	44	90
2.5	48	39	87
3.0	49	36	85
4.5	54	48	102
5.6	58	50	108
8.5	57	53	110
9.0	58	53	111
Mid-pregnancy (CRL, 10–37 cm)			
10.4	63	58	121
11.0	62	55	117
13.5	69	59	128
15.9	72	60	132
17.0	74	61	135
17.4/17.5	71	55	126
18.5	61	53	114
19.5	80	72	153
21.0	67	52	119
24.5	82	71	153
25.5	84	77	161
30.0	84	74	158
31.5–32.2	83	71	154
33–34	89	80	169
36–37	83	74	157
Late pregnancy (CRL > 37 cm)			
39.0	60	39	99
40.0	60	38	98
42.0	52	36	88
50.0	52	38	90
58.0	61	36	97
60.0	54	33	87
72.0	47	30	77

TABLE 6.11: The size of maternal cotyledons and placentomes of buffaloes

Attributes	Length, cm		Breadth, cm		Height, cm	
	Range	Mean	Range	Mean	Range	Mean
Gravid horn						
Early pregnancy, Maternal cotyledons	0.6–17	1.0	0.5–0.9	0.7	0.2–0.6	0.4
Mid pregnancy Maternal cotyledons	0.4–2.5	1.9	0.3–1.8	1.1	0.2–1.1	0.8
Placentomes	1.9–6.0	5.8	0.8–3.6	2.8	0.3–3.1	1.7

Contd.

TABLE 6.11: The size of maternal cotyledons and placentomes of buffaloes (*Contd.*)

Attributes	Length, cm		Breadth, cm		Height, cm	
	Range	Mean	Range	Mean	Range	Mean
Non-gravid horn						
Early pregnancy	0.2–1.1	0.7	0.4–0.7	0.6	0.2–0.4	0.3
Mid pregnancy						
Maternal cotyledons	0.5–2.2	1.4	0.2–1.6	0.9	0.3–0.6	0.5
Placentomes	1.0–3.8	3.5	0.8–2.3	2.1	0.6–1.9	1.4

Interplacentomal Area or Intercotyledonary Area

The space in between the placentomes is formed of intercaruncular endometrium of the maternal layers of placenta and the corresponding foestal chorionic leaves. Intercaruncular epithelium is almost flattened in early pregnancy and becomes increasingly folded and congested with the progress of gestation forming shallow crypts during mid and late pregnancy. The surface appears considerably wrinkled in late gestation and interplacentomal interval increases. The chorion layer is soft and delicate in early pregnancy, which gradually turns tough and folded with the progress of gestation period (Raja Ram and Girish Chandra, 1984).

Functions of Placenta

The placenta provides optimum environment for the normal development of the foetus *in utero*. Main functions of placenta are:

1. Transport of nutrients from mother to the developing foestus by diffusion through the placenta, by active transportation by phagocytosis and also by pinocytosis.
2. **Exchange of gases:** Oxygenated blood carried from mother to foetus through branches of the umbilical vessels. Oxygen is readily dissolved in low pH of placental fluid and released for the foetal haemoglobin. The carbon dioxide is simultaneously transferred from the foetal circulation to maternal circulation.
3. **Transfer of water:** More than three-fourth of the total substances supplied from mother to foetus is water. Water moves from mother to foestus against the osmotic gradient and low concentration of plasma proteins.
4. **Hormone synthesis:** Various hormones synthesized by the placenta are the oestrogen, progesterone and gonadotrophins. In addition to hormones some nutrients are also synthesized from the ingredients supplied by the mother.
5. **Barrier:** Placenta acts as a selective barrier and prevents the entry of many bacteria, protozoa an several harmful substances of feeds absorbed in the maternal circulation. However, unlike many species the entry of ascarid larvae through placenta to foetus has been often reported.
6. **Excretion:** The excretory products like urea is transported back in to the maternal circulation through the placenta.

▶ PARTURITION

Expulsion of foetus after the gestation period is called parturition. It is also refered as calving, natural bith or eutokia. It is a normal physiological function of the mammalian females. Although parturition is coordinated by several physical. Neural, biochemical and hormonal factors, the role of hormones has been found to be more important. At the end of the gestation period there is rise in the level of oestrogen which sensifizez uterus for the action of oxytocin release in large quantity from the posterior lobe of the pituitary gland. The level of oxytocin in the blood is very low at the onset of parturition, increases significantly during the expultion of foestus and then falls down gradually. The blood level of progesterone decreases due to gradual degeneration of the corpus luteum of pregnancy. During this period secretion of relaxin causes relaxation of the pelvic ligament to facilitate the dilatation of the pelvic outlet during the expulsion of foestus. The process of parturition is enhanced by the contraction of the abdominal and uterine muscles, the complete process is known as labour, and the intense pain experienced by the mother is called labour pain.

Symptoms of Approaching Parturition

It is difficult to determine the exact date of parturition due to considerable variation in gestation period but certain prominent changes occur in the animals while approaching parturition. The symptoms being significant increase in the size of udder and teasts, relaxation of the sacrociatic ligament and the size of vulva (Table 6.12 A,B,C). These changes are more in primiparous than in the pluriparous buffaloes . the udder and teats become voluminous, hard and tender in the last month of pregnancy. The vulva becomes voluminous, hard and tender in the last month of pregnancy. The vulva

TABLE 6.12A: Changes in the mammary glands in pregnant Murrah buffaloes approaching parturition

Month of	Size of udder (cm)			Size of teats (cm)			
	Length	Width	Depth	Length		Diameter between	
				Fore	Rear	Fore	Rear
Primiparous							
9	37.05	18.10	11.46	7.40	6.03	9.50	7.07
	+ 1.10	+ 0.30	+0.48	+ 0.34	+ 0.19	+ 0.15	+ 0.21
10	48.00	26.12	16.61	9.42	7.29	12.10	8.89
	+ 1.58	+ 0.95	+0.55	+ 0.34	+0.21	+0.32	+ 0.20
Calving day	51.38	27.91	18.04	9.50	7.50	12.79	9.40
	+ 1.64	+ 1.02	+ 0.54	+0.34	+ 0.22	+ 0.34	+ 0.20
Pluriparous I (2nd and 3rd calving)							
9	42.08	22.53	11.21	7.81	7.54	8.93	7.03
	+ 1.93	+ 1.09	+ 0.48	+ 0.36	+ 0.32	+ 0.61	+0.49
10	54.46	27.41	15.15	10.01	8.74	10.01	8.36
	+ 2.12	+ 1.46	+ 0.81	+ 0.38	+ 0.32	+ 0.41	+ 0.48
Calving day	56.59	28.40	16.71	10.48	9.18	10.55	8.86
	+ 2.14	+ 1.06	+ 0.83	+ 0.37	+ 0.31	+ 0.45	+ 0.47
Pluriparous II (4th onwards)							
9	52.28	23.14	12.75	7.61	8.02	9.08	7.18
	+ 2.29	+ 1.48	+ 0.61	+ 0.72	+ 0.65	+ 0.92	+ 0.77
10	59.82	28.14	16.78	9.05	9.20	11.12	8.61
	+ 2.22	+ 1.75	+ 0.51	+ 0.66	+ 0.63	+ 1.05	+ 0.61
Calving day	62.92	39.64	17.85	9.70	9.75	11.68	9.27
	+ 1.16	+ 1.48	+ 0.50	+ 0.62	+ 0.67	+ 0.97	+ 0.69

TABLE 6.12B: Mean relaxation (cm) in the sacrosciatic ligament of Murrah buffaloes approaching parturition

Month of	Primiparous	Pluriparous I	Pluriparous II
9	3.62 + 0.32	3.90 + 0.34	4.44 + 0.29
Relative	100	100	100
10	5.24 + 0.37	5.48 + 0.24	6.14 + 0.36
Relative	144.75	140.51	138.29
Calving day	5.86 + 0.31	5.93 + 0.24	6.18 + 0.45
Relative	161.88	152.05	153.38

TABLE 6.12C: Mean increase in the size of vulva of Murrah buffaloes approaching calving

Size of vulva (cm)	Month of pregnancy		Day of calving
	9th	10th	
Primiparous			
Length (cm)	10.35 + 0.59	13.72 + 0.92	15.60 + 0.59
Relative%	100	132.56	150.72
Width (cm)	5.61 + 0.44	8.83 + 0.48	10.12 + 0.43
Relative, %	100	157.40	180.39
Pluriparous I			
Length (cm)	11.67 + 0.77	14.25 + 0.83	15.33 + 0.81
Relative	100	122.11	131.36
Width (cm)	7.33 + 0.77	9.46 + 0.91	10.18 + 0.91
Relative,%	100	129.06	138.88
Pluriparous II			
Length (cm)	12.37 + 0.66	16.42 + 1.13	16.81 + 1.04
Relative, %	100	132.74	135.89
Width (cm)	7.70 + 0.99	10.70 + 1.42	11.68 + 1.47
Relative, %	100	138.96	151.69

becomes large, oedematous, soft and flabby. The mucous membrane is hyperaemic and secretion of mucous increases and becomes copious with the onset of parturition. Due to significant relaxation of the sacrosciatic ligament the space on either side of the sacral vertebrae appears sunken. The root of the tail appears prominently elevated. The appearance of flanks is hollow with the tense and hanging abdomen (Roy and Luktuke, 1962, Pandey et al., 1984).

The pregnant buffalo becomes slow and sluggish during the terminal month of pregnancy. The pregnant animals are reluctant to walk fast on the pasture and prefer to remain away isolated from the other animals of the herd. Hind limbs are dilated and some times mild staggering may be observed in some individuals. There may be a partial loss of appetite and irregular rumination. The animal becomes restless and anxious at the onset of parturition.

Parturition Behaviour

In normal parturition largest proportion of calves are delivered in anterior presentation. When labour pain starts the animals becomes restless with an anxious look and pupil are dilated. The parturition is completed in 3 phases i.e., (i) dilatation of cervix, (ii) expulsion of foestus and (iii) expulsion of placenta (Roy and Luktuke, 1962; Pandey et al., 1984).

i. **Dilatation of cervix:** The first stage of parturition starts from the irregular, intermittent and non-coordinated contractions of the longitudinal and circular muscles of the uterus. This is initiated by the accumulation of a contractile protein, actomycin due to sudden increase in the secretion of oestrogen (Csape, 1950). This is assisted by relaxin hormone produced in the uterus and influence of the progesterone of the corpus luteum and relaxation of pelvic ligaments takes place (Zarrow, 1950). The external genitalia becomes oedematous. After a few minutes the uterine contractions become more intense, regular and coordinated, and the animal attemts to push the foetus out of the uterus. The whole process of contraction is known as labour pain. The cervical plug is liquefied, cervix becomes soft and elastic, and opening of os uteri starts. The foestus enveloped in placenta is pushed towards the pelvic cavity by the intermittent peristaltic contractions of the uterine muscles causing opening of the os uteri. Maximumdiation of cervix takes place resulting in the formation of a continuous passage from uterus to vagina through cervix. This passage is lubricated by the copious vaginal secretion. The water bag appears at the vulval llabiae which subsequently ruptures and allantoic fluid flows from the vulva. After this amnion is pushed be the subsequent contractions into the cervix and foetus passes through the cervix and vagina. The time required for the opening of cervix is quite variable and affected by the intensity of labour pain, breed, parity and environment, etc.

ii. **Expulsion of foestus:** Anterior presentation of the foestus is prevalent in the normal delivery, because it causes least resistance in the expultion of foetus from the uterus. Both fore limbs, head and neck are extended together. In this stage hooves of fore limbs appear first which may be quickly followed by the appearance of muzzle and head in the successive contractions. The whole process may take 10 to 213 min. after this the buffalo may take a short rest before attempting the final expulsion of the foetus requiring additional time ranging from 3 minutes to more than an hour. Buffaloes normally deliver in sitting posture and then rise quickly to take care of the new born calf.

iii. **Expulsion of placenta:** In the third stage parturition is completed with the expulsion of the foetal membranes (placenta). The process is rapid in healthy animals. In this phase uterine contractions are initiated from the apex of the horns under the stimulation of oestrogen and oxytocin, and progresses towards the vagina. This helps in the expulsion of placental villi from the endometrial crypts and the physical pressure produced by the weight of membranes hanging from the vagina. The expulsion of placenta may take from half an hour to more than 8 hours, and should not be allowed to remain hanging longer than 12 hours. The expulsion of placenta is also affected by several factors like intensity of uterine contractions, breed, month of the calving, health of the dam and parity, etc.

The complete parturition in buffaloes is influenced by many factors (Table 6.13) and the owner is required to watch the calving from a remote place without disturbin the animal which may delay parturition due to the secretion of adrenaline in the frightened conditions. Important factors affecting the parturition duration are the intensity of labour pain, parity, breed and health etc. (Roy and Luktuke, 1962; Singh et al., 1966; Pargaonker, 1969; Gudi et al., 1971; Bhosrekar and Sharma, 1972; Sharma et al., 1978; Pandey et al., 1984).

TABLE 6.13: Effect of different factors on the parturition of buffaloes

Factors	Duration of parturition stages (min.)			
	Dilatation of cervix	Expulsion of foetus	Expulsion of placenta	Total time
Intensity of labour pain in Murrah				
(A) Intense	33.42	16.26	219.20	258.0
Normal	61.05	18.00	240.15	306.7
Weak	107.30	24.42	240.15	414.5
(B) Intense	49.40	7.30	50.0	270.0
Normal	111.60	9.10	282.3	396.8
Weak	211.90	11.30	286.22	430.89
Parity of calving in Murrah				
Primiparous	46.84	14.81	501.63	563.28
Pluriparous I*	62.50	13.37	450.00	252.87
Pluriparous II*	62.71	14.00	339.14	415.65
Breed of buffaloe				
Murrah	57.47	13.97	443.83	515.27
Nagpuri	38.57	185.17	392.75	461.13

Placenta at Parturition

The placenta is a leathery mass reddish grey to pale grey in colour. Its weight after expulsion varies from 2.11 to 7.50 kg in different conditions (Roy and Luktuke, 1962; Mohamed et al., 1980). The weight of placenta is affected by the breed, sex of calf, birth weight of calf and body condition of the dam.

The number of cotyledons is 108–124, and about 54 to 60% cotyledons are present on the gravid side. Three different size of placenta, i.e. small (1 < 2.5 cm), medium (2.6–6 cm) and large (> 6 cm) constitute about 13.4, 43.0 and 43.6% in the gravid, and 28.9, 47.9 and 23.8% in the non-gravid horn, respectively (Bhosrekar and Sharma, 1972).

Involution of the Uterus

Alongwith the process of parturition, regression in the size of uterus starts and the process is known as involution. The involution time may range from 15 to 64 days but in most of the normal parturition; it is 30–45 days (Roy and Pandey, 1971; El-Wishy, 1979, Mohamed et al., 1980).

Lochia

The copious uterine discharge following the parturition is known as lochia. The lochial discharge decreases gradually and ceases with 2–3 weeks period. The colour and consistency of lochial discharge changes from day to day. In the first 24 hours post-parturition it is admixture of fresh blood and becomes chocolate colour and more turbid due to the emigration of the leucocytes from the cervical mucosa. On day 4 to day 5 it becomes chocolate brown to dirty amber colour and later on light grey containing some streaks of blood. Subsequently it becomes whitish yellow with albuminous consistency. After about 2 weeks post-partum there may be scanty thick brown discharge for few more days (Sane and Desai, 1960, Luktuke and Roy, 1962).

Calving Interval

The interval between the successive calvings varies widely in buffaloes. Average calving interval has been recorded to be about 495, 461, 454, 430, 462 and 481 days in the Murrah, Surti, Bhadawari, Marathawada, Nili-Ravi and non-descript Indian buffaloes (Bhat, 1979); 488–650 days in different herds of Egyptian buffaloes (Khishin, 1951, alim and Ahmed, 1954, Asker et al., 1954; 408 days in Iraqi buffaloes (El-Wishy, 1979); 409 days in Italian buffaloes (Ferrara, 1957, Salerno, 1967); 378 days in Bulgarian buffaloes (Serra and Peiva, 1972–73); and 333–1380 days in swamp buffaloes of different south-east Asian countries and China (Jainudeen, 1977; Chantalakhana, 1979; Wang Pei Chein, 1979).

Service Period

The interval between calving and following conception is known as service period and less than 3 months service period has been found to be optimum from the production and economic point of view. The average service period ranges from 28 days to 502 days under different conditions, and it is generally more in early calvings and summer bred buffaloes (El-Sheikh and Mohamed, 1965, Rao et al., 1973, Pandey and Raizada, 1979). There may be very large variation in the animals within the herd and in a composite herd about 7.15, 18.12, 13.18, 10.00 and 7.00% buffaloes had an average 23, 46, 77, 105, 151, 240, 353 and 502 days service period, respectively (Rai, 1988).

▶ MALE REPRODUCTIVE SYSTEM

The bull is called half of the heard due to his 50% contribution in the product of conception (foetus). Since a bull is used for the breeding of very large number of buffaloes, utmost care should be taken is its selection and management. The most important physiological and behavioural functions of buffalo bull is the production of good quality semen containing potentially live spermatozoa and its deposition in the vagina of female in standing heat through natural service or in the artificial vagina for artifical insemination after necessary processing in the laboratory for increasing volume. The artificial insemination (AI) is a technique through which viable semen collected in artificial vagina (AV) is used for the insemination of larger number of buffaloes per ejaculate.

▶ REPRODUCTIVE TRACT OF BUFFALO BULL

The reproductive tract of buffalo bull is made of the primary sex organs, viz. a pair of testes placed in hanging sac of skin called scrotum. The secondary sex organs are made of duct system, i.e. the epidedymes, the vas deferens and the penis. Besides the main reproductive tract, there are few accessory organs like prostate gland, a pair of seminal vesicles and a pair of Cowper' glands or bulbourethral glands. The measurements of different anatomical parts of reverine and swamp buffalo bulls recorded by several workers (Macgregor, 1941, Asdel, 1955, Bhatnagar et al., 1955, Joshi et al., 1967) are summarized in Table 6.14.

Scrotum

The visible part of the sex organ of a bull hanging between the legs in the inguinal region is scrotum. In buffalo bull it is a 2 pouch sac developed from the invagination of inguinal skin for housing and holding the testes. It is pendulous and situated just behind the rear pair of rudimentary teasts in the inguinal region. It is apparently divided into 2 halves of almost equal size by the median vertical band slightly darker in colour than the rest of scrotal skin. The surface of scrotum is wrinkled and shrunken during cold weather and glossy bright during active phase when fully extended. The left half's is a little longer and voluminous than the right half. The scrotum of swamp buffalo bull is about 10 cm long and unlike riverine buffalo bull does not constrict at the attachment with the abdominal wall (Macgregor, 1941).

The main function of scrotum is to support the testes suspended by spermatic cord in the scrotal sac outside the abdominal cavity. It helps in he maintenance of a lower temperature of the testes necessary for normal spermatogenesis. The large number of sebaceous and sweat glands on the surface of scrotum help in the lowering of scrotal temperature during hot climate of tropical summer season. Indeed poorest semen quality improves significantly when animals are protected from the heat (Misra and Sengupta, 1965; Pandey and Raizada, 1979). The extreme environmental temperature is detrimental for the spermatogenesis. Scrotum helps in the maintenance of optimum temperature to the possible extent. During hot climate the scrotal muscles relax which provides larger surface area for the desipation of heat through increased rate of sweating. In very cold climate of winter the scrotal muscles contract and pull up the scrotum closer to the abdominal wall. The appearance of scrotum is wrinkled in winter. The tunica dortos muscle plays important role in the themoregulatory mechanism of the scrotum.

Testes

These are 2 in number present suspended in the scrotal sac by spermatic cord outside the abdominal cavity in the inguinal region. Each testis is an independent unit and separates from each other in the scrotal sac by a median septum scroti. The testes are firm and compact mass of parenchymatous tissue. In Indian buffalo bulls the average length, breadth circumference of the testes without epididymis are 7.73, 4.32 and 12.22 cm respectively. Mean weight of right testis is a little less than the left one (Verma, 1963; Joshi et al., 1967). The various measurements of testes of Indian buffalo bulls are presented in Table 6.14.

TABLE 6.14: Measurement of testis of adult Indian Buffalo bulls (Joshi et al., 1967)

Measurements	Size	
	Range	Mean
Weight (g)		
Right	38.2–116.5	74.86
Left	36.0–120.4	79.06
Length (cm)		
Right		7.60
Left		7.87
Width (cm)		
Right		4.30
Left		4.33
Circumference (cm)		
Right		12.20
Left		12.24

The main functions of the testes of an adult bull are: (i) the spermatogenesis for the production of the potent male sexual cells of reproduction (gametes), and (ii) the secretion of male hormones, the androgens (Testerone and andro-stenedione). The spermatozoa are produced by meiotic cell division of the germinal cells lining the coilrd partition of the loops of seminiferous tubules. The another type of cells. These cells secrete androgens in bulls from the onset of puberty to through out reproductive life. In buffalo bulls meiotic division of spermatogonial cells has been reported at about one year of age (Dutt and Bhattacharya, 1952). They were of the opinion that spermatogenesis in Indian buffaloes may start even earlier. The diameter of the seminiferous tubules of Indian buffalo bulls ranges from 0.17 to 0.20 mm (Bhatnagar et al., 1955). The seminiferous tubules join together to form the tubili recti which joins rete testis in the mediastinum and join together to form the tubili recti which joins rete testis in the mediastinum and join other ducts in succession to form vasa efferentia. These start as part of the mediastinum.

The main sex hormone testosterone is secreted by Leydig cells of the testis. Secretion of this hormone is regulated by the LH hormone of anterior pituitary gland. The testosterone is responsible for the development and maintenance of the functions of male reproductive tract, secondary sex characteristic and sexual behaviour. The ESH of anterior pituitary stimulates spermatogenesis. The morphological characters, voice and vigour are controlled by the male sex hormones.

Epididymis

It emeges from the joining of vasa efferentia at the dorsal part of the testis. Epididymis is a very long single duct highly convoluted to appear like a mm a mass of tubues. The duct is made of 3 parts, i.e. the head (caput), the body (corpus) and the tail (cauda). The tail of epididymis opens in the vas deference. The convoluted epididymal tube lies in a sheat of connective tissue formed from the extension of tunica albuginea. The length, breadth and thickness of the caput epididymis are 3.48, 3.90 and 0.77 cm; corpus epididymis 8.66, 0.99 and 0.29 cm; and cauda epididymis 2.41, 1.74 and 1.56 cm, respectively (Joshi et al., 1967). The mean weight of the tail piece of epidedymis has been reported 14.25 g by Verma (1963) and 15.38 g by Joshi et al., (1967).

The ductus epididymis is lined with secretary cells. The spermatozoa in the process of their development accumulate and mature during their passage through the epididymis and become capable to perform spontaneous movement and to fertilize ova when brought in contact. The epididymal sperms reserve ranges from 8.54×10^9 to 9.61×10^9 (average 9.17×10^9) in each epididymis and approximately 25.8 and 67% sperms are present in the head, body and tail segment of epididymis (Verma, 1963).

The Vas Deferens (Ductus Deferens)

The vas deferens is a tube emerging from tail segment of the epididymis. This starts from the base of the testis extending upwardand in association with spermatic cord it runs through the inguinal ring. At inguinal ring vas deferens separates from the spermatic cord, passes through abdominal cavity and enters the pelvic urethra adjacent to urinary bladder. The lumen of vas deferens is narrow and lined with mucous membrance. The wall is made of longitudinal and circular layers of involuntary muscles covered by outer layer of peritoneum. The muscles of vas deferens contract involuntarily during ejaculation of the semen and help in the expulsion of spermatozoa. The vas deferens of either side enlarges in the pelvic region to form ampulla. The ampullae have numerous glands and often spermatozoa accumulate here before ejaculation. The glands of ampullae secret fructose and citric acid in bulls (Mann et al., 1951),

Urethra

It is a muscular duct receiving semen through the openings of ampullae and the secretions of accessory sex glands. It is also the excretory passage for urine. The urethra starts near the neck of urinary bladder at the internal urethral orifice. In the urethra, spermatozoa mix with the seminal plasma from the accessory sex gland at the time of ejaculation. In the urethra of Indian buffalo bulls position of orifice of ampulla in relation to opening of the seminal vesicles was dorsal in about 55 per cent, ventral in 10% and in between in remaining 35% bulls (Joshi et al., 1967). Another study reported 40.8, 20.4, 29.2 and 9.6% in dorsal, ventral, medial and lateral sites respectively of the opening of the ampulla of vas deferens (Maurya et al., 1967).

Penis

Penis of buffalo bull extends from the neck of pelvic urethra to glans penis covered in the prepuce. The penis at rest forms an S shaped curve known as sigmoid flexer which extends greatly at the time of insemination. Shape of the penis is cylindrical with a tapering free end. It contains small amount of erectile tissue. The penis is rest is also firm and there is very little increase in shape and size or erection. The length of penis form the neck of pelvic urethra to the tip of glans range from 65.5 to 111.5 cm (average 92.11 cm). the average breadth is maximum 4.53 cm at pelvic urethral neck which decreases gradually to minimum 1.6 cm in the penile portion (Joshi et al., 1967). The penile tapering portion of penis opens at the angular end of the triangular sheath. The sheath of riverine buffaloes bulls is a pendulous triangular fold of 15–30 cm skin extending backward from the umbilicus. In the swamp buffalo bulls the sheath is tight (Macgregor, 1941). For riverine buffalo bulls sheath of 10–21 cm length and 5–10 cm circumference are preferred (Joshi et al., 1967). However, bulls with larger sheath are not uncommon.

▶ ACCESSORY SEX GLANDS (TABLE 6.15)

Accessory sex glands of the male reproductive system include the seminal vesicles, the prostate gland and the Cowper's glands or bulbo-urethral glands.

TABLE 6.15: Measurements of the different parts of the reproductive tract of Indian Riverine buffalo bulls

Organ/part		Length (cm)	Breadth (cm)	Thickness (cm)	Circum-ference (cm)	Weight (g)
Testis						
With epididymis	R	8.70–15.4 (11.21)	3.6–5.6 (4.57)	3.1–5.9 (4.09)	10.1–15.6 (12.74)	-
	L	9.20–14.5 (11.19)	3.6–5.7 (4.62)	3.2–5.2 (4.14)	10.0–16.1 (12.95)	
Without epididymis	R	6.0–8.9 (7.87)	3.3–5.3 (4.30)	- -	10.0–15.1 (12.20)	38.2–115.5 (74.6)

Contd.

TABLE 6.15: Measurements of the different parts of the reproductive tract of Indian Riverine buffalo bulls (*Contd.*)

Organ/part		Length (cm)	Breadth (cm)	Thickness (cm)	Circumference (cm)	Weight (g)
	L	5.7–9.8 (7.87)	3.3–5.5 (4.33)	-	9.0–15.9 (12.29)	36.0–120.4 (79.6)
Caput epididymis	R	2.2–4.8 (3.48)	3.0–5.2 (3.87)	0.49–1.04 (0.77)		
	L	2.2–5.6 (3.50)	2.8–5.0 (3.92)	0.5–1.2 (0.75)		
Corpus epididy	R	5.8–12.4 (8.73)	0.63–1.40 (0.99)	0.15–0.6 (0.29)		
	L	5.2–12.5 (8.59)	0.73–1.05 (0.99)	0.10–0.05 (0.29)		
Cauda epididymis	R	1.7–3.6 (2.41)	1.2–2.3 (1.69)	1.10–2.16 (1.55)	4.5–7.1 (5.45)	7.65–28.40 (15.32)
	L	1.7–3.5 (2.40)	1.3–2.9 (1.78)	1.14–2.65 (1.56)	4.3–8.0 (5.42)	7.80–28.43 (15.43)
Seminal vesicles	R	3.5–11.7 (7.14)	1.0–4.0 (3.50)	0.5–1.85 (1.14)		5.20–15.30 (11.1)
	L	3.4–11.8 (7.02)	1.5–4.1 (3.18)	0.4–1.90 (1.14)		5.17–24.66 (10.87)
Prostate		0.3–2.9 (1.52)	0.2–2.04 (0.70)			
Cowper's gland	R	2.1–4.8 (3.54)	1.0–4.15 (1.67)	0.4–1.78 (1.00)		2.02–19.20 (7.88)
	L	2.0–4.8 (3.45)	1.0–2.30 (1.58)	0.4–1.78 (1.00)		
Uterus Masculinus		1.2–4.0 (2.19)	1.2–4.0 (1.80)			
Epididymis to Inguinal ring	R	30.0–54.0 (42.79)			0.30–0.65 (0.49)	
	L	31.5–54.0 (43.19)			0.35–0.70 (0.50)	
Inguinal ring amupullae	R	17.0–42.0 (27.34)			0.12–0.45 (0.17)	
	L	19.0–37.0 (26.80)			0.10–0.44	
Convoluted part	R	1.5–15.0 (5.20)				
	L	1.4–10.0 (5.03)				
Ampullae	R	8.5–18.6 (13.80)			0.40–0.84 (0.61)	
	L	8.0–17.5 (14.05)			0.46–0.90 (0.62)	

Seminal Vesicles

Each of the 2 seminal vesicles are situated on the side of the respective ampulla. They open either above or below throw opening of vas deferens. The average length, breadth and thickness of the seminal vesicle of Indian riverine buffalo bulls are 7.8, 3.11 and 1.14 cm respectively. The weight of each vesicle ranges from 5.17 to 25.30g (Joshi et al., 1967). The seminal vesicles are lobulated and highly secretary. The secretion contains large amount of fructose and citric acid. Seminal plasma is an important carrier for the spermatozoa and also provides nutrition.

Prostate Gland

Body of the prostate gland is placed in front of the vesiculae seminalis on the dorsal surface of the pelvic urethra near the neck of urinary bladder. Average length and breadth of prostate gland are 1.52 and 0.70 cm respectively. The remaining part of prostate surrounding urethra is much lighter on the ventral surface (Joshi et al., 1967).

Prostate gland secretes a mineral rich fluid. However, it is difficult to study the chemical nature of the fluid secreted in the buffalo bulls due to very short period of ejections.

Cowper's Glands or Bulbourethral Glands

These are 2 in number weighing together 2.02 to 19.20 g (average 7.88 g) in adult buffalo bulls. They are placed distantly anterior to prostate gland on the dorsal surface of pelvic urethra. Average length, breadth and thickness was 3.50, 1.72 and 1.00 cm respectively (Joshi et al., 1967). The corresponding values 2.55, 1.76, and 1.13 cm respectively (Maurya et al., 1967) were comparable for the Indian riverine buffalo bulls.

▶ SEMEN

The male reproductive sexual fluid containing the products of seminiferous tubules (spermatozoa) of testes, excurrent duct/seminal tract (mainly the epididymis) and the products of associated secondary sexual organs drained in the urethra, is the semen. The colour of semen is creamy white to yellowish and consistency varies with the number of spermatozoa in the semen. Its volume ranges from 1.5 to 5.0 ml per ejaculate. The quality of semen is influenced by several factors, the fluctuation in temperature being more detrimental.

Semen Ejaculation

The discharge of semen in the vagina mating or AV during collection is called ejaculation. The nervous stimulation creates muscular contractions of the seminal tract which ejects spermatozoa into the penis through the pelvic urethra. The rhythmic contraction of urethra proceeds progressively in waves to force out semen through the orifice of the penis with the sudden thrust of short duration.

Sperm Reserve

Sperms reserve in buffalo bulls has been reported 7.45×10^9 spermatozoa per testis. The sperm production per g of testis ranges between 0.09 tand 0.102×10^9 (average 0.098×10^9) sperms. The epididymal sperm reserves 9.17×10^9 (8.54×10^9 to 9.61×10^9) sperms per epididymis. The sperm distribution was 25, 8 and 67% in the caput, corpus and cauda portion of the epididymis respectively. The calculated number of spermatozoa production was 2.28 billion per testis daily, and about 30 million sperms/g of testis (Verma, 1963). The size of spermatozoa decreases significantly during their passage from the testes to ejaculate. The size of head and length decreases during passage of sperms from testis to the head protion of epididymis and mid piece reduces subsequently of forward movement (Osman, 1975).

Sexual Behaviour of Buffalo Bulls

Sexual behaviour of adult buffalo bulls has been described by Johri (1960) in detail. When potential buffalo bull is brought to the female buffalo in heat, the bull normally opens his mouth drawing the upper lip and extending the neck upwards. It appears that the bull tries to inhale or suck, both through the nostrils and the mouth. The female buffalo in oestrous promptly responds and urinates. A small quantity of this urine is generally sipped by the bull. During this period the bull sometimes also licks the vulva. Simultaneously the bull makes some soft penile movements, protrudes his penis a few centimeter from the non-motile prepuce. After this bull mounths the female keeping keeping the fore legs on the back slightly clasping the female and hangs down his head. The pattern of mating is thrust coitus with quick ejaculation.

About 27.7% Egyptian buffalo bulls do not show sex response on teaser female or male animals. The sexual response is not influenced by the age or type of the teaser. The bulls teased by oestrous females usually do not respond to anoestrous female or male or male tearsers. Similarily the bulls reared isolated from females do not show response in female teaser, whereas those reared in the vicinity of females show interest in both oestrous and not-oestrous female teasers (Badaney et al., 1972).

Appearance of Sexual Activity in Bulls (Puberty)

The environment especially feeding and management practices significantly influence the sexual activity of buffalo bulls. Rearing of buffalo bull calves on subnutritional level of feeding delays growth and onset of sexual activities. The possibility of start of spermatogenesis in growing buffalo bulls of less than one year of age has been visualized by Dutt and Bhattacharya (1952) from their observation of meiotic division of the spermatogonial cells of the seminiferous tubules in an Indian buffalo bull of about 1 year age. Optimum management practices including the feeding of nutritious feeds and fodder were in adequate quantity significantly influenced the pubertal age of Surti buffalo bulls. Male buffalo calves of 4 to 19 months of age reared on scientific feeding and management were put to regular service after 13–14 months of feeding (Kodagali et al., 1970). The age and body weight of growing buffalo bulls at puberty and regular service are shown in Table 6.16.

TABLE 6.16: Mean age and body weight of Surti buffalo bulls at puberty

| | Age of Surti buffalo bulls (months) at | | Average body weight (kg) at | |
Initial	First ejaculation	Regular collection	First collection	Regular service
4	18	21	277	317
10	24	26	262	300
14	27	29	234	341
19	32	33	293	308

The first ejaculate of 7 Iraqui buffalo bulls was obtained between 16.7 and 19.5 months of age. The average volume (1.91 ml) initial motility (22.8%), count of live spermatozoa (46.4%) and density of spermatozoa (107.14 106/ml) indicated poor quality of the semen of first ejaculate, which improved significantly in the bulls of 21 months to 8 years of age (Sayeed, 1958); El-Wishy, 1978). The training of buffalo bulls for the donation of semen in artificial vagina (AV) with the use of a dummy recipient (female or male) starts at 1.5 to 2 years of age. In the cold climate of Italy and Russia the use of buffalo bulls for breeding has been reported at about 2 year of age. (Maymone, 1942; Agabelli, 1956). The mating age of Indian buffalo bulls in cold climate of Italy starts at 2.5 years of age and continues until 5–8 years of age. At traditional farms use of buffalo bulls for breeding generally ends at 4–7 years of age (de-Franciscis, 1979).

Active breeding life and duration of potency of buffalo bulls: Informations on the potency and active service life of buffalo bulls are incomplete. Although there are reports of use of buffalo bulls for breeding from 2–2.5 years of age in Italy and Russia, but in most of the buffalo breeding countries buffalo bulls are put to service at about 3 years of age indicated by the replacement of first pair of deciduous incisers by the permanent teeth. The age of active service life starts at 3.7 + 0.7 years in Egypt (El- Itriby and Askar, 1957), between 3–3.5 years in Pakistan (Majeed et al., 1961) and 3–4 years in Indian. Satisfactory semen quality and quantity has been reported in Surti buffalo bulls below 3 years of age (Gupta et al., 1980).

Loss in potency of buffalo bulls has been observed by 6–7 years of age, but desire may continue even beyond 12 years of age (Macgregor, 1941). In some parts of Indian buffalo bulls have been used for service up to 10 years of age but may remain fertile up to 19 years of age (Johri, 1960). The use of Surti buffalo bulls continues up to 9 years of age and best semen is donated between 3–7 years of age (Gupta et al., 1980). In Surti buffalo bulls largest period of service has been found 3–6 years (6–9 years of age) in about 64% bulls of artificial insemination (AI) centres in Gujarat (Kodagali et al., 1980). Most of the well managed riverine buffalo bulls do not acquire senility before 15 years of age and can serve about 100 females per year (Bhattacharya, 1974). Although most of the verterinary hospitals in India are equipped for providing AI service by free living community bulls or Government bulls (Murrah in most of the states). Non-descript stray buffalo males and entire draught buffalo males are also used for breeding due to several reasons. Some of the common reasons are the long distance of AI centre, awkward time of oestrous (mostly around mid night in winter and rainy season) and non availability of person in house capable of controlling buffalo in oestrus. Earlier at least one nominated buffalo bull was available for the buffaloes of 3–4 villages. Nowadays in India such bulls are limited to certain areas only. Free living buffalo bulls were capable of successful breeding even beyond 8–10 years of age.

Optimum Use of Breeding Buffalo Bulls

The quantity and quality of semen collected successfully up to an average 8.75 ejaculates daily were almost comparable. Murrah bulls can be classified into 3 classes on the basis of lipid, i.e. strong, moderate and weak sex drive. Average daily ejaculates per bull for the respective classes wre found to be 8.75, 5.60 and 2.90 resppectively (Saxeba and Singh, 1974). The sperm reserves in gonads and epididymis have been observed quite high (Verma, et al., 1965; Senger and Sharma, 1965; Senger and Sharma, 1965a, b Osman, 1972a, b). The calculated daily spermatozoa production capacity of bulls has been found to be 2.33–2.48 billion (Senger and Sharma, 1965; Verma et al., 1965), which showed the scope of minimum 1 service or 1 collection daily. However, it is not possible in practice due to several reasons like decreased libidi for short duration, occasional production of watery semen or aspermia etc. thus, the use of buffalo bulls for natural breeding or semen collection should be organized in a systematic order for optimum utilization. As per some old view, buffalo bulls should be used sparingly and not more than 75 times per year (Lazarus, 1945). In Egypt about 75% of services are required only during 4 months of peak breeding season annually. This means the breeding buffalo bulls should be used at least 3 times per week the peak breeding season. This works out to 48–50 services accounting about 75% of total 64–70 services per year (Asker and El-Itriby, 1958). Average annual mating at farms has been 72.17 + 19.4 with the range of 35 ot 110. Each nating comprises of 2 subsequent services with in 10–15 minutes. Increasing of semen collection frequency from once weekly to thrice weekly reduces the semen quality significantly (Sayed and Alonga, 1957). Two successive ejaculates on the day of collection have been found similar (quantitatively and qualititatively) in the buffalo bulls of north India (Semger and Sharma, 1965a, Bhosrekar, 1980). In another report best quality semen has been collected from the 3 successive ejaculates (Shalash, 1972).

The service ability of 50 Nili-Ravi buffalo bulls was found quite variable as out of total 5394 attempts only 3330 successful ejaculates (61.73%) could be collected. The collection was 67% in first and 56% in second attempt. Libido of bulls decreases between March and September and increases during November to February in the agro-climatic conditions of Pakistan. The best bull donated 167 collections out of 176 attempts in a year. This was about 95% successful and can be considered a very good collection on alternate day. The bull of lowest sex drive provided only 51 collections accounting about 29% of total 176 attempts (Wierzbowski et al., 1980). Weak sexual reflexes and and incomplete erection of penis were attributed to low level of testosterone secretion. Such bulls are not recommended for use in artificial insemination (Nour El-din, 1972). Bulls are not recommended for use in artificial insemination (Nour El-din, 1972). Bulls with good libido are uniform producers of good quality semen should be selected for breeding (Saxena and Singh, 1974).

Reaction Time

Time taken by a breeding bull for ejaculation, after it is brought to female in heat in case of natural mating or to dummy in cast of semen collection in AV, is known as reaction time. Several factors determine the reaction time of buffalo bulls. No relationship has been established between reaction time and semen quality (Prabhu and Bhattacharya, 1951). Average reaction time 43.3 seconds in the month of August was minimum and 77.5 seconds in March was maximum for Murrah bulls. Reaction time during hot (March-June), hot-humid (July-October) and cold (November-February) climate of north Indian plains ranged between 44 and 7.6, 28.3 and 58.4 andn 40.0 and 59.7 seconds, respectively (Kushwaha et al., 1955). In Murrah bulls shortest 32 seconds reaction time in February and longest 111.3 seconds in hot-humid July has been recorded. Mean reaction time during February to April, May to July, August to October and November to January had been 49.8, 89.8, 87.9 and 95.0 seconds, respectively (Tomar et al., 1966). Season variation has also been reported in the reaction time of Egyptian buffalo bulls (Sayed et al., 1962). Hot climate of summer season adversely affected reaction time and reduced libido (Misra and Sengupta, 1965).

Libido has significant effect on reaction time. A shorter reaction time has been reported on using male buffalo as dummy instead of anoestrous female buffalo (Prabhu, 1956).

Number of successive collections had adverse effect on reaction time. In successive 8 collections 75 + 11 seconds reaction time at first collection rose to 408 + 91 seconds at collection 8. the ejaculates of first 4 collections may be used for insemination (Saxena and Singh, 1971). Variable relationship has been observed between reaction time and ejaculate volume (r = 0.53 to 0.96) in different seasons (Verma, 1953). The variation in reaction time of buffalo bulls of high and medium sex drive is less than that of low sex drive mean reaction time of 8.75 (high libido), 5.60 (medium libido) and 2.90 (low libido) collections per day from one bull to each class has been 205.35 + 17.07, 179.95 + 16.70 ad 199.56 + 29.76 seconds respectively (Saxena andSingh, 1974) In Iraqui buffalo bulls of 1.75 to 8 years of age the reaction time during winter, spring, summer and autumn had been 3.4, 2.3, 2.1 and 1.6 minutes respectively. The number of ejaculates in the corresponding season was 2.2, 2.5, 1.4 and 1.4 (el-Wishy, 1978).

▶ SEMEN CHARACTERISTICS AND ATRIFICIAL INSEMINATION (AI)

Artificail insemination is a proven technique for the speedy multiplication of a species. AI technique of breeding in buffaloes was started in forties of the previous century at the Allahabad Agricultural Institute in India and first buffalo calf was born on August 21, 1943 (personal communication from late O.B. Tondon). Since the semen of eash ejaculate is extended with the use of suitable extenders (diluents) for the breeding of large number of females from the single ejaculated used for only one semen of high mating, therefore it is advantageous to use AI technique utilizing the semen of high production potential. This increases the probability of high conception and more rapid introduction of desired traits in the progeny. AI technique for the breeding of farm buffaloes has been quite popular in most of the buffalo breeding countries. The technique is also used for the cross breeding of swamp buffaloes in many countries and up grading of so called non-descript riverine buffaloes f the Indian subcontinent.

▶ COLLECTION OF SEMEN

The early method of semen collection from the vagina of cow immediately following the mating was not required to be used in case of buffaloes because the method of semen collection from cattle bull was already perfected. The same method was subsequently standardized for the buffalo bulls. AV method of semen collection is widely used for the buffalo bulls. Recently electroejaculation technique is being used at some of the places, but AV technique is more popular. Different methods of semen collection with detail description of AV methods are presented in this chapter.

1. **Ampulla massage method of semen collection:** This is done by a trained technician. The operater introduces his gloved hand per rectum of the bull tracing the male genital tract up to ampullae and seminal vesicles, and starts massaging these organs gently applying mild pressure. This causes sexual stimulation resulting in ejaculation. At the stage semen is collected by another person of buffalo bulls is very poor and they also need longer time of training. Semen volume collected by this technique is mostly small with less number of spermatozoa and pH is generally high (Singh et al., 1950, Singh, 1956). However, this method is still useful for the collection of semen from outstanding good buffalo bulls unable to mount for donation due to injuries or disorders of limbs.

2. **AV method of semen collection:** This method is widely used for semen collection and in the Indian subcontinent it is more advantageous as facilities for AI of cows

and buffaloes are provided on the same centre run by the state departments of veterinary.

a. *Things required*: The following instruments and appliances are required for semen collection:

  i. *Sevice crate:* wooden or metallic.

  ii. *Dummy animal:* This may be a sterile female or bulls may also be used for each other at the semen bank where daily collections are made from several bulls.

  iii. An autoclave for sterilizing glass wares.

  iv. Regrigerator and deep freeze depending on the requirements.

  v. Heating arrangements.

  vi. Liquid nitrogen containers of different size for the storage of semen filled straws and transportation of semen doeses to different AI centres, farms and also for export.

  vii. Arragements for uninterrupted supply of liquid nitrogen.

  viii. Gloves of latex rubber for technicians.

  ix. Artificial vagina (AV) of 40–50 cm length and 5.5 cm inner diameter.

  x. Inner lining of latex rubber for AV.

  xi. Semen collection cone of latex rubber.

  xii. Semen collection graduated tubes of glass.

  xiii. Glass cylinders, beakers, pipettes, slides, cover slip etc.

  xiv. Machine for filling, sealing and numbering of starws filled with extended semen of known bull and known quality.

  xv. Sterilized Vaseline or other suitable lubricant for the lubrication of AV.

  xvi. Semen shipment containers for short and long distance, and also storage for several days depending on the interval of semen supply at AI centres.

b. *Preparation of artificial vagina (AV):* Clean, dry and sterilized parts of AV are assembled in the laboratory under aseptic conditions. This is most important for the maintenance of semen quality. Any carelessness may cause contamination of semen and transmission of a subclinical infection (if any) from the semen of one bull to the semen of another bull. The rubber parts of AV should be washed with soap and water, and then thoroughly rinsed with hot water followed by ethylalcohol (70%) and finally with sterilized glass distilled water. After this these are dried in air in a closed dust free room. After cleaning and drying these are stored in an instrument cabinet.

At the time of semen collection AV is assembled properly. First of all inner linning of latex is inserted into the cylinder and its ends are turned back and fixed on either end of cylinder by stretching. The latex rubber cone is fixed at the distal end and then glass receptacle is attached tightly with the help of a rubber band at the end of conical funnel. Once again all joints of AV are checked after it is assembled (Fig. 6.1). Now jacket of AV is filled with hot water in sufficient quantity for developing proper pressure, the initial temperature of hot water is decided according to the season, distance between site of collection

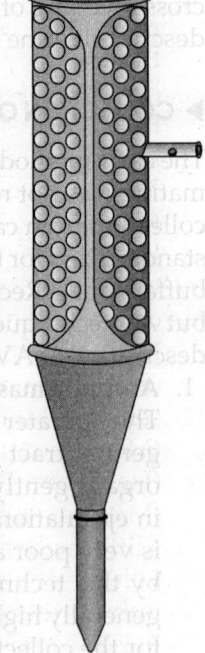

Fig. 6.1: Artificial vagina

should not vary much from 39° + 0.5°C. Destribution of spermatozoa. Considerable destruction of spermatozoa may occur at 41°C inside temperature of AV during semen collection (Mahmound, 1952). The first one-third of lining of AV is lubricated with a thin layer of sterilized Vaseline before the collection.

Collection of Semen

First of all a trained dummy animal is placed in the crate. Now an attendant brings out the buffalo bull after thorough cleaning and allow it to month. It has been observed that a false jump before actual collection increases the volume of ejaculate and the quality of second ejaculate immediately after first one is better (Senger and Sharma, 1965, Bhosarekar, 1980). In 3 successive collections also the quality of second ejaculate has been found superiore (Shalash, 1972). A restraint of 10 minutes before the collection has been found more effective than the 3 false mounts in quick succession for obtaining higher volume of good quality semen (Basawy et al., 1973). At the time of semen collection technician should hold the AV at an angle parallel to the penis so that at thrust there should not be unusual bending of the penis. The behaviour of bull must be kept in mind and operator should not be unknown person for the bull.

i. **Colour and consistency of semen:** The colour of normal semen is milky white (Shukla and Bhattacharya, 1949, Iyer, 1952). This is also referred by some workers as Jaffari buffalo bulls is quite common but in rare cases it may be yellowish milky (Kodagali, 1976). The consistency of semen collected more frequently is usually thinner than that collected at longer intervals. Semen in glass collection tube should be carefully examined for dust and other contaminations, and also for blood and pus from the infected buffalo bulls, if any.

ii. **Volume of semen ejaculate:** In practice semen is collected on alternate day at most of the centres during peak breeding season and twice weekly during rest of the year. Considerable variation has been observed in the semen volume of Indian dairy buffaloe bulls (Table 6.17). Average 1.79 + 0.38 ml per ejaculated (Prabhu and Bhattacharya, 1955) was less than 1–7–3.3 ml (Kushwaha et al., 1955) and 2.42–2.79 ml (Bhosrekar, 1980). In Murrah it is 3.8–5.1 ml per ejaculate (Sengupta et al., 1963), 3.0 ml (Abbhi, 1965), 4.5 ml (Tomar et al., 1965), 2.83 + 0.74 ml (Gopal Krishna and Rao, 1978) and 3.59 + 0.33 ml (Raizada et al., 1979). Mean ejaculate volume of Nili-Ravi buffalo bulls is Pakistan has been reported to be 1.7 ml from 3330 collections which was 2.0 ml from 1814 first ejaculated and 1.4 ml in second ejaculate of 1516 collections with minimum 0.25 ml and maximum 12.0 ml (Wirezbowski et al., 1980). In a Murrah buffalo bull also maximum 13 ml semen per ejaculate has been recorded at the Indian Verterinary Research Institute, Izatnagar (Bhattacharya, 1976). Average semen volume of Egyptian buffalo bulls is about 3.45 ml with a range of 1.2 to 6.0 ml (Mahmoud, 1952), and 3.31 ml with a range of 2.7 to 4.0 ml in other group of bulls (Hafez and Darwish, 1950). Average volume in buffalo bulls of USSR is 3.66 ml (Madatov, 1956). In China average 1.8 ml semen per ejaculate has been reported to be a little higher than that of the native swamp buffalo bulls (Cockrill, 1976). Ejaculate volume of buffalo bulls is affected by several factors like age, breed, season and nutrition etc. Average 1.19 ml first ejaculate volume in Iraqui buffalo bulls increased to 2.2–4.1 ml in mature bulls (El-Wishy, 1978). In Surti buffalo bulls of less than 3 years, 3–5, 5–7, 7–9 and above 9 years of age has been 2.2, 3.2, 3.5, 4.6 and 4.1 ml per ejaculate respectively. Effect of season and age are clearly shown in table (Gupta et al., 1980).

TABLE 6.17: Average semen volume per ejaculate in Surti buffalo bulls of AI centres of Gujarat state (Total ejaculates = 8675)

Season	Age group of Surti buffalo bulls (years)					
	< 3	3 - 5	5 - 7	7 - 9	> 0	Mean
Summer	2.6	2.9	3.1	4.1	3.3	3.3
Monsoon	3.3	3.7	4.1	5.1	4.5	4.2
Winter	3.1	2.9	3.4	4.5	3.7	3.5
Autumn	3.7	3.3	3.7	4.6	4.4	3.9
Average	3.2	3.2	3.5	4.6	4.1	**3.7**

iii. **Initial motility:** For the evaluation of semen at AI cenres of remote areas initial or mass motility is an important and quick method of quality determination. This is either judged by the movements and waves (swils) in a drop of semen under the light microscope on a 0 to 5 scale (rarely 0 to 10 scale) or by counting the total and non-motile spermatozoa with the help of a heamocutometer. The former provides an approximate estimate but later gives correct percentage of motile spermatozoa in the semen sample. The later technique is more specifically called sperm motility. Mass motility shows considerable variation evident from different values, viz., 3.6 (Kushwaha et al., 1955), 2.9 (Sengupta et al., 1963) and 3.83 (Bhosrekar, 1980) in Murrah bulls; 3.63 in Jaffary buffalo bulls (Kodagali, 1967), 3.34 + 0.02 (Kavani et al., 1973) and 2.5 (Gupta et al., 1980) in Surti buffalo bulls and 3.85 in Iraqui buffalo bulls (EI-Wishy, 1978). In Egyptian buffalo bulls it has been 7.25 on 0–10 scale (Hafez and Darwish, 1956).

Significant influence of age, season, breed and number of ejaculates has been observed on mass motility. Higher motility has been observed during spring in Murrah buffalo bulls (Kushwaha et al., 1955) which was 2.3, 2.7, 2.4, 2.9 and 4.2 in summer, rains, autumn, winter and spring season of northern plains of Indian (Sengupta et al., 1963). In Iraqui buffalo bulls it was 3.0, 3.8, 4.1 and 4.5 during winter, spring, summer and autumn season respectively (EI-Wishy, 1978). In Murrah buffalo bulls higher mass motility has been observed in first than the second ejaculate of winter season and vice-versa in the summer season (Bhosrekar, 1980). Effect of season and age on mass motility of semen of Surti buffalo bulls (Table 6.18) shows marginal variations (Gupta et al., 1980).

TABLE 6.18: Mass motility of semen of Surti buffalo bulls of different age in different season

Season	Age group of Surti buffalo bulls (years)					
	< 3	3 - 5	5 - 7	7 - 9	> 9	Average
Summer	2.2	2.4	2.4	2.3	2.5	2.36
Monsoon	2.4	2.6	2.6	2.4	2.6	2.52
Winter	2.4	2.5	2.5	2.4	2.4	2.44
Autumn	2.4	2.6	2.4	2.3	2.4	2.42
Average	2.35	2.53	2.48	2.35	2.48	2.44

Cooling arrangements during summer season of northern plains of India significantly improved the mass motility of Murrah semen (Sen Gupta et al., 1963, Singh, 1967). Preventive vaccination against foot and mouth disease has a stress period of about

45 days. Average 3.75 motility during pre-vaccination period decreased to 3.23 after vaccination and then improved progressively to comparable level with prevaccination motility after the lapse of 60 days (Tripathi and Saxena, 1976).

▶ THE MORPHOLOGY OF SPERMATOZOA

The spermatozoa are microscopic haploid germinal cells produced by testes of males. A normal spermatozoan of buffalo spermatozoa is more rectangular of buffalo is constituted of 3 distinct parts viz., head, mid piece and tail. The head of buffalo spermatozoa is more rectangular than the head of cattle spermatozoa (Mac gregor, 1941). Morphological measurements of Egyptian buffalo and cattle bulls (Mahmoud, 1952) and Murrah buffalo bulls (Venkataswami and Vedanayagain, 1962) are presented in Table 6.19.

TABLE 6.19: Average measurements of the spermatozoa of buffalo and cattle bulls

Measurements	Murrah buffalo	Egyptian buffalo	Egyptian cattle
Head length (μ)	7.40	7.44	9.13
Head breadth (μ)	4.48	4.26	4.73
Head area (μ²)	33.15	31.69	43.18
Head shape	1.65	1.75	1.93
Mid piece length (μ)	12.41	11.65	12.56
Total length (μ)	43.51	42.88	46.28

Some difference in the measurement of spermatozoa may be also observed as in another group of Murrah buffalo bulls average values of length, breadth, area and shape of head were $7.24 + 0.04$ μ, $4.41 + 0.03$ μ, $26.91 + 0.38$ μ² and $1.64 + 0.01$ respectively (Ali et al., 1978). A decrease in head length of spermatozoa in almost all types of semen extender and some increase in the head breadth in egg yolk glucose extender has been observed on the preservation of extended semen at $4 + 1°C$ for 72 hours (Nayuda, 1961). The length and breadth of head, and length of tail including mid piece decrease during travel of spermatozoa from tail to head of the epididymis.

Difference in the measurements of spermatozoa from the caput epididymis and ejaculates (Table 6.20) are non-significant (Sharma and Gupta, 1978).

Seasonal effect in the measurement of spermatozoa and dry matter content of semen (Table 6.21) has been also observed in Murrah buffalo bulls (Bhosrekar, 1980) and may not be uncommon in other types and breeds of buffaloes.

TABLE 6.20: Measurements of spermatozoa from different parts of epididymis and the ejaculated of Murrah buffalo bulls

Measurements	Epididymal spermatozoa from			Ejaculated spermatozoa
	Caput	Corpus	Cauda	
Total length (u)	71.4	70.3	67.7	69.3
Head length (u)	8.74	8.86	8.41	8.43
Head breadth (u)	5.09	5.09	4.90	-
Mid piece length (u)	12.9	13.2	13.8	13.1
Tail length (u)	49.8	48.3	45.4	47.8

TABLE 6.21: Effect of season on measurement of spermatozoa of Murrah bulls

Measurements	Winter	Summer	Monsoon
Head length (u)	6.53 + 0.07	6.53 + 0.05	6.60 + 0.04
Head breadth (u)	4.29 + 0.06	4.18 + 0.06	4.28 + 0.04
Head area (u2)	23.69 + 0.48	23.24 + 0.43	28.21 + 0.35
Mid piece length (u)	10.19 + 0.14	9.76 + 0.25	9.83 + 0.12
Dry matter in semen (g/100 ml)	5.86 + 1.01	6.30 + 1.57	6.43 + 1.45

▶ **MOTILITY OF SPERMATOZOA**

This is determined by counting the percentage of motile spermatozoa in diluted semen to contain about 20 million spermatozoa per ml. An observation shows that the transport of spermatozoa through the female reproductive tract from cervix to infundibulum is carried by oxytocin stimulated progressive contractions of the female reproductive tract. Probably sperm motility does not play any role (Van Denmark and Hays, 1954). However, later studies contradicted the observation and showed that motility helps in transport and fertilization of ovum (Wood, 1966). About 67% motility in fresh semen of non-descript riverine buffalo bull diluted with egg yolk glucose bicarbonate extender fo decreased to 40% on 5 days 30% on 8 days storage at 4–50C (Mahajan and Sharm, 1963). A large variation in the initial motility of spermatozoa from 45 to 85% in different types of buffalo bulls has been observed (Senger and Sharma, 1965, Saxena and Singh, 1974, El-Wishy, 1978, Gopal Krishna and Rao, 1978 Abhi, 1979, Chinnaiya et al., 1979, Raizada, 1979).

Several factors affecting the initial motility of spermatozoa are the composition of semen extender, duration and temperature of storage of extended semen, sex drive of bulls, season of collection, breed/type of buffalo and various stress factors (Mahajan and Sharma, 1963, Saxena and Singh, 1973, 1974, Tripathi and Saxena, 1976, El-Wishy, 1978, Chinnaiya et al., 1979, Rawat, 1979). Different magnitude of motility has also been reported in the same sample, which was 65% in fresh whole semen, 75% in fresh diluted semen and 62% in diluted semen frozen in mini straws and then thawed (Gunzel et al., 1979).

▶ **SPERM CONCENTRATION OR SPERM DENSITY**

The total count of spermatozoa without considering the shape, size and livability is called sperm concentration or sperm density. It is expressed as count or population per ml or per ejaculate of semen. Concentration of spermatozoa in buffalo semen is highly variable. Several factors like age, season of collection, frequency of collection, type /breed and size of testes etc. afftect the semen density.Spermatozoa concentration in semen of Indian riverine buffalo bulls has been reported from 600 to 1400 million per ml (Shukla and Bhattacharya, 1949; Kushwaha et al., 1955; Sen Gupta et al., 1963; Kodagali, 1967; El-Wishy, 1978; Raizada, 1979; Gunzel et al., 1979); Wierzbowski et al., 1980). Out of 4 sucessive collections also density was highest in second ejaculate and there was non-significant difference amongst the rest three collections (Prabhu and Sharma, 1953). Highest concentration has been reported during winter season in northern plains of India (Sen Gupta et al., 1963; Singh, 1967) but in north-western coastal area sperm density was highest during summer followed by monsoon and winter season in (Bhosrekar, 1980). In Egyptian buffalo bulls highest density has been recorded during the autumn followed by summer, spring and winter (El-Wishy, 1978) in descending order. Age and season effects has been noted in sperm density of Surti buffalo bulls and it is higher in young than the aged bulls (Gupta et al., 1980).

▶ LIVE AND DEAD SPERMATOZOA IN THE SEMEN

The percentage of live and dead spermatozoa is determined by counting on slides prepared by differential staining technique. The nigrosin-eosin stain (Bishop et al., 1954) is used for the differential staining of buffalo spermatozoa. The ratio of live and dead spermatozoa in buffalo semen has been found highly variable. Like other characteristics it is also influenced by factors like, age, season, breed, frequency of collection, level of nutrition, compostition of semen extender, duration and temperature of storage and mode of transportation, etc. root

Mean concentration of live spermatozoa has been reported 77.36 and 82.79%. In the first and second ejaculate of non-descript riverine Indian buffalo bulls (Prabhu and Bhattacharya, 1951). In Egyptian buffaloe also live spermatozoa percentage has been 75–86% (mean = 80.1%) in different ejaculates collected at intervals of 2 to 24 hours (Hafez and Darwish, 1956). Season significantly affected the live percentage and in Murrah bulls it ranged from 60 to 95%. Some details of breed and season effect on live count is shown in Table 6.22.

Protection of buffalo bulls from the heat stress of summer season providing simple cooling arrangements like placing a Khas (dry grass) curtain and sprinkling water on it at intervals to keep wet, direct sprinkling of water on the body of buffalo bulls 3–4 times daily for 8–10 minutes, adequate wallowing facility, shower bath etc. significantly improves semen quality. By protecting Murrah buffalo bulls with wet Khas curtains during summer season resulted in a significant increase in live sperms percentage from 69.5 in unprotected to 91.3 in protected buffaloes (Pandey and Raizada, 1979). Libido influences live spermatozoa percentage and has been found higher (58.6 + 1.70) in Murrah bulls of medium libido than 53.9 + 1.0% in bulls of low libido, and it was intermediate (55.7 + 1.5) in the bulls of high libido (Saxena and Singh, 1974).

Parentral administration of interstitial cell stimulating hormone (ISCH/FSH) also influences the ratio of live and dead spermatozoa in the semen. Administration of

TABLE 6.22: Effect of breed, season, age and protection on live spermatozoa (%)

Factors	Summer	Rains	Autumn	Winter	Spring	Reference
Murrah	64.6	82.1	90.5	84.5	95.7	Sen Gupta et al., 1963
Murrah bulls						
I. Unprotected	75.68	80.98	80.80	86.68	90.40	Singh, 1967
Protected	86.15	87.92	89.05	87.68	90.15	
II. Unprotected	75.88	81.40	82.05	87.58	90.65	
Protected	86.60	88.28	82.95	88.78	91.90	
Surti bulls (age in years)						
< 3	62.1	69.3	-	79.1	78.1	Gupta et al., 1980
3–5	74.8	74.6	-	78.1	76.4	
5–7	77.3	74.1	-	78.6	75.8	
7–9	72.4	72.2	-	77.7	77.7	
> 9	69.9	73.3	-	79.3	78.4	
Average	72.8	73.2	-	78.6	77.4	

FSH at weekly interval for 6 weeks at the doses of 500, 1000 and 1500 IU per injection resulted in the live spermatozoa count of 62.7, 77.7 and 69.8% respectively (Saxena and Singh, 1973). Stress produced by the vaccination against Foot and Mouth disease has little effect on live spermatozoa percentage in ejaculates which ranged between 87.7 and 90.2% during 0 to 90 days post vaccination against 91.3% during pre-vaccination period (Tripathi and Saxena, 1976). Very young Egyptian buffalo bulls below 20 months of age produced only 46.4% live spermatozoa in their first ejaculate (El-Wishy, 1978). An increase in live spermatozoa percentage has been recorded up to 5 years of age in Surti buffalo bulls (Gupta et al., 1980).

▶ ABNORMALITIES (%) OF SPERMATOZOA OF BUFFALO SEMEN

Different kinds of abnormalities have been observed in the buffalo semen. An apparent deviation in any part of the spermatozoa from the normal morphology is considered abnormality. The ratio of abnormal spermatozoa in the semen is used as a parameter of semen quality. Incidence of abnormalities in different sample of semen has been quite variable (Table 6.23).

TABLE 6.23: Abnormal spermatozoa in different semen samples

Type/Breed	Abnormality %	References
Indian buffalo bulls	6.60 (2.7–14.4)	Kushwaha et al., 1955
Do	4–5	Prabhu and Bhattacharya, 1951
Do	21.8 + 1.10	Saxena and Singh, 1974
Murrah buffalo bulls	15.29	Tripathi and Saxena, 1976
Egyptian buffalo	15–32	Hafez and Darwish, 1956
Iraqui buffalo	15.2–30.9	El-Wishy, 1978
Water buffaloes	20.22	Gunzel et al., 1979
USSR buffalo	1.0–11.5	Madatov, 1956

The morphology of spermatozoa is affected by several factors. About 4.88 (2.7–7.1), 8.35 (4.8–14.4) and 6.68 (5.1–8.5) per cent abnormal spermatozoa were found during hot (March-June), hot-humid (July–October) and cold (November to February) seasons respectively (Kushwaha et al., 1955). In agro-climatic conditions of Iraq highest 30.9% abnormal spermatozoa has been reported during the summer collection followed by 23.4% during autumn, 22.6% during winter and 15.2% during spring (El-Wishy, 1978).

REFERENCES

Abdel-Raouf, M. and El-Naggar, M A 1969. Zentb. Vet. Med., 16A: 838

Agarwal, K P, Raizada, B C and Pandey, M D 1978. Indian J. Anim. Sci., 49: 25

Agarwal, S K and Purbey, L N 1983a, Indian vet. J. 60: 631

Agarwal, S K and Purbey, L N 1983b, Indian vet. J., 60: 989.

Ahmed, I A and Tantawy, A O. 1956. Emp. J. Exp. Agric., 22: 213

Alim, K A and Ahmed, I A 1954. Emp. J. Exp. Agric., 22: 37

Arunachalam, T V, Lazarus, A J and Anantkrishnan, C P 1952. Indian J Dairy Sci., 5: 117

Askar, A A, Ragab, M T and Hilmy, S A 1954. Indian J Dairy Sci., 7: 135

Bagi, A S and Vyas, K N. 1983. Gujrat Agril. Uni. Res. J., 9: 52

Basirov, E B. 1964. Proc. 5th Intern. Cong., Trento, 6: 4

Basirov, E B. 1968. Trudy azarb. Nauchno-issled. Inst. Zhivot., 11: 97

Belorkar, P M, Khire, D W, Kadu, M S and Kaikini, A S. 1977. Indian vet. J., 54: 384

Bhalla, R C, Senger, D P and Jain, G C. 1964. Indian vet. J., 41: 327

Bhat, P N 1978. Proc. Indo-Soviet Symp. On Buffalo Breeding, NDRI, Karnal

Bhattacharya, P. 1954. Annual Report of AGB, IVRI, Izatnagar.

Bhosrekar, M R. 1980

Bhosrekar, M R. and Sharma, K N S. 1972. Indian J. Anim. Prod., 3: 8

Borady, A M A, Morad, H M, El-Shafie, M M, Bedier, L H and Khattab., R H. 1982. Proc. 6th Intern. Cong. On Anim. Poult. Prod., Univ. Zagazig, Egypt.

Chantalakhana, C. 1979. FAO Anim. Prod. Hlth. Paper 13: 143

Chawdhary, R A and Ahmed, W. 1979. FAO Anim. Prod. Hlth. Paper 13: 173

Damodaran, S. 1958. Indian vet. J., 35: 227.

Daneil, B., Gopakumar, N., Nair, M C and Rajgopalan, K. 1984. Indian J. Anim. Reprod., 5: 1

Dave, C N. 1983. Report on Surti buffalo herd of Agric. College, Puna.

Dave. C N. 1940. Puna Agric. College, Mag., 32: 97.

de-Franciscis, G. 1979. FAO Anim. Prod Hlth. Paper 13: 163.

El-Desouky, F and Rakha, A H. 1964. Proc. 5th Intern. Cong. Anim. Reprod., Trenta, 3: 575

El-Ghannam, F and El-Naggar, M A. 1975. Zentb. Vet. Med., 22A: 248

El-Naggar, M A and Abdel-Raouf, M. 1971. Zentb. Vet. Med., 18A: 108

El-Nauty, F E. 1971. The effect of different feeding system before and after weaning on age at puberty and age at first calving in buffalo heifers. M Sc thesis. Ain Shams University, Egypt.

El-Sheikh, A S and Abdel-Hadi, H A. 1970a. Indian J. Anim. Sci., 40: 9

El-Sheikh, A S and Abdel-Hadi, H A. 1970b. Indian J. Anim. Sci., 40: 213

El-Sheikh, A S and Mohamed, A A. 1965. J. Anim. Prod., UAR, 5: 99

El-Sheikh, A S and El-Fouly, M A. 1971a. Alexandria J. Agric. Res., 19: 159

El-Sheikh, A S and El-Fouly, M A. 1971b. Alexandria J. Agric. Res., 19: 9.

El-Wishy, 1979. Beitrage Trop. Land. Vet., 17: 77.

Fadzil, M. 1970. Kajan Vet., Singapore, 2: 159

Ferrara, B. 1957. Acta med. Vet., Napoli, 3: 203 and 255.

Gill, R S and Gangwar, P C. 1972. Indian vet. J., 49: 1164

Girish Chandra, 1979. Vet. Res. Bulletin, 2: 184

Girish Chandra, and Bhardwaj, M B L, 1981. Vet. Res. J., 4: 64

Gudi, A K, Sohoni, A D and Tatke, M B. 1971. Indian J. Anim. Sci., 41: 145

Hafez, E S E. 1963. Emp. J > Exp. Agric. 21: 15

Hafez, E S E. 1954a. Vet. Record, 66: 264

Hafez, E S E. 1954b. J. agric. Sci., Camb., 44: 165.

Hafez, E S E. 1955. Indian J. vet. Sci. and Anim. Husb., 25: 235

Hafez, E S E and Kamal, M A M. 1955. Indian J. vet. Sci. Anim. Husb., 25: 39

Hafez, F L. and Zarrow, M X. 1950. Vitamins and Hormones, 8: 151.

Jainudeen, M R, 1977. Proc. Joint conf. on Hlth. Prod. Cattle of South-East Asia, Kaula Lumper, Malaysia.

Jainudeen, M R, Sharifuddin, W and Ahmad, F B. 1983. Vet. Record, 133: 369.

Janakiraman, K. 1979. FAO Prod. Hlth Paper 13: 220

Kaleff, B. 1942. Zentb. Tierz. Zuchthiol., 51: 131.

Kamonpatana, M, Schama, D and Van de Wiel, D F M. 1979. FAO Anim. Prod. Hlth. Paper 13: 226.

Kanai, Y and Shimizu, H. 1982.

Kerur, V K and Kodagali, S B. Gujvet., 3: 27

Khishin, S S. 1951 Emp. J. Expt. Agric., 19: 185

Kodagali, S B and Deshpande, A D. 1969. Final report of scheme on infertility in Cattle, Gujrat College of Vet. Sic. and A > H>, Anand.

Leopold, J. 1968. Tierarztl. Umsch., 23: 273

Luktuke, S N and Ahuja, L D 1961. J. Reprod. Fert., 2: 200

Luktuke, S N, Roy, D J and Joshi, S R. 1964. Indian J. Vet., Sci, Anim. Husb., 34: 41.

Macgregor, R. 1941.Vet. Record, 53: 443.

Majeed, M A, Garlick, G K and Khan, L R. 1961. Agriculture, Pakistan, 12: 181.

Maymone, B . 1942. Tierzucht. Zuchthiol., 52: 1.

McRorie, R A and William, W L. 1974. Annual Rev. Biochem., 43: 777

Mehta, S N, Gangwar, P C, Srivastava, R K and Dhingra, D P. 1979. J. agric. Sci., μ K, 93: 249.

Mohammed, A, El-Ashry, M A and El-Serafy, A M. 1980. Indian J. Anim. Sci., 50: 8

Mudgal, V D . 1979. FAO Anim. Prod. Hlth. Paper 13: 247

Nambiar, K G and Raja, C K S V. 1962. Kerala Vet., 1: 75

Namboothripod, T R B and Luktuke, S N. 1978. Kerala J.Vet. Sci., 9: 293.

Ocampo, A R, 1939. Philippines Agric., 28: 286.

Pandey, M D and Roy, A. 1968. Agra Univ. J. Res. (Sci.), 17: 1

Pandey, M D and Raizada, B C. 1979. FAO Anim. Prod. Hlth. Paper 13: 235

Pandey, S K, Kharche, K G and Pandey, S K. 1984. Cheiron, 13: 19

Pargaonkar, D R. 1969. M V Sc thesis, Punjabrai Krishi Vidyapeeth, Akola.

Polding, J B and Lall, H K. 1945. Indian J. Vet. Sci and Anim. Husb., 15: 178

Polikhronov, D and Peeva, Ts. 1982. Zhivotnov dml. Nauki, 19: 12

Prasad, G, Roy, M K and Singh, L P. 1979. Indian J. Anim. Sci., 49: 184

Rai, G S. 1968. Indian vet. J., 43: 228

Raizada, B C, Agrawal, K P and Pandey, M D. 1978. Indian J. Anim. Sci., 48: 572

Raja Ram and Girish Chandra, 1979. Indian J. Anim. Hlth., 18 (2): 11]

Raja Ram and Girish Chandra, 1984. Indian vet. J., 61: 458

Rao, B R, Patel, μ G and Tamhan, S S. 1973. Indian vet. J., 50: 413

Reddy, D B. 1960. Indian vet. J., 37: 270

Rife, D C. 1959. The water buffalo of Indian and Pakistan, International Cooperá. Administration, Washington, D C.

Roy, A and Pandey, M D. 1971, Final report of ICAR scheme on causes of repord. Failure in buffaloes, Vet, College, Mathura.

Roy, A, Raizada, B C. Tewari, R B L, Pandey, M D, Yadav, P C and Sen Gupta, B P. 1968. Indian J. vet. Sci. Anim. Husb., 38: 554

Roy, D J and Luktuke, S N. 1962. Indian J. Vet. Sci. Anim. Husb., 32: 152

Salama, A, Shalash, M R and Hoppe, R. 1967. Bull. Anim. Sci. Res. Intern., Cairo, 3: 86

Salerno, A. 1967. Atti. Soc. Ital. Sci. vet., 14: 259

Sane, C R and Desai, V G. 1960. Cattle sterility report of Maharashtra state, India.

Sane, C R Kaikini, A S, Deshpande, C R, Koranne, G S and Desai, V G. 1964. Indian Vet. J., 42: 653

Sane, C R, Kaikini, A S, Deshpande, B R, Koranne, G S and Desai, V G. 1965. Indian Vet. J., 42: 591.

Serra, J L and Palva, I A E. 1972–73. Anals dos Servisos de Vet, Mojombique, 20: 21

Shalash, M R. 1956. J. agric. Sci., Camb. 51: 70

Singh, R P. 1966. Indian vet. J., 43: 820

Singh, D, Bhalla, R C and Soni, B K. 1966. Indian vet. J., 43: 812

Singh, G, Taneja, V K, Bajpai, L D and Bhat, P N. 1972. Indian J. Anim. Prod., 3: 159

Singh, G Singh, G B and Sharma, S S. 1984. Theriogenology, 22: 453

Tiwari, G P. 1972. Orissa Vet., 7: 81

Toelihere, M R 1980a. Annual report of Food Fert. Technol.Centre, Taiwan.

Toelihere, M R. 1980b. Annual report of Food Fert. Technol., Taiwan

Torres, E B, Molina, J G and Maala, C P. 1980. Philippines J. Vet. Med., 19(2): 45 Ullah, Nemat and Usmani, R H. 1985. Buffalo Bulletin, 4: 5

Vale, W G. 1983. Thesis, Tierarztliche Hochachule, Hanover, F R Germany.

Venkayya, D and Anantakrishnana, C P. 1957. Indian J. dairy Sci., 10: 123

Wahid, A. 1975. Pakistani Buffalo, Karachi University, Pakistan.

Wang Pei-Chien, 1979. FAO Anim. Prod. Hlth. Paper 13: 152.

Wang Pei-Chein, Wei Chi-Lin and Wu Hui. 1965. Acta Vet. Zootech. Sin., 8: 151

Yap, E L E. 1974. Philippines J. Vet. Med., 13: 1

7

Semen Production, Processing and Artificial Insemination

The total genital fluid discharged by the male during normal ejaculation in natural mating, artifical collection or otherwise is the semen. A large number of spermatozoa are discharged suspended in the seminal plasma. The semen is composed of (a) the spermatozoa and (b) the seminal plasma. The former are produced in the seminiferous tubules of the testes, and the later is secreted by the testes and the accessory sex glands into the urethra. The consistency of semen varies with the number of the speramatozoa.

▶ THE SEMEN EJACULATION

The process of discharging semen in the vagina of female in oestrus during mating or in the AV or by other means is known as semen ejaculation. The whole process includes the integrated sequence of the erection of penis, intromission and discharge. This is controlled by the complex nervous mechanism. Although artificially stimulated ejaculation is possible in buffalo bulls per rectum massage of ampullae or with the help of electrical stimulation.

▶ TRAINING OF THE BUFFALO BULLS FOR SEMEN COLLECTION IN AV

The morning hours before feeding and watering and after complete night rest has been found most suitable time for the training of buffalo bulls for semen donation in the artificial vagina (AV). The stomach is light and the bulls are more active during the early hours. The time of training should be marginally adjusted according to the change in environmental temperature, which may be between 5–7 AM during the summer, 6–8 AM during comfortable months and 9–10 am during the winter season.

A disease free anoestrous female preferably an experienced one or a docile male is used as a dummy. The size of dummy should be easily approachable for the young buffalo bulls put on training. The dummy should not be restless, furious and nervous. The young bulls are allowed allowed a few days to develop acquaintance with the dummy and also fro developing sexual interest, which is indicated by the muzzling of the vulva and mounting on the dummy or other animals. The bulls under training are brought in groups and one bull is put to training individually while others are kept at a distance to watch the action. Special sounds or whistling is produced by the training instructor for stimulating sex drive in the buffalo bulls. After a few days when a buffalo bull stats normal mounting and protrudes penis out the sheath in an attempt to copulation the experienced operator holding the AV should grasp the sheath and introduce the penis into the AV.

The normal temperature of vagina during the oestrous is about 39°C (Mahmound, 1949; Sharma et al., 1968). A slightly higher temperature, 40 + 0.5°C is required in the AV at the time of semen collection. A temperature higher than 41°C inside the AV may cause destruction of the spermatozoa in buffaloes (Mahmoud, 1952).

Significant difference in the psychological behaviour of buffalo bulls has been obsetved. Some of the buffalo bulls have equal reaction time with the oestrous and anoestrous females (Prabhu and Bhattacharya, 1954), while some others show quicker reaction time when males are used in place of anoestrous females (Prabhu 1956). In some rare cases bulls have specific liking for a particular dummy, and for the training of such buffalo bulls either desired type of dummy is procured or other method of semen collection is used, if the bull is highly precious and discording is not in the interest of the herd due to exceptionally high production potential.

Things Required for the Semen Collection

The following appliances are required for the collection of semen and should be readily available at the semen collection centers.

1. Service and insemination crates.
2. **Dummy animal:** It may be either a male or female animal of satisfactory body strength to bear the load of buffalo bull on mounting. Most of the buffalo bulls donate semen on male cattle or buffalo dummy. However, in some rare case a female buffalo in heat is necessary to stimulate reaction for the collection of semen.
3. Healthy buffalo bulls of known pedigree should be used .
4. Stove or heater with connections
5. Kerosene oil
6. Fish kettles
7. An autoclave
8. A hot air oven
9. Instrument cabinets
10. Artificial vagina cylinder of 35–40 cm length and 6.5 cm internal diameter.
11. Inner lining of latex rubber
12. Semen collection cone of latex rubber
13. Semen collection glass tubes preferably graduated
14. An insulating muff for semen collection tube for protecting the semen from temperature variations and sun light, and preventing the breakage of glass tube causing loss of semen.
15. Glass rod
16. Sterilized Vaseline
17. Thermometer.

Things Required for Semen Evaluation and Preservation

1. Light (Comound) microscope
2. Clean glass slides
3. Cover glass
4. Necessary stains
5. Watch glass
6. Analytical balance
7. Photoelectric colorimeter
8. Haemocytometer

9. Volumetric flastks
10. Measuring cyclinders
11. All glass distillation apparatus
12. Refrigerator
13. pH papers and pH meter
14. Pasture's pipettes
15. Graduated pipettes
16. Spirit and spirit lamp
17. Ethyl alcohol
18. Glass beakers
19. Glass funnels
20. Filter papers
21. Fresh poultry (Hen's) eggs
22. Sodium citrate (AR)
23. Sodium bicarbonate (AR)
24. Citric acid (AR)
25. Glucose (AR)
26. Fructose (AR)
27. Glycerine (AR)
28. Ether (AR)
29. Cidar wood oil
30. Liquid paraffin
31. Potassium permanganate
32. Antibiotics
33. Sulphonilamides
34. Toilet soap
35. Dettol or Savlon
36. Antiseptic cream
37. Sterilized cotton wool
38. French chalk or Talcum powder

Additional Requirements for Deep Freezing of Semen

1. Liquid nitrogen containers
2. Liquid nitrogen
3. Equipments for filling processes semen and sealing
4. Straw for filling processed semen

Things Required for Artificial Insemination (AI)

1. Thermos flasks
2. Semen shipers
3. All glass insemination catheters or disposable catheters
4. All glass syringes (1 or 2 ml) or disposable sterile syringes
5. Metalic containers for keeping insemination catheters
6. Vaginal speculum
7. Gum (Long) boot
8. Full sleeve latex gloves or disposable gloves
9. Enamel trays, jugs and buckets (other suitable type may be used).

Preparation or Assembling of Artificial Vagina (AV)

The different components of artificial vagina (AV) are cleaned, air dried and sterilized before assembling in a sterile environment in a dust free room or other suitable place. This is very important for the production of good quality semen free from contaminations and also to control the transmission of infectious diseases, if any, from one bull to the semen of another bull. All the rubber components of the AV are thoroughly washed with soap and water to make them clean and greese free. This is followed by washing with hot water, rinsing with 70% ethylalcohol and finally with glass distilled water. At some palces boiling of rubber components in water is considered better than the alcohol sterilization. Boiling is also better for rural AI centers with limited facilities and more external exposer. After this all components are dried and stored in aseptic conditions in a dust free instrument cabinet.

The AV is normally assembled a few minutes earlier than the semen collection to avoid contamination. The assembled of AV is completed in a dust free room. All works are done by gloved hands. First of all the internal latex lining is inserted into the AV cylinder and its both ends are turned back and fixed with a glass receptacle at the narrow end is fitted on the distal end of the SV cylinder fitted with the inner latex lining (Fig. 7.1). After assembling the AV all joints are rechecked before filling the jacket of AV with hot water. Sufficient amount of hot water is filled for producing proper pressure. The initial temperature of hot water is decided on the basis of atmospheric temperature, distance between the laboratory, the site of semen collection and the reaction time of the bull. The inner temperature of AV should be maintained in a narrow range of 39–40°C as destruction of the spermatozoa has been observed on 41°C inner temperature of AV at the time of collection (Mahmoud, 1952). The upper one-third paet of the inner lining of AV is lubricated with a thin layer of sterilized white Vaseline before the use for collection of ejaculate.

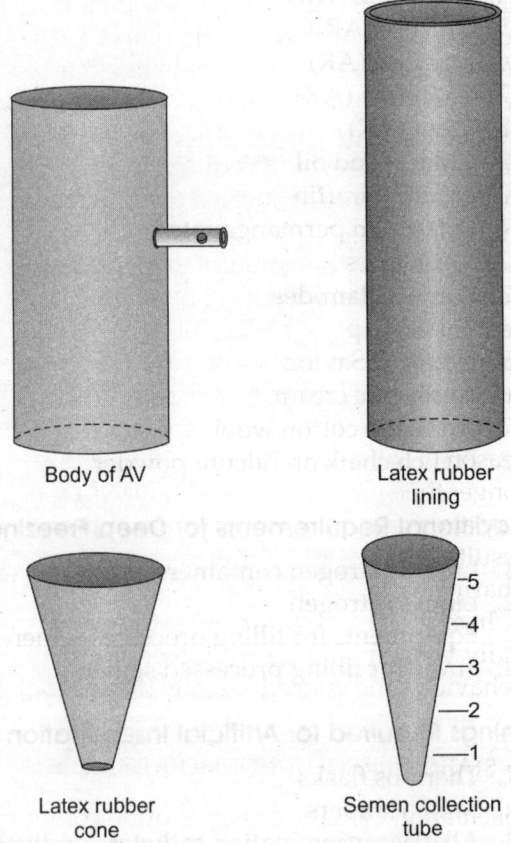

Body of AV   Latex rubber lining

Latex rubber cone   Semen collection tube

Fig. 7.1: Parts of artificial vagina (AV)

▶ COLLECTION OF SEMEN

A trained dummy animal is placed secured in a semen collection crate. Now clean buffalo bull is brought to the dummy and allowed to mount. A flash jump before the actual collection is encouraged to increase the volume of ejaculate. The quality of second ejaculate immediately following the first one has been found better (Senger and Sharma, 1965; Bhosareker, 1980). The quality of second ejaculate has also been found best in three successive collections (Shalash, 1972; Verma et al., 1983). A restraint of

10 minutes before is more effective than the three false mounts before actual ejaculation. The quality further improves on allowing three false mounts after 10 minutes restraint before the actual collection (Badawy et al., 1973).

▶ FREQUENCY OF SEMEN COLLECTION

The free living community buffalo bulls are frequently required to serve more than one buffalo daily and some times during breeding season the buffalo bulls are so exhausted that they start avoiding the females in heat. This situation is quite common during the comfortable colder months in india. In this system of natural mating many buffaloes are left empty despite 2–3 services and the cause is mainly the insemination of either seminal fluid or immature sperms in the semen. No information is available on he conception of buffaloes bred with the community buffalo bulls and other stray bulls and also the working entire buffaloes.

For good fertility, controlled use of buffalo bulls giving 3–4 days rest betweent successive service should be allowed. About 75 to 84 services per buffalo bull per year has been suggested by some researchers (Lazarus, 1946; Asker and El-Itriby, 1958). Two collections per week at an interval of 3–4 days for 3 years has no deleterious effect on the semen quality and breeding behaviour of the Murrah bulls (Bhattacharya, 1962). This works out to about 104 services per year and it will be more advantageous to use the buffalo bulls for natural service at an interval of 3–4 days for covering 90 to 120 buffaloes annually. However, it is difficult to limit the service by free living buffalo bulls unless buffalo owners are educated of the demerits of indiscriminate use of community buffalo bulls.

For the the collection of semen at the artifical insemination centers, the interval between successive collection should be 3–4 days for the production of high quality semen (Sane et al., 1960; Bhattacharya, 1962). However, some studies show that three collections per week resulted in poor semen quality associated with frequent suppression of libido (Sayed and Oloufa, 1957; Asker and El-Itriby, 1958). A study from northern plain of India recommends 3 collections per week during the peak breeding season (Tomar et al., 1968). Although some times bulls may not ejaculate or take much longer time for semen ejaculation. Normally 2 ejaculates are collected on each collection day and further increase in the number of successive donation on a collection day may result in the loss of libido, decrease in initial motility and sperm densitu (Senger and Sharma, 1965; Tomar et al., 1968; Verma et al., 1984).

In exceptional cases a few extraordinary buffalo bulls may continue to donate semen daily without significant effect on the quality and quantity of the semen, breeding behaviour and conception rate (Hafez et al., 1958).

▶ STATIC/QUIESCENT/NONMOTILE EJACULATE

Ejaculation of static semen is quite common in the buffalo bulls which gains motility either by light blow by mouth or on dilution. Initially quiescent semen is often low in quality than the initial motile semen (Table 7.1), but static semen is also able to fertilize provided active spermatozoa are present in optimum number. However, fertilization ability of quiescent semen may be somewhat lower than the fertilization ability of normal motile semen. In most of the case (Tomar et al., 1966, 1970; Joshi et al., 1967; Abhi et al., 1968; Tomer and Misra, 1971; Sengupta et al., 1977; Nema et al., 1983).

TABLE 7.1: Characteristics and composition of initially quiescent and motile ejaculates of Murrah and Surti buffalo bulls

Semen attributes	Murrah buffalo bulls		Surti buffalo bulls	
	Static	Motile	Static	Motile
Ejaculate volume (ml)	1.20 + 0.02	3.07 + 0.19	3.60 + 0.17	3.68 + 0.16
Initial pH of semen	7.66 + 0.06	6.97 + 0.02	-	-
Colour and consistency (5–0)	-	-	3.29 + 0.17	3.79 + 0.13
Sperm count (X 106/ml)	887 –5	849 + 3	899 + 47	929 + 29
Live sperm (%)	43.8 + 3.5	75.1 + 0.85	81.2 + 1.38	84.8 + 0.95
Abnormal sperms (%)	17.2 + 1.59	16.5 + 0.51	10.0 + 0.69	9.7 + 0.73
Keeping quality (days)	1.1 + 0.27	5.5 + 0.21	-	-
Initial fructose (mg/100 ml)	669 + 27	885 + 19	647 + 28	797 + 32
Fructolysis (%)	42.9 + 3.13	59.0 + 2.83	-	-
Inorganic P (mg/100 ml)	3.86 + 0.14	4.28 + 0.80	19.6 + 0.94*	15.5 + 0.64

Note: * Values in seminal plasma.

▶ FACTORS AFFECTING SEMEN PRODUCTION

Buffalo bulls reared on good feeding and management start semen donation at an early age of 9 months in Egyptian buffaloes (El-Itriby and Asker, 1957 but normally they are put to active service at 2.5 to 4 years of age, The bulls are required to maintain good libido and produce good quality semen during their active breeding life of 6–8 years of age. Some of the important factors affecting semen production have been described briefly.

1. **Hereditory factors:** Buffalo bulls with sexual anomalies in young age are discorded. A few apparently normal animals do not develop sexual interest after puberty even after repeated exposure to buffalo females in oestrus are also discorded. Such type of lack in libido, lack of interest and shyness at mating are usually hereditary defects.

2. **Effect of season** (Table 7.2): Amongst the different climatic factors hot season has been found to cause maximum deleterious effect on the semen production (Malkani, 1954; Kushwaha et al., 1955; Sengupta et al., 1963; El-Sawaf et al., 1971). The buffaloes are considered highly sensitive to hot and cold climatic changes due to their poor adaptability (Kaleff, 1942). However, during pilgrimage to Lord Kedar

TABLE 7.2: Some attribules of Murrah buffalo semen in the tropical climate of northern India (Mathura)

Semen attributes	Summer	Rains	Autumn	Winter	Spring
Ejaculate volume (ml)	3.8	3.8	4.1	4.1	5.1
	SE + 0.16	0.28	0.27	0.24	0.29
Mass motility	2.3	2.7	2.4	2.9	4.2
(0 to 5 scale)	SE + 0.14	0.09	0.09	0.09	0.09
Sperm count/ml (X 106)	1128	1065	1040	1352	1381
	SE + 81	75	71	38	100
Live sperms (%)	72.25	81.92	91.16	83.06	96.02
Initial fructose content	743	864	803	731	825
(mg/100 ml semen)	SE + 59	72	41	29	98

Nath above 7000 m in the Himalaya the author observed thousands of buffaloes alongwith bulls, calves and owners, living in open on the Bugiyals (Himalayan pastures) in the first week of May, 1999. Pwners informed normal breeding and pregnancy. Therefore, more observations are required for establishing the low adaptation ability in buffaloes. However the results in tropical conditions of western part of Uttar Pradesh in India (Sengupta et al., 1963) that best quality semen from Murrah buffalo bulls is collected during the post winter comfortable climate of the spring season.

3. **Effect of exercise:** Regular exercise of bulls is considered important for the maintenance of vitality.

    However, exercise in not essential for the loose housed bulls in capacious pen with large padock. A significant increase in the semen volume and total sperm production (Table 7.3) without considered effect of other semen traits has been observed in Murrah buffalo bulls. Exercise significantly reduces the reaction time (Matharoo et al., 1985).

TABLE 7.3: Effect of exercise on semen production in buffaloes

Semen attributes	No exercise	Standard exercise
Semen volume (ml)	2.25 + 0.22	3.29 + 0.40
Mass activity (0–5 score)	3.37 + 0.12	3.39 + 0.69
Sperm count (million/ml)	1402 + 65	1360 + 290
Total sperm production (X 106)	77, 545	1,11,941
Initial motility (%)	66.04 + 1.50	67.59 + 7.00

4. **Effect of transport:** The physica; stress caused by long distance travel of a breeding buffalo bull decreases libido and semen production for few months. Still some breeds (Murrah and Surti) could maintain though decreased libido against complete lack of libido in zebu cattle bulls (Sane et al., 1954, 1967).

5. **Effect of housing and management during stress season:** Significant improvement in libido and semen production can be achieved by providing cooling and protection from the solar radiation (Table 7.4). Simple protection of buffalo bulls with walled sheds and cooling arrangements and bath or wallow significantly improves semen production (Misra and Sengupta, 1965, Pandey and Raizada, 1969).

    However, such protection during comfortable autumn season has no significant effect and it is undesired expenditure in the climate of northern Indian plains.

TABLE 7.4: Effect of protection from hot wind and solar radiation on semen production in two seasons

Semen characteristics	Summer season		Autumn season	
	Unprotected	Protected	Unprotected	Protected
Semen volume (ml)	1.2 + 0.4	3.7 + 0.4	3.6 + 0.2	3.6 + 0.4
Mass motility (0-5 score)	0.87	1.58 + 0.3	3.7 + 0.2	3.7 + 0.2
Sperm count (X 106/ml)	1104	1527	1043	1219
Live sperm (%)	69.5	91.3	87.3	85.0

6. **Effect of nutrition:** Prolonged under feeding increases the age at puberty and thus the total semen production during the breeding life of a bull. Deficiency of some micro nutrients like vitamin A, carotenes and trace elements adversely affects the semen production (Afiefy et al., 1984) and probably non availability of green fodder

during summer season is also a major factor for significant fall in libido and semen production.

7. **Effect of frequency of semen collection:** Controlled use of buffalo bulls giving periodic sexual rest is important for the production of good quality semen and the maintenance of libido (Sayed and Oloufa, 1957, Tomar et al., 1968). For the optimum production of good quality semen two collections per week at an interval of 3–4 days is followed at most of the semen production centers.

8. **Effect of disease:** The sexual activities, semen production and semen quality are adversely affected in the clinical phases of many diseases specially those manifested by hyperthermia and weakness. The sexual activities become normal after the convalescence period in most of the cases unless there is permanent disability. Normal libido has been observed after recovery from the foot and mouth disease but semen quality was deteriorated (Sharma, 1969).

9. **Effect of preventive vaccination against infectious diseases:** Most of the preventive vaccination produces febrile reactions and stress of different duration on the body of animals. Vaccination of buffalo bulls against the foot and mouth disease has stress over a period of 6–7 weeks, which improves progressively and becomes normal after about 60 days post vaccination period (Tripathi and Saxena, 1976). However, semen motility remains poor for another 6–7 weeks.

▶ SEMEN CHARACTERISTICS

The semen characteristics are studied for the specific application in reproduction. The gross and microscopic examinations for morphological characterization are the basic requirements for the selection of good quality ejaculates before their processing and preservation for use in artificial insemination. The infromations on biochemical constituents of the semen is essential for the development of good quality semen extenders (diluents) and the proper preservation of extended semen under different facilities for storage to retain greater fertilization ability.

1. **Volume of ejaculate:** Large variation is observed in the volume of semen from different ejaculates and it is influenced by the age of buffalo bulls, libido, breed, frequency of collection, reaction time, climatic conditions, feeding, management and initial motility of the semen at the time of collection. The average volume of semen at each collection mostly ranges from 1.5 to 4.5 ml in different conditions (Hafez and Darwish, 1950; Mahmoud, 1952; Kushwaha et al., 1955; Prabhu and Sharma, 1955; Madatov, 1956; Sengupta et al., 1963; Radev et al., 1968; Clamoboy and Palad, 1967; Teipathi and Saxena, 1983; Afiefy et al., 1984). The lowest 0.25 ml and highest 12.0 ml ejaculate volume has been recorded in buffalo bulls (Singh et al., 1967; Wirezbowshi et al., 1980) > The semen is normally less in young bulls and increases gradually with the increase of age (Singh et al., 1967).

2. **Colour and consistency of semen:** The normal colour of Indian buffalo bulls is opaque milky white to yellowish and the consistency may be thin or thick depending on the density of spermatozoa (Ayyar, 1944; Shukla and Bhattacharya, 1949). The normal semen of Egyptian buffalo bulls (Mahmoud, 1852) and Surti buffalo bulls (Sane et al., 1955) is normally milky white with faint blue tinge. The colour of Murrah buffalo semen is mostly milky white but creamy appearance is also frequently observed (Hukeri, 1969).

The consistency ranges from thin to thick and average viscosity of Egyptian buffalo bulls semen is about 4.15 centripoise on the Ostwald's viscometer (Mahmoud, 1952).

Most of the buffalo bulls donate light white semen in the first collection and deeper white in the second after the long sexual rest. The viscosity of semen decreases during the hot and humid-hot season in Surti buffalo bulls (Sane et al., 1955).

3. **Hydrogen ion concentration (pH) of semen:** The normal reaction of the semen of buffalo bulls collected in optimum conditions is slightly acidic and usually ranges between 6.33 and 6.97 (Kushwaha et al., 1955; Sayed and Oloufa, 1957; Tomar et al., 1966, Singh et al., 1983). The pH of semen increases in successive ejaculates collected at short interval in quick succession (Table 7.5) and becomes alkaline from second to fourth ejaculates (Prabhu and Sharma, 1953, Senger and Sharma, 1965, Tomar et al., 1968).

The variation in semen pH due to individual bulls, breed, season and initial motility (Table 7.6) is frequently observed (Kushwaha et al., 1966, Kerur, 1971, Tomar and Misra, 1971, Toelihere, 1980b).

TABLE 7.5: Average pH of semen collected in quick succession

Experiment no.	Ejaculate number (pH)			
	1	2	3	4
1.	6.8	6.8	6.9	7.0
2.	6.8	7.1	7.4	7.6
3.	6.57	6.62	-	-

4. **Spermatozoal concentration pr sperm density or initial sperm count in semen:** The initial population of spermatozoa in the normal fresh ejaculate of buffalo semen

TABLE 7.6: Variation in buffalo semen pH due to different factors

Factors	Initial pH of fresh semen
Individuality of buffalo bulls	
Bull No. 5	6.77 + 0.08
Bull No. 102	6.87 + 0.02
Bull No. 103	6.54 + 0.18
Bull No. 109	6.94 + 0.05
Combined (mixed)	6.80 + 0.05
Breed effect	
Murrah	6.52
Surti	6.42
Jaffarabadi	6.55
Season effect	
Winter	6.90
Autumn	7.00
Summer	6.80
Spring	6.80
Over all	6.90
Age effect	
Below 3 years	6.71 + 0.04
3–6 years	6.75 + 0.02
Above 6 years	6.72 + 0.02
Over all	6.73 + 0.02
Effect of initial motility	
Initially static	7.66 + 0.06
Motile	6.97 + 0.02

usually varies between 210 and 2500 million per ml semen (Mahmoud, 1956; Singh *et al*, 1967; Verma *et al*, 1983). Such a large variation in sperm density may be due to lower adaptation ability of buffaloes to the changes in climatic conditions, feeding schedule, management and handling of bull at the time of semen collections, feeding schedule, management and handling of bull at the time of semen collection. In normal conditions the sperm density is 600–1200 million per ml (Shukla and Bhattacharya, 1949; Prabhu and Bhattacharya, 1953; Hafez and Darwish, 1956; Radev et al., 1966; Yassen et al., 1975; Nema et al., 1986). The sperm density in semen is affected by age if the buffalo bulls (Radev et al., 1966; Kerur, 1971), seasonal changes (Sengupta et al., 1966; Porwal et al., 1972; Tripathi and Saxena, 1983), protection from the harsh climatic conditions (Pandey and Raizada, 1979; Chalapathy and Rao, 1981), frequency of semen collection (Senger and Sharma, 1965b; Yassen et al., 1975). Nutritional variations (Prabhu and Bhaya, 1965a, b; Afiefy et al., 1984), sex drive and reaction time of buffalo bulls (Prabhu and Bhattacharya, 1954; Prabhu and Sharma, 1955; Prabhu, 1956, 1957) and use of hormones and other stimulating drugs (Goswami, 1962; Afiefy et al., 1984; Umashanker et al., 1984).

5. **Initial motility or mass activity of the spermatozoa:** The activity of spermatozoa is judjed by the initial motility in fresh semen at the time of collection. Generally 2 scales (0 to 5 or 0 to 10) are used for the determination of mass activity of spermatozoa by visual appraisal with the help of a compound microscope. The initial motility of spermatozoa in the normal ejaculates generally ranges from + 3 to + 4.5 on the 5 points scale or + 6 to + 9 on a 10 point scale, and similar to other species it is also affected by the bull's sex drive, breed, frequency of collection, number of successive ejaculates on the day of collection, season, nutrition and use of sex stimulating ejaculates on the day of collection, season, nutrition and use of sex stimulation agents etc. (Prabhu and Bhattacharya, 1953; Prabhu and Sharma, 1953; Prabhu and Bhaya, 1962a; Sengupta et al., 1963; Tomar et al., 1968; Tripathi and Saxena, 1983). In buffaloes static semen is frequently collected which gains motility after dilution in most of the ejaculates and used satisfactorily although quite often static semen ejaculates are poorer than the normal motile ejaculates (Abhi et al., 1968; Tomar et al., 1970; Nema et al., 1983).

6. **Travel of spermatozoa:** The information available on the speed of travel of buffalo spermatozoa suspended in the egg yolk-citrate extender revealed 1.65 mm per minute in vitro (Mahmoud, 1952). This is less than half of the 4 mm per minute in the cattle bulls of Bos Taurus species (Gallein and Roux, 1948).

7. **Progressive motile spermatozoa:** The concentration of the progressively motile spermatozoa determines the initial or mass motility in the fresh semen. The progressive motility of spermatozoa is generally high in the fresh semen and thereafter gradually decreases on storage at 4 to 6°C. Average progressive motility of spermatozoa in normal semen varies from 48.5 to 69.9%, and it is influenced by several factors like post pubertal maturity, sex, drive, frequency of semen collection, number of successive ejaculates per collection, season and breed etc. (Prabhu and Bhattacharya, 1951; Senger and Sharma, 1965; Rodev et al., 1996; Singh an Saxena, 1968; Singh and Misra, 1975; Yassen et al., 1983; Tripathi and Saxena, 1983; Tripathi and Saxena, 1983). Initially static semen often becomes motile on dilution (Abhi et al., 1968). Some times different motility of sperms is observed in the same sample of semen. An average 65% progressive motility in fresh whole semen is increased to 75% in fresh diluted semen which remains 62% in the diluted semen frozen in mini

straw and then thawed (Gunzel et al., 1979). Semen extenders had also significant influence on the motility of spermatozoa (Rawat, 1979).

8. **Population and ratio of live and dead spermatozoa in the semen:** The semen evaluation for the content of live and dead spermatozoa is required for the assessment of dilution rate and quality of the semen. The average percentage of live spermatozoa usually varies between 60 and 90 in the buffalo bulls maintained under optimum management (Prabhu and Bhattacharya, 1951; Hafez and Dorwish, 1956; Oloufa et al., 1959; Tomar et al., 1966; Gupta et al.,1980; Tripathi and Saxena, 1983). In some exceptional buffalo bulls the percentage of live spermatozoa may be higher than 90 (Singh et al., 1983). The ratio of live spermatozoa in the semen is influence by the age of buffalo bulls, breed, sex drive, frequency of collection, number of successive ejaculates at the time of collection, seasonal and climatic changes, nutritional factors, protection from the extremes of hot and cold season, etc. (Hafez and Dorwish, 1956; Prabhu and Bhaya, 1962a; Sengupta et al., 1963; Tomar et al., 1968; Kerur, 1971; Saxena and Singh, 1971; Gupta et al., 1980; Chalapathy and Rao, 1981). The percentage of live spermatozoa is usually less in the static semen than in the motile ejaculates (Abhi et al., 1968; Tomar and Misra, 1971).

9. **Abnormal spermatozoa in the semen:** The abnormal spermatozoa in the fresh semen of buffalo bulls may very from as low as 3% to more than 32% (Prabhu and Bhatacharya, 1951; Hafez and Dorwish, 1956; Madotov, 1956; Senger and Sharma, 1965a; Saxena and Singh, 1974; Tripathi and Saxena, 1976; El-Wishy, 1978; Gunzel et al., 1979). Different factors responsible for the occurrence of abnormal spermatozoa in the semen are breed, frequency of semen collection and level of nutrition etc. influence the percentage of abnormal spermatozoa in the semen (Kushwaha et al., 1955; Sayed and Oloufa, 1957, Senger and Sharma, 1865, Tomar et al., 1968). The different types of sperm abnormalities are megahead, microhead, oyriform head, elongated head, double head, proximal droplets, distal droplets, acrosomal granules, abaxial attachment of mid piece, swellon mid piece, double formation of mid piece, neck fracture, coiled tail, bent tail, tailless, double tails etc, (Prabhu and Sharma, 1954; Heuer et al., 1982).

▶ BIOCHEMICAL CONSTITUENTS OF THE BUFFALO SEMEN

The semen contains many organic an inorganic substances normally needed for the maintenance of the viability and normal functions of the spermatozoa which are essential for the fertilization. These constituents are required for the maintenance of osmotic pressure, supply of nutrients to the spermatozoa and metabolic activities of the live cells. Generally great variation is observed in the concentration of different biochemical constituents of the semen (Table 7.7) which is influenced by several factors like age, frequency of semen collection, breed, nutrition, and season etc. (Roy et al., 1950a, b, 1960; Pal et al., 1956; Oloufa et al., 1959; Misr et al., 1969; Alamy et al., 1976).

1. **Carbohydrates in the semen:** The average content of total reducing substances in the buffalo semen has been found 700 to 875 mg per 100 ml which is 85 to 90 fructose (Roy et al., 1950a; Pal, 1957). The initial fructose content in the semen (Table 7.8) is significantly influenced by the concentration of spermatozoa in the semen (Roy et al., 1950b), interval between the collection period and the successive ejaculates (Misra et al., 1969; Abdou et al., 1977), age of the bulls (Alamy et al., 1976), initial motility of the spermatozoa (Tomar and Misra, 1971; Nema et al., 1983). Other carbohydrates present in very small amount are glucose and hexosamine (Anand, 1973).

TABLE 7.7: Biochemical constituents of the buffalo semen

Biochemical constituents	Range	Mean value	Source
Total reducing matters (mg/100ml)	370 - 1650	700 + 52	Roy et al., 1950 a
		743 + 37	Roy et al., 1960
	375 - 1480	875 + 51	Pal, 1957
Initial fructose		880	Eapan et al., 1946
	253 - 1075	615 + 30	Royy et al., 1950a
	325 - 1423	782	Pal, 1957
	800 - 1000		Anand, 1973
		643 + 24	Abdou et al., 1977
		946 + 114	Dhanotiya and Srivastav, 1979
Total Nitrogen	381 - 525	485	Pal, 1957
	605 - 703	649 + 12.8	Chaudhuri and Ganguli, 1977
Non Protein Nitrogen	85 - 140	109	Pal, 1957
	107 - 127	116 + 2	Chaudhuri and Ganguli, 1977
Creatinine	4.09		Oloufa et al., 1959
Ascorbuc acid		14.4	Eapan et al., 1946
	1.04–6.09	3.7 + 0.37	Roy et al., 1950a
		8.6 + 0.37	Abdou et al., 1977
		3.3 + 0.36	Tomar and Misra, 1973
		6.2	Banerjee and Ganguli, 1973
Sialic acid		133.2 + 4.3	do
Citric acid		441	do
	322 - 820	489	Pal. 1957
	411 - 632	507 + 14	Chaudhuri and Ganguli, 1977
Total phosphorus		103.8 + 8.9	Roy et al., 1960
	110 - 131	121 + 5	Chaudhury and Ganguli, 1977
Inorganic phosphoru	14 - 25	17	Pal. 1957
		6.4 + 0.6	Roy et al., 1960
		5.4	Banerjee and Ganguli, 1973
		12.86 + 0.49	Abdou et al., 1977
Organic phosphorus	55 - 999	68	Pal, 1957
Acid soluble phosphorus		72 + 3.9	Roy et al., 1960
Calcium	35 - 62	42	Pal, 1957
		40 + 2	Roy et al., 1960
Chloride		369	Sayed and Oloufa, 1957b
		373 + 55	Roy et al., 1960
Copper (ug per 100 ml)		229 + 37	Rawat, 1979
Lipid contents			
Total lipids	483.52		Iqubal et al., 1984
Total cholesterols	85.5 + 14.22		Rawat, 1979
Free cholesterols	43.0 + 9.68		Do

TABLE 7.8: Effect of various factors on initial fructose content in buffalo semen

Factors	Initial fructose (mg/100 ml)
Concentration of spermatozoa (million per ml)	
394 + 13.6	1015 + 50
737 + 16.1	855 + 35
1149 + 26.1	729 + 60
Collection interval,	
8 days	812.4
72 hours	940.3
48 hours	885.7
24 hours	828.0
Successive ejaculates	
First	719 + 33
Second	591 + 39
Third	554 + 59
Age of buffalo bulls	
Young	525.5
Adult	620.5
Old (aged)	412.7
Initial motility	
Static	669.2 + 26.6
Motile	885.3 + 18.8

2. **Nitrogenous constituents of semen:** The average content of nitrogenous compounds in the semen has been found to range from 485 to 649 mg per 100 ml. These values include 109 to 116 mg non protein nitrogenous compounds (Pal, 1957; Chaudhury and Ganguli, 1977). Climate has also some effect on the nitrogenous substances (Table 7.9). The electrophoresis of seminal plasma revealed 8 components forming about 3.33, 33.5, 19.0, 17.0, 9.0, 4.3 and 3.0% of the protein content. Out of these 5 were anodic and 2 cathodic. The migration behaviour of 3 major and 5 minor protein fractions was almost similar to that of alpha and beta-globulins of the blood serum (Agar et al., 1965). Total 9 amino acids, viz. alanine, arginine, aspartic acid, glutamic acid, glycine, lysine, histidine, serine and tyeosine have been identified in the seminal plasma of the Murrah bulls (Rawat, 1979) and 13 amino acids, i.e. alanine, arginine, cystein, cystine, histidine, leucine, isoleucine ornithine, phenylalanine, praline, serine, threonine and valine have been observed in the seminal plasma of the Surti buffalo bulls (Ghosal et al., 1984).

TABLE 7.9: Total nitrogen and non protein nitrogen (NPN) content in seminal plasma

Season	Total nitrogen (mg/100 ml)	Non protein nitrogen (mg/100 ml)
Rauny season (Mid April–Mid July)	605 + 13.5	107 + 4.9
Autumn (Mid July–Mid November)	703 + 31.8	111 + 4.9
Winter (Mid November–Mid February)	668 + 33.3	127 + 5.1
Spring (Mid February–Mid April)	621 + 36.2	120 + 5.5

3. **Organic acids in the semen:** Several organic acids viz. acetic, propionic, lactic, formic, succinic, malonic, glycocolic, malic, citro-isocitric, butyric and some long chain fatty acids are reported in the semen of cattle bull (Ramsey et al., 1963) are likely to be present in the buffalo semen. Few informations available on the lipid groups in buffalo semen needs more exploration. A great variation has been observed in the concentration of ascorbic acid and citric acid (Table). The lactic acid content in fresh semen of buffaloes is 34.52 + 2.11 mg per 100 ml (Singh et al., 1983).

4. **Lipids of semen:** Some lipids and fatty acids have been found in the semen, spermatozoa and seminal plasma of buffalo bulls (Guraya and Sidhu, 1975; Jain and Anand, 1975, 1976a, b; Sarmah et al., 1983; Iqubal et al., 1984). The average lipids contents of the spermatozoa is much higher than the content in seminal plasma (Table 7.10) and the glyceraldehydes constitutes largest fraction followed by the neutral lipids. Average value of dry matter contents 5.93 + 0.18 and 4.73 + 0.14% in the semen and seminal plasma respectively are much less than 18.46% present in the spermatozoa.

TABLE 7.10: Lipids concentration in spermatozoa and seminal plasma

Constituents	Spermatozoa (mg per 109)	Seminal plasma (mg/ml)
Fresh weight	50.093	1019.100
Dry weight	9.247	48.203
Total lipids	1.147	1.500
Neutral lipids	0.286	0.439
Unsaponifiable matter	0.106	0.176
Glycolipids	0.397	0.581
Phospholipids	0.548	0.594
Gangliosides	0.015	0.010

The fatty acids are important components of the membranes structure and play important role in endogenous respiration. Average content of polyunsaturated fatty acids in the triglycerides of the spermatozoa and seminal plasma is 54.6 and 60.7% respectively. Arachidonic acid is the main unsaturated fatty acid of the triglycerides, diglycerides and cholesterol esters. Stearic acid is the major component of saturated fatty acids in most of the neutral lipids, and palmitic acids is a little higher than the stearic acid in most of the neutral lipids, and palmitic acid is a little higher than the stearic acid in the 1,2-diglycerides and cholesterol esters of the neutral lipids. In the phospholipids also stearic acid is main except in the sphingomyelin, choline and ethanolamine, plasmalogen, sperm phosphatidyl choline and ethanolamine. Oleic acid is the major component of the choline and the ethanolamine plasmalogen. The docosahexaenoic acid is the major fraction of sphingomyeline sperm phosphatidyl choline and ethanolamine. The saturated fatty acid fraction of the phospholipids is formed of mainly stearic acid followed by palmitic acid (Jain and Anand, 1976b). SA significant loss in the content of total lipids and phospholipids occurs after the cold shock and freezing, which is more in the later treatmen (Sarmah et al., 1984).

Large variation has been observed in the total cholesterol and free cholesterol content of the semen of Murrah, Surti and Nili-Ravi buffalo bulls (Mohan et al., 1977; Rawat, 1979; Nema et al., 1983; Iqubal et al., 1984). Significant increase occurs in the total cholesterol content during the summer season (Table 7.11).

TABLE 7.11: Cholesterol content in the semen of buffalo bulls

Factors	Cholesterol content (mg per 100 ml) in-	
	Whole semen	Seminal plasma
Total cholesterol		
Murrah bulls	85.5 + 14.22	53.0 + .88
In winter season	92	-
In summer season	142	
Surti buffalo		62.2 + 4.04
Motile ejaculate		64.1 + 6.88
Static ejaculate		117.83
Nili-Ravi buffalo bulls		
Free cholesterol in Murrah bulls	43.0 + 0.68	16.6 + 3.97
Surti buffalo bulls		
Motile ejaculate		28.85 + 2.63
Static ejaculate		30.61 + 3.86

5. **Enzymes of semen:** Many enzymes are present in the semen of buffalo bulls are required for the various metabolic activities of the spermatozoa. These are acid phosphatase, alkaline phosphatase, transaminase, acetylcholinesterase, hexakinase, aldolase, phosphoglyco-isomerase, lactic dehydrogenase, malate dehydrogenase, succinic dehydrogenase and deoxyribonuclease (Roy et al., 1960; Misra et al., 1969; Tomar and Misra, 1971; Abdulla et al., 1973; Abdou et al., 1974, 1977, 1978; Chauhan et al., 1975; Daader et al., 1982; Dube et al., 1982; Dhanda et al., 1983; Sidhu and Guraya, 1979). The enzymes of spermatozoa involved in the fertilization of ovum have been differentiated as (i) hyaluronidase, (ii) corona penetration enzyme, and (iii) acrosin (Ganguli, 1979). The other important enzymes of semen, seminal plasma and acrosomal preparations are the hyaluronoglucosaminidase, B-N- acetylglucosaminidase and aryl-sulphatase (Anand, 1979), adenosine triphosphatase and fructose–1,6 diphosphatase (Dhanotiya and Srivastava, 1979) and glutamate oxalacetate transaminase (Gupta and Srivastava, 1981).

6. **Inorganic constituents of semen:** The bulk of inorganic constituents of semen includes sodium, potassium and calcium followed by phosphorus and sulphur. Chloride is the main anion in semen. Trace elements are copper, zinc and manganese.

▶ METABOLISM OF SPERMATOZOA

For the maintenance of viability of the spermatozoa continuous supply of biological energy is essential. The main source of energy in the semen is fructose though other sugars are also present in very small quantity. Fructolysis occurs in the semen through intermediary metabolism catalyzed by the enzyme hexakinase and the high energy adenosine tri phosphate (ATP). A decrease in ATP content of bull semen has been found associated with the impaired motility of the spermatozoa (Mann, 1945). Metabolism takes place bu both aerobic and anaerobic pathways.

▶ FRUCTOLYSIS

The rate of fructolysis in buffalo semen varies from 25.3 to 59.01% in 3 hours at 37°C. It is influenced by several factors like temperature, concentration of inorganic phosphorus, ionic concentration, osmotic pressure, pH, sperm density and collection interval (Roy et al., 1950b; Misra et al., 1969; Tomar and Misra, 1971; Abdou et al., 1977; Rawat, 1979).

▶ FRUCTOLYSIS INDEX

The measure of glycolytic capacity of the spermatozoa is known as fructolysis index. The quantity of fructose in milligram (mg) utilized by 1 billion spermatozoa during the 1 hour incubation period at 37°C in conditions approaching anaerobiosis is expressed as fructolysis index (Mann, 1948). The average fructolysis index of the buffalo spermatozoa ranges from 1.523 to 2.20 in different bulls during the first hour of incubation and reduces significantly during the second and third hour of the incubation period (Table 7.12). Fructolysis index is also influenced by the age of bulls and sperm density in the semen (Roy et al., 1950b; Alamy et al., 1976; Abdou et al., 1977b).

TABLE 7.12: Fructolysis index of semen at different hours

Fructolysis index	Incubation period at 37°C		
	1 hour	2 hour	3 hour
Young buffalo bulls	2.066	1.196	-
Adult buffalo bulls	1.833	1.285	-
Old (aged) buffalo bulls	1.523	0.875	-
Overall average	1.723	1.133	-
Mixed semen samples	2.200	1.400	0.800

The metabolic acitivities of the spermatozoa as determined by oxygen uptake, fructose utilization and lactic acid balance at different intervals in different seasons show significant different (Table 7.13, 7.14 and 7.15). The oxygen uptake is significantly influenced by the season, pH, osmolarity of the suspending medium and concentration of the potassium and calcium ions (Rawat, 1979).

TABLE 7.13: Average oxygen uptake (micro litre), fructose utilization (microgram) and lactic acid (microgram) balance per 5 X 108 washed spermatozoa of Murrah buffalo bulls

Factors	Incubation interval in minutes				
	30	60	90	120	150
Season	Oxygen uptake (microlitre)				
Winter	34.28	51.59	67.43	81.18	99.33
Spring	28.98	47.12	57.98	70.81	94.29
Summer	17.53	26.58	33.12	43.47	50.64
Autumn	27.73	36.10	47.45	62.36	79.08
	Aerobic fructose utilization (microgram)				
Winter	341	766	1220	1377	1648
Spring	352	600	755	983	1175
Summer	275	425	575	700	925
Autumn	525	950	1125	1325	1450
	Lactic acid balance (micro-gram)				
Winter	320	428	562	528	508
Spring	214	329	405	391	390
Summer	28	133	194	233	283
Autumn	155	225	315	375	313

TABLE 7.14: Effect of different factors on Oxygen uptake per 5 X 108 washed spermatozoa of Murrah buffalo bull

Factors	Incubation interval in minutes				
	30	60	90	120	150
Initial pH of suspending medium					
5	23.24	36.63	48.39	59.98	69.18
6	22.78	36.96	49.28	63.09	75.11
7	19.01	32.24	42.77	55.72	64.74
8	16.05	27.96	38.83	50.39	50.59
Osmolarity expressed as milli osmoles of Sodium chloride					
150	12.53	28.76	48.58	64.47	78.31
256	20.79	36.30	51.97	69.01	85.54
308	17.72	31.23	45.24	63.47	76.64
375	13.28	24.27	35.73	49.38	60.32
436	11.56	19.68	29.69	42.11	50.92
Initial K^+ ion content in medium (mg%)					
120	21.16	34.64	43.53	55.31	65.65
200	18.57	31.61	39.33	51.59	60.68
280	16.68	30.11	41.56	54.48	62.77
380	18.00	29.43	38.43	50.08	50.08
Initial Ca^+ concentration (mg%)					
25	14.26	29.70	46.45	58.53	97.89
35	16.14	34.75	51.94	62.72	79.11
45	15.87	33.14	50.42	60.89	73.16
60	15.89	32.42	48.82	60.08	73.49

TABLE 7.15: Average oxygen uptake (milli litre), fructose utilization (mg) and lactic acid balance (mg) per 5 × 108 washed spermatozoa after 150 minutes incubation under different conditions

Factors	Condition of the incubation medium			
Initial pH	5.00	6.00	7.00	8.00
Shift in pH	5.23	5.71	6.67	7.39
Fructolysis (µg)	305	470	600	730
Lactic acid balance (µg)	264	445	468	455
Initial osmolarity	150	236	375	436
Fructolysis (µg)	985	1435	1247	1335
Lactic acid balance (µg)	330	456	451	467
Initial K^+ content (mg%)	120	200	280	360
Fructolysis (µg)	1330	1320	1275	1310
Lactic acid balance (mg%)	297	281	307	365
Initial Ca^+ content (µg)	25	35	45	60
Fructolysis (µg)	1655	1705	1860	1840
Lactic acid balance (mg%)	339	365	355	347

▶ MICROBIAL CONTAMINATION OF SEMEN

The normal glandular secretions of healthy buffalo bulls are free from the microbial contaminations. The common sources of semen contamination are the seat if non clinical mircrobial multiplication in the urethral canal, prepuce and sheath. The most common route of infection is the penile orifice. The sheath and prepuce are freely exposed to the external environment and frequently come into contact with ground, excreta, dirt, soiled bedding and other contaminated materials. Carelessness in the proper sterilization of the components of artificial vagina is another important source of microbial contamination of the semen may not be always pathogenic, indeed necessary precautions should be observed to keep them at the lowest level as far as possible. Several groups of bacteria and fungi have been isolated from the fresh and stored semen samples. Use of contaminated fluids in the semen extenders further increase the intensity of contamination of the semen after dilution (Mahmoud, 1953; Singh, 1962; Kodagali., 1973, 1979; Naidu et al., 1982).

▶ BACTERIA IN SEMEN

Buffalo semen has been found to be contaminated by several types of bacteria even at the time of collection if buffalo bulls are not maintained under hygienic environment. These are mostly Gram positive and Gram negative organisms in the semen and prepuce of the Egyptian buffalo bulls. The microorganisms have been identified as Diptheriods, Basillus fusiformis and Smegma bacilli. Mixing of a suitable sulph drug and penicillin and broad spectrum antibiotics during the process of dilution significantly reduces the microbial count in the semen (Mahmoud, 1953). The presence of different types of bacteria in the fresh semen samples and sheath (Table 7.16) in the somewhat semi-arid tropical climate of the north-west India (Singh, 1962) and identification of about 275 isolates (Table 7.16) from the semen samples and diluents in the hot and humid hot tropical climate of the Deccan platueau of India (Naidu et al., 1982) shows the need of more hygienic measures of management for reducing the bacterial contamination of the semen.

TABLE 7.16: Occurrence of bacteria in the semen and sheath of buffalo bulls (%)

Type of bacteria	Semen sample	Sheath
Staphylococci	50.0	25.0
Staph. aureus	11.4	-
Staph. album	34.2	25.0
Staph. citricum	15.2	12.5
Micrococcus	3.0	-
Streptococci	30.0	39.5
Strep. pyogenes	3.8	1.5
Strep. uberis	7.6	-
Strep. acidominimus	15.2	25.0
Enterococci	15.2	-
Corynebacteria	30.4	-
Coryn. pyogenes	15.2	-
Non-haemolytic	19.0	-

Contd.

TABLE 7.16: Occurrence of bacteria in the semen and sheath of buffalo bulls (%) (*Contd.*)

Type of bacteria	Semen sample	Sheath
Bacillus sp.	50.0	62.5
B. subtilis	26.6	25.0
B. mycoides	22.8	37.5
B. cereus	15.2	-
B. sphericum	15.2	-
Untyped gram +ve	22.8	12.5
Proteus	19.2	-
P. vulgaris	7.6	
P. mirabilis	3.8	
P. speciosus	11.4	
Bacterium	15.2	12.5
B. coli	3.8	
B. alkaligenes	11.8	12.5
Aerobactor	11.4	12.5
Pseudomonos aurogenosa	26.6	25.0
Untyped gram –ve rods	7.6	-

Incorporation of penicillin in the diluted semen helps in the reduction of microbial loads either by killing or by inhibiting their further multiplication. The action of penicillin is gradual and most effective at about 72 hours storage of the diluted semen under standard conditions in the refrigerator. About 33.37, 77.23 and 93.79% increase in the microbial count has been recorded on the storage of diluted semen without the addition of antibiotics for 24, 48 and 72 hours respectively. On the use of antibiotics in the diluted semen a significant reduction occurs in the bacterial count. The mean reduction in bacterial count in a study was about 47.4, 55.4 and 63.5% at 24, 48 and 72 hours storage respectively. (Table 7.17)

TABLE 7.17: Bacterial load (X 103) in the neat and diluted semen samples of buffalo

Semen and storage time	Range	Mean
Neat semen	9.833–24.266	15.662
Diluted semen without antibiotics after,		
24 hours	16.555–26.222	20.888
48 hours	19.388–33.888	27.758
72 hours	21.555–39.277	27.758
Diluted semen containing penicillin,		
24 hours	3.888–12.111	8.240
48 hours	3.666–9.444	6.985
72 hours	2.888–8.777	5.723

▶ FUNGAL CONTAMINATION OF SEMEN

Contamination of semen with several species of fungi has been also reported (Kodagali, 1973, 1979). The fungi identified in the fresh semen are Candida tropicalis, C. stellectoides, Aspergillus, Fusarium, Penicillium, Mucor and Yeast cells. The preputial sac has been found infested with fungi and prevalence is high during the humid hot season in camparison to other months of the year.

▶ SEMEN EXTENDERS/DILUTERS

The number of spermatozoa in each viable ejaculate are much higher than the requirement for successful conception. Therefore, technologies have been developed for the dilution of semen at each collection to facilitate the breeding of more buffaloes from the semen of each ejaculate. This technology significantly reduces the number of bulls for breeding, increases the use of pedigreed buffalo bulls for the breeding of much larger number of females for the improvement of production potential and also the use of preserved semen for breeding the buffaloes at a far away place with in the country and other countries. Cryopreservation technique has provided apportunity for the use of semen for breeding even after the death of the bull. A number of semen extenders have been developed for extending the buffalo semen (Ayyar, 1952; Srivastava et al., 1971; Yassen and El-Kamash, 1972; Ganguli et al., 1973; Rawat, 1979; Gupta and Tripathi, 1983). Some of the buffalo semen extenders developed and used are listed as follows:

1. Egg yolk glucosem bicarbonate
2. Egg yolk, citrate, glucose
3. Milk or skim milk diluents
4. Citric acid, whey diluent
5. Tris buffer based diluents
6. Cornell University diluent

▶ DILUTION RATE OF BUFFALO SEMEN

Although there is scope of dilution of high quality semen with more than 80% motility to the extent of more than 50 times but in practice buffalo semen is diluted in 1: 10 or 1: 20 ratio depending on the initial motility and concentration of the live spermatozoa. Dilution rate of 1: 25 of optimum quality semen at collection has also given good results (Vierzboski et al., 1980).

▶ PRINCIPLE OF SEMEN FREEZING

High storage temperature including the room temperature in tropical countries is not suitable for the semen preservation because it spoils rapidly the quality of semen due to fast metabolic processes. Therefore, freezing is necessary for the long time storage of useful semen. The semen for freezing is first diluted in a suitable extender which is practically not affected by the process of freezing. This buffer based extenders have been found to provide good protection to spermatozoa from the damaging effect of freezing.

▶ SEMEN SHIPERS

Following types of semen shipers are mostly used for the safe transportation of extended and processed semen.

1. Semen shiping box fitted with inner lining of cord board
2. Semen shiping box with inner lining of suitable synthetic material
3. **IVRI container:** It is made of a double walled copper can with space in the center for placing the semen vials. The can is then filled with clean and sterilized water and

then frozen. After this semen filled vials are wrapped in cotton wool are placed in the central space. Felt paddings are provided at the top and bottom of the copper can. Now this container is placed in an insulated container of rexin or canvas bag. The total final weight of this semen shiper is about 4.5 kg.

4. **Mathura container:** It was developed at the U P College of Veterinary Science and Animal Husbandry, Mathura. It is made of a rectangular metal case for holding the wide mouth thermos flask. A piece of felt is rolled in between the glass flask and metal case of the thermos flask. An inner lining of 6 mm thick foam rubber is placed in the glass flask for preventing the jerk during transporation. The diluted semen vials filled up to rim are put into a polythene or glass jar providing cotton wool packing for reducing agitational damage during the transportation. The diluted semen vials filled up to rim are put into a polythene or glass jar providing cotton wool packing for reducing agitational damage during the transportation. Small cubes of ice are filled in the space between the flask and semen container, and the thermos flask jar closed tight with a cork and plastic cap. In this container inside temperature is about 1–2°C even after 52 hours of storage and fall in the progressive motility is about 2.6 to 18.4% after 52 hours (Sengupta and Roy, 1968). The weight of container is 2 to 2.5 kg and it withstands rough handling during transportation even up to 100 km.

5. **Bangalore container:** It is made of an aluminium case with a handle. The inner side of case is lined with 1.25 cm thick sponge rubber for providing shock proof condition for the thermos flask. The container is suitable for a courier and its packed weight is about 2.25 kg.

6. **Poona container:** It is a 20 cm × 20 cm rectangular box of teak wood 30 cm in height. It is provided with handle on either side and on the top. There is locking arrangement for safe delivery. It can hold a thermos flask of 1.5 litre capacity and total packed weight is about 5 kg.

▶ MODES OF SEMEN TRANSPORTATION

Processed and properly preserved semen can be transported in a suitable semen shipment container by any of the available transport facility, viz.

1. **Pedestrian:** For transportation in th hilly areas lacking other transports.
2. Bicycle is used for short distance of 10 to 20 km daily run at AI centers where facilities are not available for the storage of semen. This is also used by the local inseminators covering animals in a radius of about 5–6 km.
3. Motor cycle is used by the inseminators of semen bank for covering the buffaloes in a radius of 10–16 km or at places where buffaloes ar scattered in small number with the farmers.
4. Jeep or bus is used for the shipment of semen from semen back to AI centers having refrigerator. The consisignment with the marked containers are booked in the bus or carried in a jeep or other suitable four wheel motor van for the shipment for long distance of 30 to 50 km or even longer.
5. Railway trains are used on the connected routes and also for longer distance exceeding 100 km.
6. Steamer and boats are used on water routes.
7. Aeroplanes are used for very long distance and also for international consignments.

▶ **METHODS OF ARTIFICIAL INSEMINATION (AI)**

The AI techniques used for the cows have been adopted for the buffaloes and cervical insemination techniques have been found to be more effective for AI.

1. **Vaginal insemination:** This is a very simple technique of AI. This is used by less experienced inseminators and also at a time when sterilized catheters are not available. The extended semen is taken in a sterilized all glass syringe of 2 ml capacity and deposited in any part of the vagina.

2a. **Cervical insemination with the help of a speculum:** The vaginal passage of the buffalo in standing heat is dilated by inserting a sterilized speculum into the vagina to make the os cervix visible. The insemination catheter is inserted into the os cervix by gentle pressure and extended semen or straw loases with semen is pumped into the cervix with the help of air pressure created by a sterilized glass syringe attached with insemination catherter. This method is more simple and effective than the vaginal insemination technique. It is essential to clean and sterilize the glass catheters and speculum after each use. Any laxity may cause reproductive problems.

2b. **Cervical insemination by recto-vaginal technique:** In this method the inseminator puts his hand in a long sleeve glove and placed his hand deep enough in the dung evacuated rectum to palpate and catch hold the cervix. The sterilized insemination catherter placed into the vagina and then its tip is guided by the fingers of inserted gloved hand to be palced into the os cervix by applying gentle pressure and then extended semen in a 2 ml sterilized all glass syringe or semen containing straw is pumped into the cervix by putting air pressure through few injections of air in the catherter.

   A non irritant lubricant is applied on the glove before inserting the hand into the rectum and air is allowed to enter at the time of inserting the hand. This helps in evacuating the rectum due to which force is not required for the removal of dung. This method provides an opportunity for the examination of the genitalia and also activate the uters somewhat similar to that of natural mating.

▶ **SITE OF INSEMINATION**

Although it is possible to deposite semen in the uterine horn, in practice it is deposited into the cervix to avoid traumatic injury of uterus and uterine cornua from the movements of the buffalo. There is no significant advantage of insemination in the uterus or uterine cornua but there is definite advantage of insemination in cervix as trauma is avoided.

▶ **DOSE OF EXTENDED SEMEN FOR A I**

Earlier 1.5 to 2.0 ml extended semen containing about 50 million motile spermatozoa were used for the deposition in the cervix of receptive buffaloes. Now the volume has been drastically reduced to put 0.2 ml extended semen in the straws used for A I.

▶ **SPEED OF TRAVEL OF THE SPERMATOZOA IN THE FEMALE GENITAL TRACT**

The survival time of the spermatozoa in the genital tract of female buffalo is 22 to 49 hours (Rao et al., 1960, Basirov, 1964). The spermatozoa rakes about 190 and 200 seconds to reach the anterior part of the fallopian ture after artificial insemination in the cervix and natural mating respectively (Rao et al., 1960).

▶ CONCEPTION RATE (CR)

Great variation occurs in the conception rate of buffaloes ranging from as low as 20% to more than 92% under different systems of management. The various factors affecting the C R are age of the buffalo, season of breeding, quality of the season, stage of oestrus, composition of semen extender, storage condition of semen, quality of feed and hygienic condition from the time of semen collection to inseminatuin. The number of service per conception may very from 1 to 4. Average service per conception in tropical conditions has been found to very from 1.39 + 0.31 to 2.38 + 0.27 in different studies in different studies in different breeds of buffaloes (Hafez, 1952, 1953; Bhattacharya and Prabhu, 1955; Oloufa, 1960; Wangi pei Chien, 1979; Mohemad et al., 1980; Chantalakhana et al., 1981).

REFERENCES

Abdou, M S S, El-Guiadi, M M, Mostafa, M A. El-Wishy, A R, Farhat, A A. 1974. Zentl. Vet. Med., A 21; 759–767.

Abdou, M S S, El-Guindi, M M, El-Menoufy, A A and Zaki, K.1977a. Zeitst. Fierz. Zuchthiol. 94; 8–26

Abdou, M S S, El-Guindi, M M, El-Fayoumi, M T. 1977. Zentl. Vet. Med., A24'636–641

Abdou, M S S, El-Guindi, M M, El-Menouf, A A and Zaki, K. 1978. Zentl. Vet. Med. A25; 222–230.

Abdulla, A., El-Guinid, M M and Mostafa, M A. 1973. Zentl. Vet. Med., A20; 567–570

Abhi, H L, Sengupta, B P, Roy, A and Sahni, K L 1968. Indian J. Vety. Sci. Anim. Husb., 38; 253–257

Afiefy, M M, Idris, A A and Yousef, H L 1984. Proc. 10th Intern.Cong. Animal Reprod. AI, Illinois, USA

Agar, N S, Rawat, J S and Roy, A 1965. Indian J dairy Sci., 18; 101–103

Alamy, M A, Alim, S O, Danesoury, M S and Olufa, M.1976. Indian J. Anim. Sci., 46; 163–166

Ali, H H, Ahmad, I A and Yassen, A M. 1981. Alexandria J. Agric. Res., 29; 47–57

Anand, S R. 1973. J. Reprod. Fert., 32; 93 - 100

Anand, S R. 1979. FAO Anim, Prod. Hlth. Paper 13' 284–291

Asker, A A and El-Itriby, A A. 1958. Alexandria J. Agric. Res., 6; 25–28

Ayyar, R V. 1944. Indian Vet. J., 20; 253–260

Badawy, A B A, El-Sawaf, S A and El-Wishy, A R. 1972. J. Egyptain Vet. Med. Assoc., 32; 81–90

Banerjee, A K and Ganguli, N C. 1973. J. Reprod. Fert., 33; 171–173

Barr, M A S, El-Hashim, S and El-Desouky, F. 1964. Proc. Intern. Cong. Reprod. Toronto, 4; 298–306

Basirov, E B. 1964. Proc. 5th Intern, Cong. Anim. Reprod., Toronto, 6; 4–10

Bhattacharya, P. 1962. Artificial insemination in the Water buffalo. Communication No. 15, Commonwealth Agric. Bureaux, England.

Bhattacharya, P and Prabhu, S S. 1955. Indian J. Vet. Sci. Anim. Husb., 25; 263–291.

Bhosrekar, M R. 1980

Bhosrekar, M R and Ganguli, N C. 1966

Chalapathy, P V and Rao, A R 1981. Indian J. Anim. Sci., 51; 761–765

Chantalakhana, C. 1981

Chaudhary, K C and Gangwar, P C. 1977. I. Agric. Sci., U K, 89; 273–277

Chauhan, R A. 1973

Chauhan, F S, Dwaraknath, P K and Vyas, K K 1973. Indian Vet. J., 52; 12–13

Chinnaiya, C P, Kakar, S S and Ganguli, N C 1979. Zntl. Vet. Med.,

Clanohoy, L L and Palad, O A. 1967. Philippines Agric., 51; 341–347

Daader, A H, Fayaz, L, Merai, M and Maar, A S. 1982. Proc. 6th Intern. Cong. Anim. Poult. Prod., Uni. Zagazig, Egypt, 1; 198–209

Dhanda, O P, Madan, M L and Razdan, M N. 1983. Indian J. Anim. Sci., 53; 1069–71

Dhanotiya, R S and Srivastava, R K. 1979. Zentl. Vet. Med., A 26; 810–814

Dube, G D, Pareek, P K, Dwaraknath, P K and Vyas, K K 1982. Indian J. Dairy Sci., 35; 80–82

Eapan, K J, Srivatava, P N and Raza Nasir, M M. 1964. Indian Vet. J. 41; 284–286

Prabhu, S S and Sharma, U D. 1953a. Indian J. vet. Sci. Anim. Husb., 23; 383–387

Prabhu, S S and Sharma, U D. 1953b. Indian J. Vet. Sci. Anim. Husb., 34; 273–277

Prabhu, S S and Sharma, U D 1955. Indian J. Vet. Sci. Anim. Husb., 25; 89–97

Radev, G, Danov, D and Mezinov, P. 1966 Nauchi Trud. Vissh 'Sel Inst. Georgia, Dimitrov Zootekh., Fak., 16; 341–352

Rahman Ali, N E D A 1962. Zivotnovodstovo, 24(8); 65–67

Ramsey, H A, Lodge, A R, Graves, C N and Salisbury, G W. 1963. J. Dairy Sci., 46; 1132–1134

Rao, A S P, Luktuke, S N and Bhattacharya, P. 1960. Indian J. Vet. Sci. Anim. Husb., 30; 178–190

Rawat, J S. 1979. FAO Anim. Prod. Hlth. Paper 13; 272–283

Roy, A, Kaenik, Y R, Luktuke, S N, Bhattacharya, S and Bhattacharya, P. 1950a. Indian J. Dairy Sci., 3; 42–45

Roy, A, Luktuke, S N, Bhattacharya, S and Bhattacharya, P. 1950b. Indian J. Dairy Sci., 3; 161–172

El-itriby, A A and Asker, A A 1957. Emp. J. Exp. Agric., 25; 156–160

El-Sawaf, S A, Badawy, A B A and El-Wishy, A B 1971. Zeitst. Tierzuch. Zuchthiol., 88; 222–230

El- Wishy, A B 1978.

Gallein, L and Roux, P 1984. Artificial Insemination in Domestic Animals. Press's University, Paris, France.

Ganguli, N C 1979. FAO Anim. Prod. Hlth. Paper 13; 292–303

Ganguli, N C, Bhosreker, M R and Jose Stephan 1973. J. Reprod. Fert., 35; 355–358

Gopalkrishna, and Rao, 1978

Goswami, S B 1962. Indian Vet. J., 39; 637–648

Gunzel, A R, Boenke, H J, Valencia, J. And Fischer, H 1979. Zuchthyg., 14; 181–184

Gupta, R S and Srivastava, R K 1981. Cellular Molc. Biol., 27; 539–541

Gupta, H P and Tripathi, S S 1983. Indian J. Anim. Sci., 53; 756–758

Guraya, S S and Sidhu, K S 1975. J. Reprod. Fert., 42; 373–376

Guselnov, G G, Guselnov, M A and Salmonov, Z M. 1969. Kend. Teserruf. Elmi Kheberieri Ves. Sel. Khoz Nauki, 3; 21–23

Hafez, E S E 1952. Proc. 2nd Intern. Cong. Physiol. Path. Animal Reportd. And A I, Copenhagen, 1; 97–100

Hafez, C, Bader, H and Bajwa, M A 1982. Pakistan Vet. J. 2; 155–160

Hukeri, B V 1969. Ph. D yhesis, Nagpur University, Nagpur

Iqubal, M, Samad, H A, Yakub, M and Najib-Ur-Rehman 1984. Pakistan Vet. J., 4; 158–160

Jain, Y C and Anand, S R 1975. J. Reprod. Fert. 42; 129–132

Jain, Y C and Anand, S R 1976a. J. Reprod. Fert., 47; 255–260

Jain, Y C and Anand, S R 1976b. J. Reprod. Fert. 47; 261–267

Joshi, S C, Tiwari, R B L, Sahni, K L and Rawat, J S 1967. Indian Vet. J., 44; 319–322

Kaleff, B 1944. Zeitst. Tierz. Zuchthiol., 51; 131–178

Kerur, V K 1971. Indian J. Anim. Hlth., 10; 199–121

Kodagali, S B 1973. Report on infertility in cattle in Gujrat, Gujrat Vetcol, Anand

Kodagali, S B 1979. Indian Vet. J.., 56; 807–809

Kushwaha, N S, Mukherjee, D P and Bhatacharya, P. 1955. Indian J. Vet. Sci. Anim. Husb., 25; 317–328

Lazarus, A J 1946. India Farming. 7; 247–250

Madatov, M R 1956. Truchy Azerb. Nauch. Issled Inst. Zivotn., 1; 129–144

Mahajan, S C and Sharma, U D 1961. Indian J. Vet. Sci. Anim, Husb., 31; 24–28

Mahmoud, L N 1952. Bulletin No. 15, Faculty of Medicine, Foud Uni., Egypt

Mahmoud, L N 1953. Indian J. Dairy Sci., 6; 197–200

Malkani, M 1954. M Sc. Thesis, Bombay University, Bombay

Mann, T 1948. J. Agric. Sci., Camb., 38; 323–331

Matharoo, B S Indian Farming

Misra, M S and Sengupta, B P 1965. Indian J. dairy Sci., 18; 130–133

Misra, B S, Singh, B P and Tomer, N S 1969. Indian J. Dairy Sci., 22; 202–203

Mohan, G, Madan, M L and Razdan, M N 1977. Trop. Agric. 54; 21–28

Naidu, K S, Rao, A R and Rao, V P 1982. Indian Vet. J., 59; 91–95

Nema, S R. Kodagali, S B, Janakiraman, K and Prabhu, G A 1983. Indian J. Anim. Reprod., 3; 5–8

Oloufa, M M 1960.Bulletin No. 214, Cairo university

Oloufam M M, Sayed, A A and Badreldin, a L 1959. Indian J. Dairy Sci., 12; 10–17

Osman, A M 1971. J. Egyptian Vet. Med. Assoc., 31; 55- 76

Pal, K 1957. Current Science, 26; 212–213

Pal, K, Luktuke, S N, De, S K and Bhattacharya, P. 1956. Indian J. Physiol. Allied Sci., 10; 67–75

Pandey, M D and Raizada, B C 1979. FAO Anim. Prod. Hlth. Paper 13; 253–246

Porwel, M L, Khan, F H and Karandikar, G W 1972. Indian Vet. J., 49; 491–495

Prabhu, S S 1956. Indian J. Vet. Sci. Anim. Husb., 26; 21–33

Prabhu, S S 1967. Indian J. Vet. Sci. Anim. Husb., 37; 107–117

Prabhu, S S and Bhattacharya, P 1953. Indian J. Vet. Sci. Anim. Husb., 21; 357–262

Prabhu, S S and Bhattacharya, P. 1953. Indian J., 30; 122–128

Prabhu, S S and Bhattacharya, P. 1954. Indian J. Vet. Sci. Anim. Husb., 24; 35–50

Prabhu, S S and Bhaya, K D 1962. Indian J. Vet., Sci. Anim. Husb., 29; 97–105

Prabhu, S S and Bhaya, K D 1965a Indian J. Vet. Sci. Anim. Husb., 32

Prabhu, S S and Bhaya, K D 1965b. Indian J. Vet. Sci Anim. Husb.,

Roy, A, Pandey,M D and Rawat, J S 1960. Indian J. dairy Sci., 13; 112–118

Roy, A, Srivastava, R K and Pandey, M D 1955. Current Science, 24; 246–247

Sane, C R, Gokhale, D R and Diwakar, K V 1954. Annual report of A I Centre, Poona

Sane, C R, Gokhale, D R and Diwakar, K V 1955. Annual Report of A I Center Poona

Sane, C R, Gokhale, D R, Diwakar, K V and Kaikini, A S 1960. Report on Cattle Sterlity Scheme, Maharahtra, Bombay

Sarmah, B C Kaker, M L and Razdan, M N 1983.Theriogenology, 20; 521–257

Saxena, V B and Singh, G 1971.J. Anim. Morph. Physiol., 18; 195–202

Sayed, A A and Oloufa, M M 1957. Indian J. Dairy Sci., 10; 167–169

Senger, D P and Sharma, U D 1965a. Indian J. Dairy Sci., 18; 54–60

Senger, D P and Sharma, U D 1965b. Indian J. Dairy Sci., 18; 61–64

Sengupta, B P and Roy, A. 1968. Indian J. Vet. Sci. Anim. Husb., 38; 288–297

Sengupta, B-P, Misra, M S and Roy, A. 1963. Indian J. Dairy Sci., 16; 150–165

Sengupta, B P, Singh, L N and Roy, A. 1969. Indian J. Anim. Sci., 49; 281–293

Sengupta, B P, Singh, L N and Roy, A. 1969. Indian J. Anim. Sci., 49; 281–293

Sengupta, B P, Singh L N and Rawat, J S. 1977

Shalash, M R, 1972. Zootech, Vet., 27; 71–76

Sharma, N C, 1969. M V Sc thesis, Bombay University, Bombay

Shukla, D D and Bhattacharya, P. 1949. Indian J. Vet. Sci. Anim. Husb., 19; 161–171

Sidhu, K S and Guraya, S S. 1979. J. Reprod. Fert., 57; 205–208

Singh, S P and Dutt, M 1964. Indian J. Dairy Sci., 17; 109–112

Singh, G and Saxena, V P. 1968. J. Anim. Morpj. Physiol., 15; 53–59

Singh, B., Singh, B P, and Tomer, N S. 1967. Indian J. dairy Sci.; 20; 81–85

Singh, B., Mahapatra, B B and Sadhu, D P. 1969. J. Reprod. Fert., 20; 175–178

Singh, B., Singh, H O and Sadhu, D P. 1974. Indian J. Anim. Hlth., 13 (1); 5–10

Singh, B and Sadhu, D P. 1978. Indian vet. J., 55; 296–303

Singh, M P, Sinha, S N and Balraj Singh, 1983. Indian J. Anim. Hlth., 22; 152–153

Srivastava, P N, Prabhu, S S and Bhattacharya, P. 1953. Gurrent Science, 22; 152–153

Stoev, P, Doiceva, M and Apostolov, N. 1966. Zhivostnovudatvo, 20 (3); 41–43

Toelehere, M R 1980. Biological aspect of reproduction and artificial insemination of the swamp buffaloes. Proc. Small Farms. Food Fort. Technol. Center, Taiwan

Tomar, N S and Misra, B S 1968. Indian Vet. J; 45; 702–705

Tomar, N S, Pande, R and Desai, R N 1964. Indian J. Dairy Sci., 17; 104–106

Tomar, N S, Misra, B S and Johri, C B. 1966. Indian vet. J., 43;

Tomar, N S, Sharma, O P and Singh, B P. 1970. Indian Vet. J., 47; 552–555

Tripathi, S S and Saxena, V B. 1976.

Tripathi, S S ans Saxena, V B 1983.Cheiron, 12; 193–199

Uma Shanker, Benjamin, B R and Agarwal, S K. 1984. Indian J. Anim. Sci., 54; 38–40

8

Mammary Glands and Lactation

▶ **INTRODUCTION**

Like other ruminant mammalians buffaloes posses mammary glands (udder) in the inguinal region. These are modified cutaneous glands for the highly specific function of milk production, which is the natural food of the new born calf. The cellular differentiation of mammary glands occurs in early pre-natal stage from the dermal cells on the ventral surface of embryo in the inguinal region. During the process of foetal development the mammary cells aggregate to form 4 distinct mammary buds, that is 2 on either side of the mid line. The formation of glands is almost similar in both sexes except that the development of teats in pre-natal growth is much slow in male foetus. The development of non-glandular portion consisting of connective tissue and fat pad is almost complete by the time of birth. Active development of mammary glands takes place at a much higher rate than the over all body growth in the early post-natal life. Larger portion of mammary ducts grow before conception and the formation of alveoli starts with the conception, which gradually replaces the pad of adipose tissue of the udder. In normal situation secretion of milk starts immediately after the birth of calf, but in excesptionally high milk producing buffaloes it may start a few days earlier than the calving date.

▶ **ANATOMY OF UDDER**

The mammary glands are collectively known as udder. Buffalo udder contains 4 mammary glands placed 2 on either side parallel to mid line in the inguinal region. The two lateral halves of udder has clear external demarcation in the site of median suspensary ligament, which is distinct on viewing form the rear through the gap between the hind limbs. The front attachment of udder is fused with abdominal wall and rear is folded and placed high between the hind limbs. Udder of dairy type riverine buffaloes is much larger and voluminous than their wild ancestors and draught type swamp buffaloes the 4 quarters of udder of dairy buffaloes should be well developed and almost similar in shape and size for convenient milking particularly for the machine milking. The length, width and girth of udder, udder score and type of udder significantly affect the milk yield (Taneja and Bhatnagar, 1958; Saxena and Prabhu, 1970; Saxena, 1973; Saakova, 1979a; Turadov and Abullave, 1979; Hafeez and Naidu, 1981; Tsankova, 1983). Usually, fore quarters are less voluminous with smaller teats than the rear quarters, and also yield significantly less milk in most of the animals (Polikhronov and Tosev, 1970; Ragab et al., 1971; Tsankova and Tosev, 1980; Pandey et al., 1981; Alim et al., 1982; Tripathi and Sarswat, 1982). Normally there is an increase in milk yield during the subsequsent lactations but udder characteristics remain almost unchanged (Hafeez and Naidu, 1981).

In the process of milking or suckling by the calf the milk flows out of the mammary glands through the teat canal. In most breds of buffaloes front teats are shorter than the rear teats (Saakova, 1979b). Supernumerary teats are often present but they are non-functional in almost all cases, and had no relationship with milk yield, lacation length and reproductive traits (Dwivedi and Prabhu, 1970; Ludri and Sarma, 1981; Verma et al., 1984). An exceptional instance of the fusion of left fore and rear teats, and another female with 5 functional teats has been reported in swamp buffalo (Fischer, 1962). Author detected one Nili-Ravi female with only 3 functionally developed quarters and teats and a yearling heifer with only 2 teats, one on either sude of midline.

▶ PART OF UDDER

The udder consists of external and internal supportive structures, circulatory vessels, lymph vessels, nervous net work and glandular parenchyma with lacteal canals opening into the cistern. All parts of udder play important role in milk production.

Skin

The skin of udder is thinner and soft than rest of the skin and encapsulates the mammary glands. Besides providing support it protects glands from external injuries and invasions of microorganisms. The skin is connected with abdomen with a coarse connective tissue.

Suspensary Apparatus

The suspensary apparatus of udder is formed of 2 layers of lateral and 2 layer of median suspensary ligaments (Katiyar and Girish Chandra, 1983). The suspensary ligaments are the most important supporting components of udder.

Larteral Suspensary Ligaments

Two layers of lateral suspensary ligaments are present on either side of the udder. These emerge from the sub-pelvic and prepubic tendons. Immediately after origin, the lateral suspensary ligaments are divided into a thin superficial and a thick deeper sheet. The superficial part is attached to semi-membranous and abductor muscles. Thicker layer is larger than the thinner superficial part which extends downward and forward covering the convex lateral surface of udder. A large number of lamellae from the thicker layer penetrate in interior of the glands forming interstitial septa for providing additional support. The ligaments are composed of elastic and collagenous fibres of connective tissue. The fibres are mostly arranged longitudinally and transversely with few oblique arrangements. Elastic fibres are thicker in outer and middle, and thinner in the inner zone of the lateral suspensary ligament (Katiyar and Girish Chandra, 1983).

Median Suspensary Ligament

These are the main supporting tissue of udder. These extend between right and left halves of udder and separated from each other after running a short length from their origin. The median suspensary ligaments are formed by the reflection of 2 lamellae of the yellow elastic fibres originating from the abdominal tunic at some distance posterior to umbilicus and have firm attachement with the mid line near the centre of gravity of the udder. Posteriorly they extend nearer to the ischial arch. These ligaments are mainly composed of elastic fibres which are thicker than the fibres of lateral suspensary ligaments. The fibre arrangements are oblique and transverse in the outer and inner zones, and longitudinal in the middle zone. Numerous lamellae of median suspensary ligaments extend into the gland parenchyma and form sling like supporting arrangements by joining with the lamellae of lateral suspensary ligaments. In addition to suspensary ligaments the abdominal tunic is also attached firmly on the dorsal convex surface of the mammary glands of buffalo.

Vascular System

Largest volume of oxygenated blood from the heart is supplied to the mammary glands by paired external pudic arteries arising from the posterior aorta in the inguinal region (Hossain et al., 1980, Badawi et al., 1985). The other sources of blood supply are the right and left common iliac arteries and the external iliac arteries. The external pudic arteries emerge through the external inguinal ring and then extend as the mammary arteries. Great variation may be seen in the branching pattern of mammary arteries among the animals. Branchig is more extensive in high milk producing buffaloes. Immediately after entering the udder mammary artery of each lateral half is divided into 2 main branches, viz. cranial mammary artery and caudal mammary artery. In large size udders of high milk yielders 2 additional off shoots of caudal mammary artery are given off before the origin of the main caudal mammary artery. The additional caudal mammary arteries of almost equal diameter to that of the main caudal mammary arteries branch extensively and supply the posterior part of the udder. Cow like pattern of branching of mammary arteries is also observed in many buffaloes. In such cases the cranial branch of mammary artery travels about two-third of the gland and then bifurcates into the cranial mammary artery supply to fore teats and udder. The main trunk extends forward as subcutaneous abdominal artery and terminates in front of the base of udder (Katiyar and Girish Chandra, 1983).

a. **Cranial mammary artery:** This extends forward after the branching of caudal mammary artery. It runs cranio-ventrally, continues distally and terminates on the cranio-lateral aspect of the fore teats as papillary artery. In its course numerous small branches arise and enter into the fore quarters of udder.

b. **Caudal mammary artery:** It travels almost ventrally in the hind quarters of udder forming an arch. The convexity of caudal mammary artery is directed cranially. The ventral course gives rise to a large branch extending downward and forward in the glandular parenchyma of the hind quarters of udder, and finally terminates in the lateral wall of the rear teats. The posterior branch of caudal mammary artery ramifies in the posterior part of mammary glands.

c. **Subcutaneous abdominal artery:** In many buffaloes, the subcutaneous artery anextension after the branching of the cranial mammary artery. It runs cranially in the glandular tissue near the lateral basal border and ramifies in the ventral abdominal wall in front of the base of udder. Severl lateral, medial and ventral branches of subcutaneous abdominal artery supply the glandular mammary tissue.

d. **Perineal artery:** A branch of posterior aorta at the ventral commissure of the vulva is called perineal artery which extends ventro-cranially under the skin in perineal region. Near the caudo-ventral region of the mammary gland several branches emerge to supply the mammary fascia of rear quarters. Usually no branch extends into the mammary glands.

The supra-mammary lymph glands are supplied by a thin branch of mammary artery which emerges before its bifurcation into the cranial and caudal branches. The vessels are more larger and tortuous in the voluminous udder of high milk yielding buffaloes.

The intermediate layer of wall of teats is the vessels zone of an extensive network of blood vessels. In the teats of virgin buffaloes the arteries are almost straight and muscular. The blood vessels increase in number and size with the advance of pregnancy. The arteries supplying lactating teats are highly thickened and tortuous is their course due to an increase in fibreo-muscular tissues aroud them. The blood flow of teat arteries is controlled by valves like arterial bolsters of different types Moussa, 1982).

At the point of termination of capillaries, origin of venules takes place which subsequently anastomose with each other to form the mammary veins that drain blood from the udder. The veins of udder traverse almost adjoining with the mammary arterial system. The blood flows through external pudic veins, external iliac and perineal veins into the posterior vena cava.

Second channel for the return of blood for the return of blood comprises of two subcutaneous abdominal veins commonly known as milk veins. These emere at the anterior border of udder. Flow of blood is directed towards udder in the region posterior to the umbilicus in young animals. The valves of veins become ineffective in lactating buffaloes and can flow either way, that is towards anterior vena cava as well as the udder.

Flow rate of blood in the udder is one of the most important factor for regulating the milk production in lactating animals. An increase in blood flow towards he udder and decrease n uterine circulation is observed during early post-partum period. Probably this condition plays an important role in the initiation of milk secretion by increased flow of milk precursors and lactogenic hormones into the mammary glands. The flow rate of blood towards udder continues to rise up to the peak yield period and thereafter starts a gradual decline.

Lymphatic System

Lymph is a colourless body fluid originating from the fileration of blood. Its composition is similar to that of blood except that the lymph is devoid of blood cells and contains lower concentration of proteins. Exchane between the constituents of blood plasma and interstitial fluid largely contributes in the production of lymph. The mammary glands are traversed by an extensive proliferation of lymph vessels. The mammary glands are traversed by an extensive proliferation of lymph vessels. The mammary glands are drained by superficial and deep sets of lymph channels. The superficial vesselsare are spread all around the surface of mammary glands beneath the cover of skin, fasciae and a thick layer of adipose tissue, while majority are in direct contact with the glandular parenchyma. Anastomoses occur between the lymphatics of fore and rear quarters of sma side but not with the other side. This plays significant role in controlling the infections from one side to other side. Many minor superficial lymphatics arise from the glandular parenchyma at the ventral border of mammary glands and around the base of teats. They run tortuosly upwards on the lateral surface of the body of mammary glands (Corpus mammae). In their course some of the lymph vessels dorsally receive lymphatics draining the glandular parenchyma. All the lymph canals terminate as different vessels on the ventral border of the supramammary lymph node.

Lymphatics on the caudal surface of mammary glands run a tortuous course dorsally and cranillay, and terminate as afferent ducts of the mammary lymph node. The others unite with lymphatics of lateral surface and then terminate on the ventral border of mammary lymph gland. Lymph vessels of the mammary lymph gland. The deep parenchyma of mammary glands is drained either directly or coalesced with superficial lymphatics into the mammary lymp gland.

The mammary lymph glands (nodes), 2 in number are situated on either side of the mid line near the caudal aspect of base of the udder beneath the thick layer of adipose tissue. A notch on the dorsal border of mammary lymph gland represents the hilus. Mammary lymph nodes are flattened and oval or somewhat triangular in shape. Its length ranges from 5 to 7 cm and width 3 to 5 cm.

The efferent lymph vessels of mammary lymph node are 6–7 in number of which 2–3 vessels of cranial group after arising from the hilus run cranio-dorsally in a tortuous shape and cross the mammary vessels. After this they run dorsally to enter the inguinal canal along the cranial border of external pulic vein beneath the cover of external oblique muscle of abdomen. These lymphatics then cross the vein near ventral aspect of the body if ilium to turn abruptly posterior and ventral to enter into the ilio-femoral lymph node. The caudal group of efferent lymph vessels are larger in diameter and more tortuous than the cranial group. After leaving the hilus of lymph node they move dorsally and enter the inguinal canal, where they intend posterior to external pudic ertery for a short distance and cross it beneath the ilium before termination at the lateral surface of ilio-femoral lymph node, also known as deep inguinal lymph gland. This gland is situated under the body of ilium in the angle formed by external iliac and circumflex iliac arteries. The shape is oval, length ranges from 7 to 9.9 cm and width from 4 to 7 cm (Barnwal and Dhingra, 1978).

▶ NERVE SUPPLY

Mammary glands are supplied with afferent (Sensory) and efferent (Motor) nerves of the sympathetic nerve fibres. These nerves arise from the ventral lumbar, inguinal and perineal branches of central nervous system (CNS). Sensory nerves are important in milk ejection mechanism. Motor nerves regulate blood supply and inervate the smooth muscle around the milk collecting ducts and the teat sphincter. Since nerves of the mammary glands are situated in the connective tissue and not in the direct contact with the alveolar cells of the parenchyma, there seems to be no direct effect of nerve supply on hormone, epinephrine, which has vaso-constriction property and has inhibitory effect on milk secretion. Massage, temperature and suckling of teats stimulate the secretion of oxytocin from the pituitary gland, which induces let down of milk.

▶ MAMMARY DUCT SYSTEM

A series of ductules draining from the alveoli through larger channels into the teat cistern and ending at the streak canal form the mammary duct system. The ductules and secretory lobules are supported by intralobular and interlobular connective tissue septa. The quantity of connective tissue is more in low milk producing animals, whereas mammary glands of high milk producing buffaloes contain greater proportion of alveolar tissue and ductular tissue with minimum amount of connective tissue. In Egyptian buffaloes the ratio between glandular and non-glandular tissues of high yielding buffaloes reported 1.79 was almost double than 0.82 observed in low milk yielders (Nosier, 1972). The opening of streak canal of teats is controlled by strong sphincter muscles and streak canal is the continuation of teat cistern. The teat cistern continues as the gland cistern at the base of udder. The gland cistern is poorly developed in buffaloes because there is no accumulation of milk before milking in the gland cistern of buffaloes (Aliev, 1964). A series of branches of mammary ducts arise from the gland cistern and ramify through sub-branching into the alveolar tissue and at the end forming terminal ductules for draining milk from each alveolus.

▶ DEVELOPMENT OF MAMMARY GLANDS

Milk production in animals is mainly influenced by the amount of milk synthesizing cells, the alveoli. The proportion of alveolar tissue is much higher than the connective tissue and other non-glandular tissues in high milk producing buffaloes (Nosier, 1972).

a. **Pre-natal development of mammary glands:** The cellular differentiation of mammary tissue takes place in early embryonic life of 3 to 5 weeks post conception from the dermal cells in the inguinal region. Aggregation of mammary cells occurs during the foetal development of non-glandular tissue, viz. connective tissue and fat pads is almost complete at the time of birth and glandular part is rudimentary.

b. **Post-natal development up to puberty:** At birth although formation of glands and teat cisterns is complete, the mammary duct system is still short and limited to the region of gland cistern. Growth of udder is slow in early post-natal life up to 6–7 weeks and then increases steadily to a much faster rate than the body growth. In Egyptian buffalo heifers significant development in length and diameter of teats and the circumference of udder has been observed between 45 to 900 days of age, when the mammary glands reached functional stage (Nosier et al., 1973). About 2–3 months before the onset of first oestrous a rapid proliferation of mammary parenchyma occurs. Cyclic change exhibited by the accumulation of secretion in the lumen of smaller mammary ducts occurs during the oestrous cycle and some regression is observed later in the oestrous cycle.

c. **Mammary growth during pregnancy:** In the early phase of pregnancy more proliferation of mammary ducts occurs in the young heifers. Formation of interlobular ducts takes place and alveoli grow to replace adipose tissue in udder. Growth of glandular parenchyma is rapid through out the gestation period but in heifers it becomes consipicuous usually after 3–5 months of pregnancy. The size of alveoli increases significantly during the terminal phase of pregnancy when udder becomes distended, smooth and bright in appearance.

d. **Mammary growth during lactation:** The multiplication of cells of mammary the glands continues in early phase of lactation, probably up to peak lactation. Therefore, the alveoli are densely packed in the udder. During declining phase of lactation the degeneration of glandular cells exceeds the formation of new cells. The maintenance of multiplication of mammary cells is maintained at a steady rate for longer duration in high milk producing buffaloes with longer lactation length.

e. **Mammary growth during dry period:** Wide variations occur in the mammary glands of buffaloes during dry period because it varies from less than 40 days to more than a year or so. Under normal breeding the buffaloes should be given a minimum 60 days of lactation rest otherwise milk production will be adverseluy affected in the following lactation. Partial to complete involution of udder occurs during the dry period depending on the length of dry period. Involution of udder is incomplete in females that conceive during the lactation period because the growth of mammary glands is stimulated by the hormones produced during pregnancy.

▶ HORMONAL REGULATION OF THE DEVELOPMENT OF MAMMARY GLANDS

Almost all the hormones required for the regulation of normal reproduction are also play significant role in the growth of mammary glands. This is evident from the fact that greater growth of mammary glands takes place during puberty, pregnancy and a short period after calving. The hormones involved in mammary development are produced by anterior pituitary gland, ovaries, adrenal glands, thyroid glands and placenta.

a. **Anterior pituitary (hypophysis):** The growth hormones and prolactin stimulate the growth of mammary tissues and also had synergestic effect on the udder development stimulation of ovarian hormones, the oestrogen and progesterone.

b. **Ovaries:** The ovarian hormones, oestrogen and progesterone regulate the growth of mammary glands during puberty and pregnancy. The oestrogen stimulates proliferation of mammary duct system while its combination with progesterone is required for the multiplication of glandular parenchymal cells of the udder.

c. **Adrenal and thyroid glands:** The stimulatory effect of administration of adrenal steroids and thyroxine is perhaps related with their general stimulatory effect on metabolic activities in the body. The effect of these hormones on mammary growth is probably secondary.

d. **Placental hormones:** Oestrogen and lactogen are the important hormones of placenta which impart synergestic effect on the mammary growth alongwith hormones of anterior pituitary gland and ovaries.

▶ UDDER CONFORMATION

The shape and size of udder influence the lactational characteristics like milk ejection, milking time, rate of milk flow and also the milk yield (Polikhronov and Tosev, 1970; Nosier, 1972; Saxena and Prabhu, 1972; Sidhu and Pal, 1978; Turabov, 1982).

a. **Shape of udder:** The shape of buffalo udder has been distinguished into 3 to 5 types on the basis of their appearance in the lactating buffaloes. Commonly described 3 types of udder are bowl or trough shaped, round or globular shape and goat type (Saxena and Prabhu, 1072; Saxena, 1973; Turabov and Abuliaev, 1979; Turabov, 1982). Pendulous type udder (Singh and Bhatnagar, 1977) and sub grouping of round udders into bath-shaped, narrow-round shape and primitive type udders (Sankova, 1979) have been also identified in small herds of Indian and Caucasin buffaloes. Bowl shaped udder is prevalent and found in 70–75% Indian dairy buffaloes followed by round shape in 14–18% and goat type in 8–12% animals of the organized herds. Round shaped udder is more in Caucasian buffaloes followed by bowl shape and goat type.

b. **Size of udder:** The length, width and depth of udder and milk yield continue to increase up to third and fourth lactations after that there is gradual decrease in milk yield without any significant change in the size of udder (Saxena, 1973; Hafeez and Naidu, 1981). Udder size is also significantly influenced by the stage of lactation and the number of lactation (Sidhu and Pal, 1978). The size of developed udder of Murrah type, Egyptian and Caucasian buffaloes is presented in Table 8.1

The size of udder significantly decreases after milking (Alim, 1983). The growth of alveolar cells of mammary glands is very rapid in the early lactation period and a gradual increase in udder size associated with the corresponding increase in milk yield is observed up to the peak yield and thereafter gradual involution of udder and decline in milk yield take place.

TABLE 8.1: Mean size of udders of different types of dairy buffaloes

Udder traits (cm)	Murrah type (Saxena, 1973)	Caucasian (Saakova, 1979)	Egyptian (Alim, 1983)
Circumference		85.50 + 0.30	86.61 + 0.53
Length	54.81	32.46 + 0.74	
Width	49.60	23.68 + 0.32	
Depth	15.29	13.05 + 0.03	
(i) Fore udder			15.91 + 0.10
(ii) Rear udder			14.41 + 0.09
Udder score			1330.67 + 14.09

A little difference has been observed in the udder shape of Murrah type buffaloes at the Military dairy farms in India showing a preference for bowl shaped udder. Almost linear increase in udder size and milk yield has been observed up to fourth lactation without a significant difference between the fourth and fifth lactations of the Murrah group of buffaloes at there organized dairy farms of India (Saxena, 1973). The length and width of udder showed a declining trend in the fifth lactation but depth continues to increase (Table 8.2).

TABLE 8.2: Effect of lactation number on udder size and test milk yield in Murrah type buffaloes

Traits			Lactation number		
	1	2	3	4	5
Udder traits (cm)			**Jabalpur dairy farm**		
Length	49.30	53.22	55.25	58.00	58.09
Depth	44.64	48.88	50.66	52.46	51.04
Width	13.18	14.67	15.39	16.09	16.22
Milk yield (kg)	5.06	6.22	6.41	6.73	6.86
			Meerut dairy farm		
Udder, Length	51.00	55.15	56.84	60.67	58.51
Depth	49.23	50.36	53.24	57.01	53.61
Width	12.64	13.83	14.35	15.23	15.52
Milk yield (kg)	6.65	7.13	7.46	8.40	8.47

Somewhat similar trend is observed in Egyptian buffaloes. Significant fall in circumference and score of udder has been observed during different lactation stages being highest during the first 2 months of lactation (Table 8.3) in Egyptian buffaloes (Alim, 1983).

TABLE 8.3: Measurements of buffalo udder

Traits	Udder measurements (cm)			
	Front depth	Rear depth	Circumference	Udder score
Lactation number				
First	14.26	12.53	73.74	1004.02
2nd to 4th	17.34	15.63	97.75	1613.43
Stage of lactation (month)				
1st and 2nd	16.17	14.63	98.09	1537.15
3rd and 4th	15.75	14.10	88.85	1334.71
5th and more	15.89	14.05	79.96	1229.19

c. **Topography of udder:** Udder of buffaloes is situated in the inguinal region. In dairy type reverine buffaloes well developed udder is placed just behind the umbilicus and may be as high as up to thirl beneath the lower vulvar commissure. The teats hang almost vertical in line with the ground surface. In swamp buffaloes mostly small size udder is placed posteriorly between the hind limbs and provides convenient disposition for calves to suckle from rear side through the space between the hind legs. Rear suckling is quite common in swamp buffaloes. In Murrah type buffaloes distance from ventral end of vulva to rear attachment of udder then to rear teat is 31.24 and 4.80 cm; from front ventral end of udder is 12.36 cm. udder length is 53.47 + 6.66 cm and distance from ground to udder is 59.00 + 5.45 cm in a herd of organized farm (Mangurkar and Desai, 1981). The length of udder increases and the distance from ground decreases in subsequent lactations. Chamge in other measurements may be inconsistent (Table 8.4).

TABLE 8.4: Udder measurements in different lactation of Murrah type buffaloes

Udder measurements (cm)	Lactation number					
	1	2	3	4	5	6
Distance from ventral end of vulva to rear attachement	12.36	11.84	12.23	12.03	11.75	12.80
Distance from rear attachment of udder to rear teats	27.31	29.24	30.33	31.92	33.26	33.28
Distance from front attachment of udder to fore teats	9.86	10.74	11.31	10.94	11.99	12.34
Udder length	47.15	50.90	52.23	53.71	56.65	57.86
Distance from ground to lowest end of teat	61.41	59.04	58.31	57.82	55.49	56.73

▶ **TEATS**

The teat is a tubular terminal continuation of each quarter of udder and its main function is to provide passage for the ejection of milk from udder at the time of suckling and milking. Flow of milk is controlled by strong sphincter muscles around the streak canal. The teat is formed of external epidermis which is thicker towards the orifice. Middle layer of chorium is formed of dense connective tissue with numerous blood white fibrous tissue, elastic fibres and a few bundles of smooth muscle fibres. The teat skin is free from hair follicles as well as sweat and sebaceous glands. The teat cistern starts narrow from the streak canal and widens upwards to continue as poorly developed udder cistern. The tunica epithelialis of teat canal is formed of a single layer of cuboidal cells resting on a basement membrane. Numerous folds project from the mucosa (Fahmy et al., 1969).

a. **Shape of teats:** Three types of teats are found in the Indian riverine buffaloes. These are cylindrical, conical and funnel shaped. The first 2 types are more common and found in 70–80% of buffaloes (Bhosrekar and Nagpaul, 1971; Saxena and Prabhu, 1972; Singh and Bhatnagar, 1977). Variation in the shape of teats of fore and rear quarters of the same buffalo is quite common.

b. **Size of teats:** Moderate type evenly placed teats provide convenient disposition both for hand milking and machine milking. Rear teats are usually longer and voluminous than the fore teats. Various factors like age, number of lactation and stage of lactation significantly affect the size of teats (Nosier et al., 1973; Sindhu and Pal, 1978; Saakova, 1979b; Alim, 1983). Mean length and diameter of teats in a herd of Caucasian buffalo has been 6.64 cm and 1.60 cm for the fore teats, and 8.03 and 1.93 cm for the rear teats, respectively (Saakova, 1979). These measurements of corresponding teats in Murrah buffaloes are 7.50 + 7.03 and 2.65 + 0.04 cm, and 8.50 + 0.13 and 2.83 + 0.04 cm (Sindhu and Pal, 1980). Milking has significant effect on the size of teats (Table 8.5). Usually, length increases and diameter decreases after the milking of buffaloes which return to original form before the next milking time (Aliev et al., 1965; Alim, 1983). A large variation in the teat length of less than 6.64 cm and diameter below 1.60 cm are generally not suitable for machine milking (Gotsiridze and Saakova, 1980).

TABLE 8.5: Changes in size of teats after milking

Milking effect	Teat length (cm)		Teat circumference (cm)	
	Fore	Rear	Fore	Rear
Left side				
Before milking	7.86 + 0.04	8.87 + 0.06	3.30 + 0.02	3.34 + 0.02
After milking	8.58 + 0.03	9.23 + 0.04	2.83 + 0.02	2.90 + 0.02
Right side				
Before milking	8.02 + 0.06	9.12 + 0.05	3.14 + 0.02	3.49 + 0.02
After milking	8.78 + 0.03	9.58 + 0.04	2.90 + 0.02	3.09 + 0.02

c. **Placement of teats:** Like length and diameter there is also great variation in the placement of teats. Even size squarly placed teats are convenient for milking. Distance between the four teats is greater when udder is distended before milking, which comes closer after milking due to sunkenning of the udder (Table 8.6). Distance between the fore teats and between rear teats is usually adequate but mostly less between the opposite teats for efficient milking (Alim, 1983). Average

TABLE 8.6: Distance between the teats of Egyptian buffaloes before and after milking

Attributes		Distance between teats (cm)
Fore teats	Before milking	13.71 + 0.077
	After milking	11.39 + 0.067
Rear teats	Before milking	9.23 + 0.061
	After milking	7.95 + 0.053
Left side	Before milking	7.41 + 0.049
	After milking	6.39 + 0.044
Right side		7.42 + 0.066
		6.46 + 0.042

distance between the fore teats and between the rear teats in a herd of Murrah buffaloes has been recorded to be 13.44 + 0.14 cm and 8.96 + 0.13 cm respectively (Sindhu and Pal, 1980).

▶ ANOMALIES OF UDDER AND TEATS

Different kinds of structural anomalies have been observed in buffaloes and these are more common in dairy type reverine buffaloes.

a. **Anomalies of udder:** An unique case of hypoplasia in twin buffalo heifers born in Sumatra presented satisfactory evidence of mirror imaging requirement of the monozygous twins. One heifer lacked a teat on right fore quarter and the other on left fore quarter, and both had unilateral hypoplasia of the udder on different sides (Fischer, 1956). In a mixed herd of 66 Murrah, 380 Murrah grades and 184 non-descript female buffaloes the incidence of udder anomalies was about 4.91%. This included about 1.58, 1.75 and 1.58% of hypoplasia, cloven udder, and hypo and hypermastis respectively (Rao and Murthy, 1984). Prevalence of udder anomalies had been much higher in Murrah group of buffaloes.

b. **Anomalies of teats:** Various teat anomalies encountered in buffaloes are the fused teats, pouched teats, blind teats, supernumerary teats and deficit teats. A case of fusion of fore and rear teats of left side without any sign of existence of right fore teat was observed by author in a Murrah grade durig 2001. An example of 5 functional teats has been reported in Thialand (Fischer, 1962). Incidences of about 4.91% fused teats, 1.93% pouched teats and 2.28% supernumerary teats have been recorded in mixed herd of 630 female buffaloes comprising of Murrah, Murrah grades and non-descript animals (Rao and Murthy, 1984). Great variation ranging from 2.28 to 37.9% has been observed in the incidence of supernumerary teats in the Indian riverine buffaloes (Dwivedi and Prabhu, 1970; Ludri and Sarma, 1981; Verma et al., 1984). The incidence of supernumerary teats in herds of Murrah, Mehsana, Jaffarabadi, crossbred and graded buffaloes has been found about 2.60, 1.34, 2.33, 8.65 and 2.67% respectively, which was lowest in Mehsana breed. Occurrence of intercalary (between the normal teats) position is more tha the caudal and ramal positions. About 1.8% supernumerary teats had been found functional. Incidence of single supernumerary teat is more (2.25%) than the two supernumerary teats (0.34%) in Murrah type buffaloes (Dwivedi and Prabhu, 1970).

▶ LACTATION

The process of milk secretion from the mammary glands is known as lactation. The milk constituents are partly contributed by the blood and largely produced by the alveoli of the mammary glands. There is no significant difference in the osmotic pressure of milk and blood, but there is significant difference in their composition. The milk of buffaloes is white in colour whereas normal blood is bright red. The concentration of proteins in milk is lower than the blood but that of sugar, lipids, calcium, phosphorus and potassium is much higher. Sodium and chloride contents are also less in milk but increase considerably during the declining phase of lactation. Milk proteins are largely casein with small amount of albumins and globulins. The later are much higher in the first milk, colostrums. On the other hand albumins and globulins are the main proteins of blood. The milk fat is largely triglycerides while principal components of blood lipids are cholesterol and phospholipids.

Under normal conditions lactaction in buffaloes starts immediately after parturition when stimulated by suckling of calf or mild manipulation applying light pressure by the milker. The first milk is colostrums which contains very high percentage of fat, proteins including immunoglobulins and minerals, and low level of lactose in comparison to normal milk. In dairy buffaloes, milk secretion increase steadily to attain peak yield at 3–10 weeks of lactation period in different breeds (Maymone, 1945; Kumar and Bhat, 1979; Chowdhary and Chaudhary, 1981).

Following terminologies are commonly used for describing different events of lactation, i.e.

i. Lactation or galactopoiesis is the complete process of secretion and removal of milk from the udder.

ii. Initiation of lactation or milk formation is referred to the lumen of albeoli.

iii. Milk ejection or let down of milk is the process of milk removal from the udder due to contraction of the myoepithelial cells surrounding the alveoli. This function is initiated by the action of oxytocin hormone either liberated intrinsic from the posterior pituitary gland or injected pharmaceutical preparations.

iv. Milk removal involves both active action of oxytocin and passive removal by suckling calf or milking.

▶ HORMONAL CONTROL OF LACTATION

Although several hormones are associated with the initiation and maintenance of milk secretion, the precise mechanism of action is not yet fully known. Milk production capacity of buffaloes depends on the ratio of glandular and non-glandular tissues in the mammary glands, which is wider in high yielders (Nosier, 1972). Oestrogen stimulates the growth of mammary duct system and in combination with progesterone the growth of lobulo-alveolar tissue (Shalash et al., 1961; Ferrera et al., 1966; Sud and Singh, 1974). For the complete development of mammary glands, pituitary hormones are also necessary alongwith oestrogen and progesterone. Prolactin and adenocorticotropic hormone (ACTH) are important for the initiation and maintenance of lactation. ACTH maintains the required levels of different milk precursors in the blood. Thyroxine has temporary effect on increasing the production of milk but it is not essential for galactopoieses (Asker et al., 1954; Aliev, 1962). The pituitary hormone, oxytocin is responsible for milk ejection and frequently used for the let down of milk in difficult animals (Chandiramani et al., 1966; Jadhav and Khambhata, 1967; Hanna et al., 1979). Oxytocin stimulates the contraction of the myoepithelial cells around the alveoli and along the mammary ducts and milk secretion starts.

▶ INITIATION OF LACTATION

At the time of parturition level of prolactin and ACTH increases and that of oestrogen and progesterone decreases. This marked change in the levels of different hormones is responsible for the initiation of lactation.

▶ MAINTENANCE OF LACTATION

Maintenance of lactation in buffaloes is influenced by the hormones and the husbandry practices like optimum balanced feeding, adequate water supply for drinking and wallowing or shower batn, maintenance of good health and regulation in milking.

In buffaloes gentle massage of udder and teats with warm water in weaned and suckling in nursing buffaloes stimulate the release of hormones. Unlike cows there is noaccumulation of milk in the cistern and thus, thesuppression of lactation due to high intra-mammary pressure may not be important in buffaloes (Aliev, 1962). However, suppression of lactation due to engorgement of mammary ducts may not be ruled out. The ratio between secretary cells at the stage of formation, the actively functioning cells and the cells under process of involution varies during different stages of lactation period. The ratio of cells are maximum during the peak lactation. It is assumed that the individual groups of secretary-motor complexes of the mammary glands (Olenov, 1954). These secretary-motor complexes are functionally different from one another due to which milk of different fat percentage is obtained in the consecutive portions of a single yield of buffaloes (Table 8.7).

TABLE 8.7: Fat percent in different portions of milk of a single milking during different stages of lactation

Portion of milk	Fat content (%) at different month of lactation		
	1st month	4th month	7th month
1	6.02	9.97	9.10
2	5.19	9.20	10.60
3	4.77	7.13	12.40
4	4.95	7.90	14.61
5	6.35	9.50	-
6	7.72	11.20	-
7	10.76		

▶ MILK EJECTION OR LET DOWN OF MILK

The mechanism of transfer of milk from functional alveoli into themammary ducts and its subsequent flow from the mammary glands through the orifice of teats is known as milk ejection or let down of milk. This process lobe of the pituitary gland. Oxytocin is quickly transported in blood to the mammary tissue, where it produces contraction of the myoepithelial cells surrounding the alveoli. The milk is expelled from the alveoli into duct system to finally enter in cisterns of the udder and teats. This causes sudden rise of internal pressure in the cisterns. At this stage milk is easily removed by suckling calf or by milking. The complete process is governed by afferent motor nerve and the hormone, oxytocin, and this relax action is known as neuro-hormonal or neuroendocrine reflex.

In the dairy buffaloes this reflex becomes conditional and can be stimulated by the specific sound of ratling milk pails, the sound of milkers, the application of teat cups in case of machine milking, the washing of udder, movement to milking byre, massage of udder by milker and suckling of calf. Significant changes in surroundings disturbing the animal may greatly influence the let down of milk. In case of suckling when calf is tied away from the normal practice of keeping near the dam, the buffalo gets agitated and milk let down is incomplete and secretion of fat in different portions of milk is irregular (Aliev, 1971). Oxytocin is effective for a very short period of 3–10 minutes (Shafie et al., 1971; Gupta et al., 1974; Dass et al., 1976; Alim, 1983; Roy and Nagpaul, 1984).

▶ INDUCED LACTATION

Infertility and sub fertility are the serious reproductive disorders of buffaloes in most of the countries. Such animals are mostly called for slaughter in active productive life or maintained barren for many years without any return except the swamp buffalo females are used for draught power in agricultural operations. Establishment of active lactation in such buffaloes can be helpful in obtaining the large amount of milk going waste in these buffaloes. Various degree of udder growth and lactation has been achieved by hormonal treatments in barren buffaloes. Treatment with administration of oestrogen and progesterone stimulates the growth of mammary glands and teats, initiates milk production and maintains lactation for various duration (Shalash et al., 1961). Biopsy of udder shows different stages of alveolar growth, i.e. resting parenchyma, various stages of growing parenchyma and milking lobuls and acini (D' angelo and De Franciscis, 1966). The response of hormonal induction of lactation has been poor in young buffalo heifers of 15–18 months of age (Shalash et al., 1966a, b_, but encouraging results have been obtained in adult infertile heifers of 4–6 years and buffaloes of 6–13 years of age (Sud, 1979, Rao et al., 1982; Atheya and Sud, 1985).

As usual the composition of milk of induced lactation animals becomes normal after 5 days (Table 8.8). In case of virgin heifers the milk fat content has been found less than the normal milk (Minieri et al., 1966) and in adult buffaloes it was higher than the normal milk (Atheya and Sud, 1985). In five such studies residual oestrogen in milk could not be detected by the vaginal smear and uterine weight methods using ovareectomized albino rats (Shalash et al., 1964).

TABLE 8.8: Chemical composition of milk from normal and induced lactation

Milk constituents (%)	Young buffalo heifers			Adult buffaloes	
	Induced 1st milk	Last milk	Normal milk	Induced milk	Normal milk
Milk fat	5.80	6.80	7.48	8.71	6.42
Protein	20.05	4.60	3.95	4.13	4.24
Lactose	0.65	3.42	4.90	4.40	4.53
Ash	3.18	0.85	0.08	0.73	0.73
Casein	7.73	3.68	3.16	ND	ND
Solids not fat	23.88	8.87	9.65	8.53	8.30

For the artificial induction of lactation in barren and sub fertile buffaloes, hormones are administered by subcutaneous injection or as a subcutaneous implant in the neck region followed by subcutaneous injection after 6 weeks or alongwith udder infusion of diethylstilboestrol of milk for human consumption. Some quacks are practicing in may parts of India and there is urgent need of legistation for the use of this technology, if it does not has harmful effects on human health.

▶ HORMONAL STIMULATION OF LACTATION

Thyroxine and various iodinated proteins like thyroidin, thyroprotein and iodinated casein have shown stimulatory effect on the lactation in buffaloes (Asker et al., 1954; Maqsood, 1956; Aliev, 1962). An increase up to 19% in milk yield and 42% in milk fat may occur due to administration of thyroxine. Administration of thyroxine in the beginning of lactation mainly stimulates the secretion of milk, at the peak of lactation both milk and fat, and during the declining phase it limits the drop in milk yield, and increases fat percentage in milk. It has complicated effects on the secretion of milk proteins, which is primarily affected by the stage of lactation. In beginning there is no change in protein percentage but total production is high due to increased milk yield. At the peak of lactation both protein percentage and milk yield are increased. During the declining phase of lactation small doses of thyroactive substances do not have significant effect but administration of larger doses increased protein content (Aliev, 1971). Administration of thyroprotein should be accompanied with the feeding of the higher level of available energy. The use of thyroactive substances for increasing milk production for increasing milk production to milk is not in most of the animals. Adverse effects of feeding methylthiouracil on lactation and accelerated involution of secretary cell sof the mammary glands has observed. It causes sudden drop in milk yield but increases milk fat percentage (Aliev, 1971).

▶ BIOSYNTHESIS OF MILK

The milk is made of water, milk fat, proteins, lactose, minerals and vitamins. Some leucocytes, shaded mammary cells and enzymes are also present. The biosynthesis of milk depends on the extraction of nutrients from blood by the mammary cells, conversion of nutrients in blood into milk constituents and discharge of milk from the alveoli into the alveolar lumen.

▶ SECRETARY CELLS OF THE MAMMARY GLANDS

Each functional state of mammary glands is characterized by the development pattern of secretary cells, which are at different stages of differentiation. The ratio betweensecretary cells and non-secretary tissue is very wide in the non-lactating growing heifers up to about 31 months of age and it becomes narrower due to faster proliferation of the glandular tissue during puberty (Table 8.9). The right half of udder contains more

TABLE 8.9: Mean area (cm²) of secretary (S) and non-secretary (NS) tissues of Developing mammary glands at different age in buffalo heifers

Part of Udder	Age of buffalo heifers (months)				
	13	18	24	31	37
Left fore; S	14.5	14.9	14.9	18.5	17.6
NS	228.5	259.3	239.8	249.3	226.3
NS: S ratio	15.74	17.40	16.9	13.48	12.86
Right fore; S	15.0	20.6	16.3	18.5	23.7
NS	233.5	247.7	254.0	231.7	253.6
NS: S ratio	15.57	12.02	14.85	12.52	10.70
Left rear S	16.4	16.5	20.0	15.8	22.3
NS	270.4	252.9	254.0	230.2	192.6
NS: S ratio	16.49	15.33	12.70	14.57	8.64
Right rear; S	21.2	25.6	22.6	20.6	21.5
NS	226.5	247.3	243.7	248.1	217.6
NS: S ratio	10.68	9.66	10.78	12.04	10.12
Whole udder; S	16.8	19.4	18.7	18.4	21.3
NS	236.7	251.6	2449	239.8	222.5
NS: S ratio	14.09	12.97	13.10	13.03	10.45

glandular tissue than the left half. This is either due to difference in blood supply to 2 sides of the udder or due to characteristic of buffaloes (El-Sheikh and Sultan, 1977). The ratio between glandular and non-glandular tissues changes significantly in the functional udders due to many fold quantitative and qualitative increase in the glandular tissue. The ratio of glandular tissue is much higher in the high milk yielding buffaloes than the low yielding buffaloes (Nosier, 1972). It is assumed that the individual group of secretary cells at different stages of their development constitute qualitatively different secretary-motor complexes of the udder. These complexes are distinguished from one another on the basis of their synthesis ability of different milk constituents, the nature of secretary processes and the ability to discharge the synthesized milk (Olenov, 1954).

The mammary cell is highly active during lactation with very high rate of metabolism for the systhesis of varius milk constituets (Patton, 1969). Functional mammary cells obtain large quantity of milk precursors like glucose, acetate, amino acids and minerals from the blood. During active lactation phase high milk yielding animals may loose body tissue to meet the high nutrients requirements of the mammary glands.

▶ STRUCTURE OF SECRETARY CELL OF MAMMARY GLAND

The epithelial cells in alveoli are the secretary cells. A functional secretary cell is sutuated on the basement membrance of outer connective tissue alongwith blood capillaries and inner layer of myoepithelial cells (Fig. 8.1). Each cell is encapsulated in a plasma membrane in addition to a well defined nucleus. Various cytoplasmic inclusions are the mitochondria, golgi apparatus, endoplasmic reticulum, lysosome, fat droplets and protein micelles.

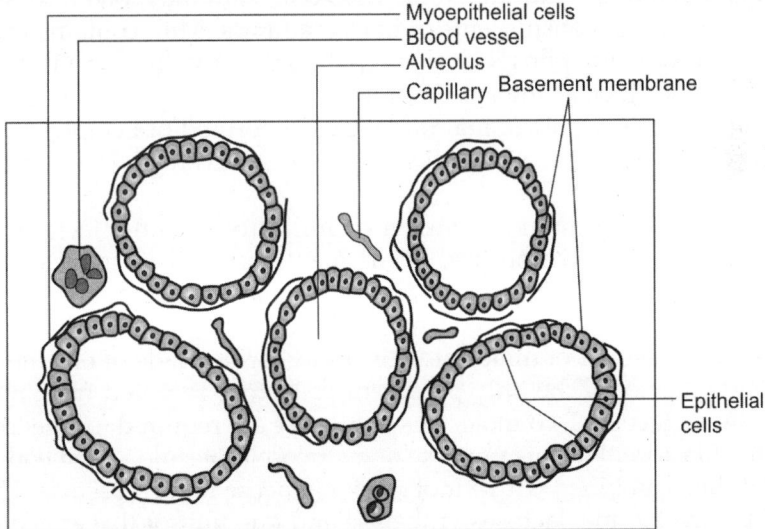

Fig. 8.1: Diagramatic representation of lactating mammary cell

Nucleus: the nucleus of mammary cells is responsible for the transmission of inherent lactation characteristics in genes for the systhesis of milk proteins and certain enzymes required for the catalysis of many biochemical reactions in the secrtary cells. Deoxyribonucleic acid (DNA) in chromosome of nucleus possesses genetic information, which is passed on to ribonucleic acid (RNA). The RNA carries information to endoplasmic reticulum through the fine pores in the nuclear membrane.

Endoplasmic reticulum: The specialized organelle found in the basal part of cytoplasm in a secrtary cell is made of a canal system. The RNA moves with specific message from the nucleus to the endoplasmic reticulum and transmits information for the linkage of different amino acids for the synthesis of milk proteins and enzymes in the mammary cell. The surface of some of the canals of endoplasmic reticulum is lodged with the RNA protein combination known as ribosomes. Synthesis of milk proteins from the linkage between peptide bonds of amino acids in various sequence occurs in the ribosome.

Golgi apparatus: The packaging of proteins like combination of calcium and phosphorus with the casein micelles takes place in the Golgi apparatus. After synthesis, milk proteins emerge out of Golgi apparatus in small vacuoles which fuse with the plasma membrane. Lactose synthesis also occurs in the Golgi apparatus.

Mitochondria: Several mitochondria are present in the active secretary cells of mammary glands. These organelles generate energy for the synthesis of milk proteins and fats in the secretary cells.

Lysosomes: These are membrane bound particles and the integrity of lysosomal membrane is maintained by hormones. Leakage of degradative lysosomal enzymes into the cytoplasm activates the digestion and removal of cell from the body. The lysosomes are more active during the involution of glandular tissue of the mammary glands, which occurs with the end of lactation extending to early dry period.

Cellular membrane: Each secretary cell of mammary gland is encapsulated in the plasma membrane. The various organelles in the cytoplasm are enclosed in separate membranes, which are very specific for the passage of chemicals into various compartments of the cells. Although milk is isotonic with the blood but there is great difference in the normal consitituents of both the fluids. Milk contains much higher level of fat, sugar, calcium, phosphorus and potassium, and lower amount of sodium and protein than the blood of the same animal.

Cytoplasm: the greater part of mammary cells is formed of cytoplasm. It contains soluble and colloidal from of many nutrients, enzymes and other cytoplasmic inclusion bodies.

Milk proteins: The primary proteins of milk are caseins, lactoalbumin and lactoglobulins. These are synthesized in the mammary cells form free amino acids received from blood. The other group of proteins comprising of immunoglobulins and milk serum albumin are also received from the blood and remain unchanged in milk.

Lactose: The main sugar of milk lactose is disaccharide made of one molecule each of glucose and galactose. The only precursor of lactose received from blood in the mammary cells is glucose. Two molecules of glucose are required for the formation of one molecule of lactose. For this purpose one glucose molecule is first converted into galactose and then combined with a molecule of glucose to form lactose. The reaction is catalysed by an enzyme, lactose synthetase and one unit of this enzyme is alpha-lactalbumin.

Milk fats: The milk fats are mostly mixed triglycerides (triacylglycerol) containing high proportion of satured fatty acids. The short chain fatty acids are synthesized in he secretary cells of mammary glands from the volatile fatty acids, i.e. acetic and butyric acids produced during the microbial digestion of dietary carbohydrates in the rumino-reticulum and obsorbed in the body pool. Most of the long chain fatty acids of milk fat are contributed directly by the dietary lipids. Fatty acids of plant origin are almost unsaturated long chain fatty acids, which undergo various degree of saturation in the rumen. These saturated long chain fatty acids are absorbed from the intestine into the lymphatic system. In the lymph lacteals fatty acids bind with a protein and then transported in the blood stream and carried to mammary glands. The secretary cells of mammary glands absorbed these fatty acids from the blood which ultimately form the part of milk fat.

Vitamins and minerals: The entire amount of vitamins and minerals in the secretary cells of mammary glands are obtained from the blood through the selective permeability. These are not synthesized in the mammary glands.

Water in milk: Milk water is derived from 2 sources, i.e. (i) the blood and (ii) high potassium intracellular fluid of the alveolar cells. The synthesis of lactose, fat and protein in the secretary cells stimulates the flow of water from blood for the maintenance of osmotic equilibrium between the milk and the blood. Buffalo milk contains about 82% water.

▶ MILKING OF BUFFALO

Systems of milking: Head milking is extensively followed for buffaloes, but on some organized farms machine milking is also practiced. However, machine milking could not be popular due to high variation in the teat size not only between the breeds but also with in the breed. Dairy buffaloes are normally milked two times daily at almost equal interval. Low milk yielding swamp buffaloes are generally milked once daily in the morning before releasing for frazing alongwith calves. The calves are let loose with dams after 2–3 months of age. Machine milking is more common in mediterinian buffaloes.

Hand milking: Two methods of hand milking i.e. (i) full hand milking, and (ii) stroping are common in most of the tropical countries. A third milking method known as fisting or knuckling is also practiced by some of the milker. This method is highly undesirable because it is injurious for the teats and tissue damage may predispose the teats for infection leading to mastitis.

i. **Full hand milking:** In this method the teats are hold with the thumb and first finger and milk is drawn out by applying adequate pressure with palm and fingers starting at the base of teats along with some lowe part of udder and sqeezing down the tip. The process is repeated at a very fast rate in quick succession.

ii. **Stripping:** In this method teats are stripped with the help of thumb and first finger. It is rarely used for milking of dairy buffaloes because their teats are long and voluminous for convenient holding in palm for full hand milking. However, in case of some swamp buffaloes teats are quite small and stripping is practiced.

iii. **Knuckling or fisting:** This method is undersirable and banned at the organized farms. In this method teat is hold with palm and inward half bend thumb for applying high pressure on the teat white stripping.

Precautions to be observed at Milking

1. Milking pail and byre should be clean and free from flies, other insects and offensive odours. Milk absorbs odour from environment very quickly.
2. Buffaloes should be washed clean before sending in the milking byre.
3. Milker should use clean cloth and cap covering the hair. He should wash hands clean and rinse with dilute solution of potassium permanganate.
4. Udder is washed clean and wiped dry with a clean cotton before milking.

5. First milk streams are drawn on strip cum for clinical examinations.
6. Knuckling or fisting of udder should not be permitted.
7. Strangers should not be allowed to avoid holding of milk.
8. Animals should be handled gently and should not be annoyed by threatening or otherwise. A disturbed buffalo may hold milk and may not release before the next milking. Person responsible for ammoying the buffalo should keep away for few days or behave gently to pacify the animal.
9. In case of suckling for let down the calf should be guided to suckle all the teats in quick succession.

▶ MILKING DURATION

The total time of milking includes pre-milking stimulation either by hand or by suckling calf and milking duration.

i. **Milk let down or pre-milking stimulation:** It ranges from 30 seconds to 300 seconds in different buffaloes and it is influenced by several factors (Dass et al., 1976; Gangwar et al., 1980; Alim et al., 1982; Roy and Nagpur, 1984). Some of the following factors affect let down of milk.

   a. *Milking schedule*: Twice a day milking at regular interval of 12 hours is the normal milking schedule in buffaloes. Milk let down time in Murrah type buffaloes is 0.5 to 4.0 minutes (Gupta et al., 1974; Dass et al., 1976; Ludri, 1980; Roy and Nagpaul, 1984). In Egyptian buffaloes it is 2.72 + 0.89 minutes at morning milking and 2.82 + 0.92 minutes at the evening milking when udder is gently massaged with a warm clothe sqeezed in hot water at 104–105°F (40+ °C) (Alim et al., 1982). Any significant change in milking schedule may increase let down time.

   b. *Frequency of milking*: Milk let down time is increased significantly in Murrah type buffaloes from 113 + 7.36 seconds in case of twice daily milking to 137 + 10.04 seconds on thrice daily milking at equal interval between the milkings (Dass et al., 1976).

   c. *Stage of lactation*: Let down time of milk may slightly decrease in third month of lactation and then again increases significantly in Murrah type buffaloes. However, it varies greatly between the animals and has been reported 50–256 (mean, 123) seconds during 31 to 60 days of lactation period, 32–210 (mean, 120) seconds between day 61 to 90, 32–318 (mean, 146) seconds between day 91 to 120, and 50–300 (mean, 146) seconds between day 121 to 150 in Murrah type buffaloes kept under the standard farm management (Ludri, 1980).

   d. *Effect of weaning*: Early weaning of buffaloes increases the milk let down time and it has been reported 133–172.5 seconds in early weaned, 86.4–100 seconds in late weaned and 97.5–104 seconds in unweaned Murrah type buffaloes (Gupta et al., 1974).

   e. *Effect of environmental cooling and season*: Environmental cooling arrangements like shower bath and wallowing during the dry-hot and humid-hot seasons significantly increases the milk let down time. Average milk let down time has been found to be 3.105, 3.683 and 4.154 minutes in buffaloes without bath, with shower bath and wallowing respectively during the dry season. Corresponding figures for humid-hot season were 3.089, 3.501 and 3.608 seconds (Gangwar et al., 1980).

f. **Effect of udder massage:** Gentle udder massage before milking with a cloth sqeezed in hot water at 104–105°F increases pre-milking stimulation time in Egyptian buffaloes. Mean let down time is about 4.39 + 1.30 minute on dry hand massage and 5.31 + 1.51 minute on wet massage with warm cloth for 2 times daily milking (Alim et al., 1982).

g. *Effect of temperament:* Average milk let down time in docile buffaloes is about 120.83 seconds and it increases significantly to 295.32 seconds in nervous buffaloes yielding 9.81 and 7.89 kg milk per day respectively (Roy and Nagpaul, 1984a).

ii. **Actual milking duration:** Actual milking duration varies from 5 to 13 minutes in different types of buffaloe (Shafie et al., 1971; Turabov and Abullaev, 1979; Gangwar et al., 1980; Tsankova and Tosev, 1980; Alim et al., 1982; Roy and Nagpaul, 1984b). Almost equal time is required on machine milking (Aliev et al., 1971; Gotsiridze and Saakova, 1980). Following factors affect the time of actual milking in buffaloes.

a. *Time of milking:* Milking duration is normally longer in morning than in the evening, which is mainly due to more milk secretion in morning (Shafie et al., 1971; Alim et al., 1977, 1982).

b. *Effect of lactation number or parity:* Milking duration increases significantly up to the third lactation. In a report average machine milking time was 6.39, 8.47 and 10.26 minute at the milking rate of 0.74, 0.77 and 0.99 kg per minute in first, second and third lactation respectively (Gotsiridze and Saakova, 1980). In a hand milking herd of Caucasian buffaloes average milking duration in corresponding lactations at a flow rate of 0.56, 0.61 and 0.67 kg per minute and milk yield 4.13, 5.37 and 6.35 kg has been 7.08, 8.30 and 9.46 minutes (Turabov, 1982).

c. *Effect of udder shape:* Udder shape has marked effect on milking duration. The bowel shaped and round udders yield more milk than the goat type udder, and require much less time for complete milking (Saakova, 1979; Turabov and Abulaev, 1979; Turabov, 1982). Milking duration may vary from 6.27–8.97 minutes for bowel shaped, 8.72–9.64 minutes for round and 8.19–13.67 minites for goat type udder.

d. *Effect of udder quarters:* Milking of fore quarters of udder requires less time than the milking of rear quarters, because fore quarters secrete less milk (30–42 % of total) at the particular milking (Polikhronov and Tosev, 1970; Tsankova and Tosev, 1980; Pandey et al., 1981; Alim et al., 1982).

e. *Effect of udder massage:* Wet massage with a clothe sqeezed in warm water at 104–105°F and dry massage take almost equal time for milking (Alim et al., 1977, 1982). Light massage of udder during milking reduces the duration of milking. Udder massage also affected the flow rate and higher contribution of milk from the fore quarters of udder (Gotsiridze and Kitoshvili, 1981).

f. *Effect of environment cooling:* Shower bath increases milking duration due to significant reduction in flow rate of milk. However, wallowing has little effect (Gangwar et al., 1980).

g. *Effect of temperament:* Docile buffaloes require less time than the nervous buffaloes for the milking of equal quantity of milk, because flow rate of milk in nervous buffaloes is usually low (Roy and Nagpaul, 1984; Gupta et al., 1985).

▶ MILK FLOW RATE OR RATE OF MILKING

The flow rate of milk from udder during the time of milking is an important factor in milking management specially for machine milking. Great variation occurs in the flow rate of milk. This is influenced by several factors. It varies from 0.21 to 0.99 kg per minute in different animals being maximum in bowel shaped and round udders and lowest in goat type udder (Ragab et al., 1971; Alim et al., 1977, 1982; Gangawar et al., 1980; Gotsiridze and Kitoshvili, 1981; Turabov, 1982; Kapoor and Ludri, 1984; Roy and Nagpaul, 1984).

a. **Effect of number of laction or parity:** Linear increase in milk flow rate occurs with the increase in lactation number. Average milk flow rate may differ amongst the different herds of buffaloes depending on the milking skill of milker, type of animals and system of milking. Mean milk flow rate in a herd of Caucasian buffaloes on machine milking had been 0.74, 0.77 and 0.99 kg per minute in the first, second and third lactation respectively (Gotsiridze and Saakova, 1980). In the same order of lactation mean milk flow rate in a hand milked herd was 0.56, 0.61 and 0.67 kg per minute (Turabov, 1982).

b. **Effect of udder shape:** Milking of bowel and round shaped udder is more easy and efficient both by hand milking as well as machine milking (Turabov, and Ablaev, 1979; Turabov, 1982), The goat type udder is difficult to milk and has been unsuitable for the machine milking (Gotsiridze and Saakova, 1980).

c. **Effect of udder quarters:** Milking rate is invariably higher for the rear than the fore quarters. This is probably due to higher percentage of total milk yield from the rear quarters (Alim et al., 1982).

d. **Effect of milking frequency:** Twice daily milking at an interval of 12 hours is the common practice and milk flow rate is normally more at the morning than the after noon milking (Alim et al., 1982). On increasing milking frequency from twice daily to thrice daily at 8 hours interval resulted in about 15.5% decrease in milk flow rate (Dass et al., 1976). However, such trend may not be considered common as milking of Murrah buffaloes at an interval of 4, 8, 12 or 16 hours interval had no significant effect on milk flow rate (Kapoor and Ludri, 1984).

e. **Effect of udder massage:** Pre-milking gentle massage of udder significantly increases milk flow rate up to 25.7% and also the total milk yield as well as the length of lactation period (Gotsinidze and Kitoshvili, 1981). However, system of massage does not have significantly effect on milk flow rate (Alim et al., 1977, 1982).

f. **Effect of body cooling and season:** A marginal increase in milk flow rate occurs in buffalows allowed wallowing before the milking but shower bath had adverse effect on milk flow rate during dry hot season. However, in himid-hot season wallowing increases milk flow rate (Soni, 1975).

g. **Effect of temperature:** Contrary to very high increase in let down time of milk in nervous and aggressive buffaloes only little slower milk flow rate occurs when compared to docile buffaloes (Roy and Nagpur, 1984; Gupta et al., 1985).

h. **Effect of milking machine:** The type of milking machine significantly affects the milk flow rate. A machine with an arrangement of mechanical udder stimulation mechanism through gentle massage gives best results (Aliev et al., 1971). The pulsation rates and the pressure in machine during the time of milking also influence the milk flow rate. At the rate of 60 pulsation per minute at 40 cm Hg pressure the performance of 'Stimul' machine has been found superior (Aliev and Kuliev, 1965).

▶ RESIDUAL OR COMPLEMENTARY MILK

A small amount of milk remains in udder after the normal milking and it is known as residual or complementary milk. Since the cistern milk is almost negligible in buffaloes, very little amount of milk is left in unstripped in the udder (Aliev et al., 1965). Residual milk may be obtained by administration of 10 IU oxytocin hormone. Amount of residual milk is usually less than half litre (Aliev, 1966; Jadhav and Khambata, 1967; Ludri, 1980). Residual milk contains very high percentage of milk fat. Administration of oxytocin by subcutaneous or intramuscular route has no significant effect on its let down effect (Hanna et al., 1979) and due to this reason oxytocin and posterior pituitary injections are indiscriminatory used in many countries by the buffalo owners for let down of milk in difficult buffaloes.

▶ INVOLUTION OR REGRESSION OF UDDER

Regression of the glandular parenchyma in lactating buffaloes is a slow and gradual process. Due to this characteristic buffaloes have longer lactation length ranging from 270 to 352 days in Murrah type, about 350 day in Surti and 276 days in Bhadawari breeds (Bhat, 1979). In Egyptian buffaloes, lactation length ranges from 245 to 362 days in different herds (Ragab, 1979) and in draught type swamp buffaloes of Thialand from 210 to 333 days (Chantalakhana, 1979). In very rare animals lactation length of about two years has been reported by the owners during survey in Tarai region of India by author. The involution or regression process of udder starts after the peak lactation, during declining phase of lactation. The process of involution is enhanced by pregnancy, late weaning and irregular milking schedule.

▶ AN UNUSUAL CASE OF SPONTANEOUS LACTATION IN A VIRGIN BUFFALO

An unbred buffalo heifer developed functional udder without mating, calving or any other treatment at about three and half years of age and started milk secretion. The heifer was milked for 5 years and yielded about 5–6 seers of milk equivalent to about 4.5 to 5.5 kg (Bali, 1962). Instance of milk production without breeding and also for 2–3 years after first calving are heard in the village of dairy buffalo tract of India but such reports are mostly unrecorded where say.

REFERENCES

Aliev, M G 1962. Doki.Akad. Nauk., Azerb. 18 (6); 67
Aliev, M G 1964. Baku Izdateijstvo Akademli Nauk, Azerb. 188 pp.
Alive, M G 1971. Dairy Science Abstract, 33; 175
Aliev, M G and Kuliev, K M 1965. Trudy Sekt. Fiziol., Baku, 8; 55
Aliev, M G, Kuliev, K M and Mamedov, N G 1965a. Trudy Sekt. Fiziol., Baku, 8; 46
Aliev, M G, Kuliev, K M and Mamedov, N G 1965b. Trudy Sekt. Fiziol., Baku, 8; 67
Aliev, M G, Kuliev, K M and Abbasov, S 1971. Tekhnika sel'khoz. Mosk., 31 (5); 28
Alim, K A 1983. World Rev. Anim. Prod., 19 (3); 13
Alim, K A, Barbari, A and Badran, A 1977. World. Rev. Anim. Prod., 13 (2); 27
Alim, K A, Barbari, A and Feel, F M 1982. World Rev. Anim. Prod., 18 (1); 33
Asker, A A, Ragab, M T and Kamal, T H 1954. Indian J.Dairy Sci., 7; 36
Atheya, U K and Sub, S C 1985. Indian J. Anim. Sci., 55; 236
Badawy, H, Ahmed, A K, Misk, N A and Makady, F M 1985. Assuit Vet. Med. J., 14 (27); 19
Bali, B D 1962. Indian Vet. J., 39; 351

Barnwal, A K and Dhingra, L D 1978. Indian J. Anim. Sci., 48; 753

Bhat, P N 1979. FAO Anim. Prod. Health Paper 13; 129

Bhosrekar, M R and Nagpaul, P K 1971. Indian J. Dairy Sci., 24; 208

Chandiramani, S V, Gautam, A N and Luktuke, S N 1966. Indian J. Dairy Sci., 19; 143

Chantalakhana, C 1979. FAO Anim. Prod. Health Paper 13; 143

Chowdhary, M S and Chaudhary, A L 1981. Indian Vet. J., 58; 203

D'angelo, A and De Franciscis, G 1966. Atti Soc. Ital. Sci. Vet., 20; 371

Dass, P C, Basu, S b and Sharma, K N s 1976. Indian J. Dairy Sci., 29; 113

Dwivedi, J and Prabhu, S S 1970. J. Remount Vet. Corp, 9 (2); 14

El-Sheikh, A S and Sultan, Z A 1977. Indian J. Anim. Sci., 47; 630

Fahmy, MFA, Morcos, MB and El-Gafary, M. 1969. Indian Vet. J., 46; 856

Ferrara, B, Badolato, F, Minieri, L and De Franciscis, G 1966. Atti Soc. Ital.Sci., Vet., 20; 363

Ferrer, B, De Franciscis, G, Interieri, F and Rendian, N 1966. Atti. Soc. Ital. Sci. Vet., 20; 367

Fischer, H 1956. Berl. Munch. Tierarztl. Wschr., 69; 89

Fischer, H 1962. J. Malay Vet. Med. Assoc., 3; 110

Gangawar, P C, Soni, P L and Mehta, S N 1980. Indian J. Nutr. Dietet., 17; 302

Gotsiridze, N K and Kitoshvili, I 1981. Zhivotnoodstvo, Uchebno Issled Intst. Tbilsi, U S S R.

Gupta, S C, Gangwar, P C and Kooner, D S 1974. Indian J. Anim. Sci., 44; 334

Gupta, S C, Handa, M C and Sahoo, G 1985. Indian J. Dairy Sci., 34; 45

Hafez, A and Naidu, K N 1981. Indian J. Dairy Sci., 34; 49

Hanna, A K, Hassan, A, Yaseen, a and Badawy, A 1979. Alexandria J. Agri. Res. 27; 567

Hossain, M I, Mia, M A, Khan, M A B and Talukdar, A H 1980. Bangladesh Vet. Journal, 14; 25

Jadhav, D S and Khambata, F S 1967. Indian Vet. J., 14; 25

Kapoor, M and Ludri, R S 1984. Indian J. Anim. Sci., 54; 153

Katiyar, R S and Girish Chandra, 1983a. Indian Vet. J., 60; 347

Katiyar, R S and Girish Chandra, 1983b. Indian Vet. J., 60; 709

Kumar, R and Bhat, P N 1979. Indian J. Dairy Sci., 32; 156

Ludri, R S 1980. Indian J. Anim. Sci., 50; 891

Ludri, R S and Sarma, PA 1981. Indian J. Dairy Sci., 34; 352

Malossini, F. 1967. Annali Inst. Sper. Zootec., Roma, 11; 91

Mangurkar, B R and Desai, R N 1981. Indian Vet. J., 58; 392

Maqsood, M. 1956. Agric. Pakistan, 7; 77

Maymone, B 1945. Z. Tierz., Zuchtbiol., 52; 1

Minieri, L, Interieri, F and Romano, M 1966. Atti Soc. Ital. Sci. Vet., 20; 374

Moussa, M H G 1982. Anatomischer Anzeiger., 152; 129

Nosier, M B 1972. Egyptian J. Vet. Sci., 9; 81

Nosier, M B, Shalash, M R, Zaki, K m and Affiefy, M N 1973. Atti del VII Simposio Intern. Di Zootecnia, Milano, April 15 –17, 1972

Olenov, Yu M 1954. Doki. Akad. Nauk,SSR, 97 (2); 361

Patton, S 1969. Milk Science, America, 221; 58

Pandey, H S, Kumar, S and Katpatal, B G 1981. Indian J. Anim. Sci., 51; 105

Polikhronov, D and Tosev, A 1970. Zhivots. Nauk., 7 (3); 11

Ragab, M T, 1979. FAO Anim. Prod. Health Paper 13; 155

Ragab, M T, Shafie, M M and Kilani, M 1971. J. Anim. Prod., UAR, 9; 67

Rao, A V N and Murthy, T S R 1984. Indian J., 61; 311

Rao, A V N, Sreemannarayan, O and Rao, P V 1982. Livestock Adviser, 7(12); 29

Roy, P K and Nagpaul, P K 1984a. Indian J. Anim. Sci., 54; 566

Roy, P K and Nagpaul, P K 1984b. Indian J. Dairy Sci., 37; 74

Saakova, L I 1979a. Trudy gruz. Zootekh. Vet. Nauchno Issled Inst., 108 (42); 141

Saakova, L I 1979b. Trudy gruz. Zootekh. Vet. Nauchno Issled Inst., 108 (42); 135

Saxena, S C and Prabhu, S S 1970. Indian J. Anim. Prod., 1; 97

Saxena, S C and Prabhu, S S 1972. Indian J. Anim. Prod, 2; 24

Shafie, M M, Ragab, M T and Kilary, M. 1969. J. Anim Prod, UAR, 9; 211–219

Shalash, M R, Salama, A A and Mousa, A 1961a. Proc. VIII Intern. Cong. Anim Prod, Hungry, 1: 217

Shalash, M R, Salama, A A and El-Guindi 1961b. Emp. J. exptl. Agric., 29; 45–48

Shalash, M R, Salama, A A, Nawito, N and Mousa, A. 1964. Proc. 5th Intern. Cong. Anim Reprod and A.I.. Trento,Vol II; 250–262

Sindhu, M S and Pal, R N. 1978. Haryana Agric Uni. J. Res, 8; 131–135

Singh, M and Bhatnagar, D S 1977. Indian Vet. J., 54; 377–383

Soni, Ph 1975. M. Sc. Thesis, Punjab Agril. Uni, Ludhiana

Sud, S C 1979. Indian J Anim Sci., 49; 229–231

Sud, S C and Singh, RV 1974. Indian J. Anim Sci, 44; 335–356

Taneja, G C and Bhatnagar, D s 1958. J Vet Anim Husb, Res, Mhow, 3; 86–89

Tripathi, M D and Garswat, B L 1982. Asian J Dairy Res, 1; 227–230

Tsankova, M 1983. Zhirotsnov dni Nauki, 20 (5); 39–44

Tsankova, M and Tosev, A. 1980. Zhivostnov' dni Nauki. 17 (7); 16–22

Turabov, T 1982. Molochinei Myasnoe Skotodstve No. 5; 19–22

Turabov T and Abllaev, M G 1979. Molochine I Myasnoe Skotovodstve No. 3; 25–30

Verma, G S, Tomer, S S and Tomer, 05 1984. Indian Vet J, 61; 521–522

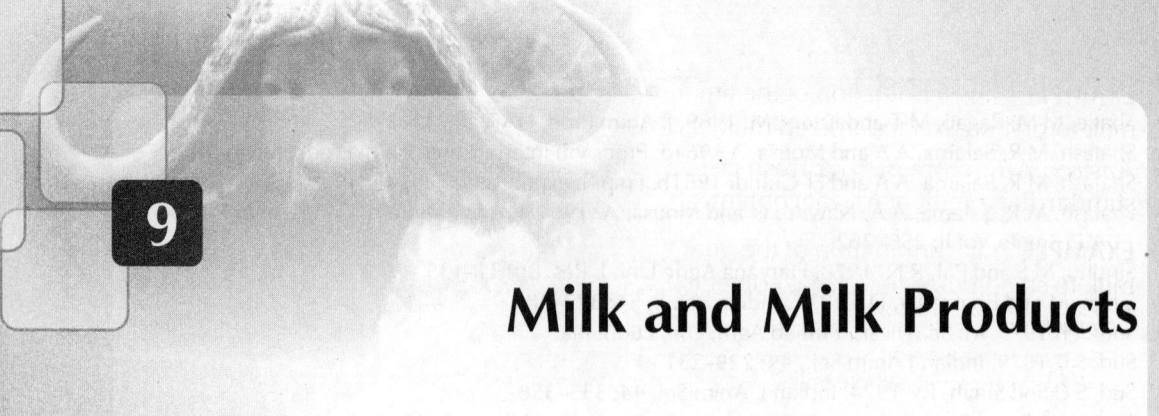

Milk and Milk Products

Buffalo is a triple purpose animal providing milk, power and meat for human requirements. The primary contribution of riverin e breeds is the milk production, while swamp buffaloes are the famous draught animals in the paddy growing countries. All types of buffaloes are slaughtered for meat production nomally after their utilization as milch and draught animals. Intensive fattening for meat production is praticed I some Mediterranean countires of Europe and Asia, Egypt, Brazil, West Indies, Thailand and Philippines, etc.

▶ MILK

Milk is the normal secretion of mammary glands, secreted after parturition for the nourishment of the new born calves. It is fluid complex system presenting different phases, viz., (i) Continuous phase is consisting of water and water soluble milk constituents like lactose, salt and water soluble vitamins, etc (ii) Colloidal phase is consisting of minute particles of caseins, albumin, globulins and enzymes dispersion. (iii) Emulsion phase is consisting of larger globules of milk fat, phospholipids, cholesterol, fat soluble vitamins and small quantity of associated minerals in the form of organic compounds.

Whole Milk

Normal milk secretion of a healthy udder after about 7–10 days of calving is known as whole milk.

Separated or Skim Milk

The fluid milk residue left after the removal of cream is known as separated or skim milk. It contains about 0.1% milk fat.

Standardized Milk

The adjustment of milk fat and or solids-not fat percentage of milk according to the Prevention of Food Adulternation (PFA) rules is known as the standardization of milk. This is done by the addition of skim milk in case of high fat milk and fresh cream in case of low fat milk. The amount of skim milk or fresh cream required to obtain the desired fat percentage in milk is calculated by the Pearson's square on weight basis.

EXAMPLE 1: Determination of the amount of 40% fresh cream to be mixed in 5% whole milk to prepare a standardized milk of 6% milk fat content.

Answer: A mixture of 1 kg fresh cream (40% fat) and 34 kg milk (5% fat) will gave a standardized milk of 6% fat content.

EXAMPLE 2: Determination of the quantity of 0.1% skim milk for mixing with 7% whole milk to standardize for 6% fat content.

Calculations:

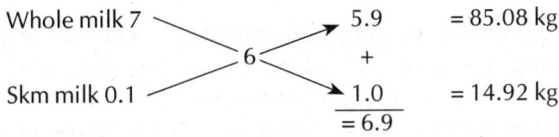

Answer: A mixture of 1kg skim milk and 5.9 kg milk will provide a standardized milk of 6% fat content.

Homogenized Milk

The whole milk processed in a homogenizer for reducing the size of fat globules to such an extent that no apparent layer of cream appears on the surface of milk even after 48 hours undisturbed storage. The size of fat globules in homogenized milk is mostly less than 2 microns in diameter. Homogenization of milk is affected by two factor 5, i.e.

i. The temperature of homogenization which should be preferably 65–70°C. A temperature range of 38–49°C should be avoided during and after homogenization to control the lipase activity in the milk.

ii. **Pressure of homogenization:** A single stage pressure of 2000–2500 psi is adequate for the homogenization of milk containing less than 6% milk fat. For higher fat percentage, two stage homogenization is required. In first stage pressure is mentained at 2000 psi followed by 500 psi in the second stage.

Toned Milk

The milk containing 3% milk fat and 8.5% solids-not fat obtained by mixing water and skim milk powder in whole milk is known s toned or single toned milk.

Double Toned Milk

The milk adjusted with the addition of water and skim milk powder to contain 1.5% milk fat and 9% solids-not fat is known as double toned milk.

Humanized Milk

The modification of buffalo milk through the addition of water, sugar and or skim milk powder to resemble the human milk in chemical composition is known as the humanization of buffalo milk and the milk, thus obtained is called humanized milk.

Reconstituted Milk

The fluid milk prepared by dispersing whole milk powder in water in the ratio of 1:7 or 1:8 is known as reconstituted milk. Spary dried milk powder is preferred for the preparation of reconstituted or rehydrated milk because it is more easily dispersible and leaves little sediment.

Recombined Milk

The fluid milk prepared by the mixing of butter oil, skim milk powder and water in the proportion present in whole milk or toned milk as per the requirement.

Sterilized Milk

The milk heated at 100–110°C for about 30 minutes is known as sterilized milk. The sterilized milk has longer storage life at room temperature and it is free from the pathogenic and other harmful microorganisuns except the heat resistant spore forming bacteria, if any present in the raw milk. Sterilization of milk result into significant loss of vitamin C and B complex.

Pasteurized Milk

The fluid milk heated at 63°C or 145°F for 30 minutes, or at 72°C (161°F) for 15 seconds and then quickly cooled below 5°C (41°F) is known as pasteurized milk. The pasteurization of milk is a common practice in the organized dairies for the supply of safe milk for human consumption.

Market Milk

The whole milk sold to consumers is usually called as market milk. It may be milk of a single cow or buffalo, a cow herd, a buffalo herd or mixed whole milk of cows and buffaoes.

Composition of Buffalo Milk

The constitutens of buffalo milk are similar to normal mammalian milk. Main constituent of whol milk are water, milk fat, protein, lactose and inorganic matter or ash. The composition of milk in dairy terminology is given as milk-fat, total solids, solids-not fat and ash. The other components of milk are phospholipids, sterols, enzymes, vitamins, pigments and dissolved gases (Ling, 1948). The various constituents of milk may be illustrated in Table 9.1.

Chemical Composition of Buffalo Milk

The average chemical composition of milk of different types of buffaloes shows significant variation (Table 9.1). The milk fat is most variable component of the milk, which is normally higher in draught type swamp buffaloes than the dairy type riverin buffaloes except the Bhadawari breed found in the south west parts of Uttar Pradesh and adjoining areas of Madhya Pradesh in India.

Factors Affecting the Chemical Composition of Milk

The chemical composition of milk is quite variable and it is influenced by several factors. The milk constituents are almost common but their proportion differ significantly

TABLE 9.1: Variation in composition of buffalo milk

Breed	Location	Number of samples	Milk fat	Protein	Total solids	Solids-not fat	Lac-tose	Reference
1	2	3	4	5	6	7	8	9
Murrah	Lucknow	294	7.19	-	-	9.43	-	Mc Mohan et al., 1932
	Allahabad	308	7.16	3.78	16.41	3.25	4.88	Schenider et al., 1948
	Bangalore (a)	37	6.56	3.88	15.75	9.19	5.23	Basu et al., 1948
	(b)	35	6.60	-	9.10	-	-	Paul et al., 1954
	(c)	80	6.80	-	-	9.31	-	Bhimsen and Dastur, 1985
	(d)	127	6.80	3.91	16.41	9.61	4.70	Ghose and Ananakrishnan, 1963
	Poona	50	7.80	-	-	10.68	-	Kulkarni and Dole, 1955
	Karnal	-	6.87	-	-	9.91	-	Basu et al., 1979
	Lushiana	72	6.79	-	-	-	-	Tiwana et al., 1980
	Bombay	10	7.40	3.94	-	9.39	-	Sharma et al., 1980
	Izatnagar	221	7.05	4.32	17.15	10.02	4.66	Pandey, 1981
	Bulgaria	18	8.23	4.78	18.60	10.37	4.80	Shalichev and Polikhronov, 1969
Bhadawari	Jansi	-	12.00	-	-	-	-	-
Surti	Poona	50	7.09	-	-	10.77	-	Kulkarni and Dole, 1956
	Udiapur	50	7.05	-	15.68	-	-	Bhargava and Murdia, 1980
Mehsana	Bombay	10	7.40	3.92	-	9.31	-	Sharma et al., 1980
Jafarabadi	Bombay	10	7.40	4.01	-	9.52	-	Do
Non-descript	Bombay	10	7.30	4.01	-	9.52	-	Do
	Calcultta	20	6.70	-	-	10.6	-	Stewart and Banejee, 1930-31
	Allahabad	496	7.60	3.80	16.99	9.39	-	Schneider et al., 1948
Bulgarian	Bulgaria	-	7.50	4.10	17.38	9.88	4.78	Grigarov et al., 1962
Bulgarian X	Murrah							
	F1 Bulgaria	98	8.14	-	-	-	-	Polikhronov et al., 1978
	F2 Bulgaria	17	7.48	4.28	-	-	5.03	Shalichev et al., 1975
Farmbred	USSR (a)		9.25	-	-	-	-	Akhundov,-
	(b)		8.10	4.32	18.00	9.90	4.96	Merzamatov, 1965
	(c)		8.00	4.45	18.45	10.45	-	Dilanyan et al., 1971
	(d)		7.60	4.17	16.98	-	-	-do-
Local	Egypt (a)	700	6.37	3.87	17.40	10.03	-	Asker et al., 1957
	(b)	72	6.53	3.78	-	-	5.00	Abd-El-Salam and El-Shibiny, 1966
Farmbred	Iraqi	193	7.46	-	17.07	9.61	-	Alsafar and Juma, 1970
Local	Mesopotamia	49	8.28	-	18.33	10.05	5.17	Dalaly et al., 1976
Nili-Ravi	Pakistan	330	6.70	-	15.80	9.10	-	Ishaq and Shah, 1975
Farm bred	Italy (a)	132	7.22	3.95	16.86	9.64	4.88	Minieri et al., 1965
	(b)	65	7.19	3.82	17.34	10.15	6.60 (ash)	Minieri et al., 1967
Carabao	Philippines (a)	307	8.80	-	19.10	10.22	-	Alim, 1975
	(b)	-	8.00	-	18.83	10.83	5.29	Trung and Conzales, 1978

between the animals. The variation decreases with the increase in the size of herd and greatest variation is observed in the fat percentage of milk. The following factors are found to be responsible for the difference in the chemical composition of milk.

1. **Variation due to breed and type:** Great variation in chemical composition of the buffalo milk of different genetic groups is apparent in (Table 9.2 and 9.3). Such difference is also found is different breeds of buffalo from the same agro-climatic condition. The chemical composition of milk is relatively less variable between the breeds of same place (Rao and Nagarcenkar, 1977; Sharma et al., 1980).

2. **Variation due to stage of lactation:** Almost all milk constituents are significantly affected by the stage of lactation. Milk fat, protein and casein percentage increases while lactose decreases with the progress in up to peak yeld and thereafter show rising trend (Basu et al., 1948; Singh et al., 1961; Salerno, 1967; Kumar et al., 1980). Most of the milk constituents showed inconsistent monthly variation in the Egyptian buffaloes (Abd El-Salam and Shibiny, 1966) but definite trend (Table 9.4 and 9.5) in Murrah buffaloes (Pandey, 1981).

TABLE 9.2: Variation due to type and breed

Breed/Type	Composition of milk (%)					
	Total solids	Solids-not fat	Fat	Protein	Lactose	Ash
Dairy type buffaloese						
Bulgarigan	17.44	9.94	7.50	4.33	4.80	0.81
Caucasian	1.34	9.76	7.58	4.05	4.05	0.71
Egyptian	17.91	9.95	7.96	4.16	4.16	0.78
Hungarian	16.21	8.99	7.22	3.65	3.65	0.78
Italian	18.06	10.21	7.85	4.28	4.28	-
Mehsana	16.71	9.31	7.40	3.94	3.94	0.72
Murrah (India)	17.24	9.86	7.38	3.60	3.60	0.78
Rumanian	18.25	10.02	8.23	4.76	4.76	0.76
Russian	18.96	10.40	8.56	4.76	4.76	0.86
Zafarabadi	16.62	9.52	7.40	4.01	4.01	0.73
Swamp type buffaloes						
Carabala	21.54	11.19	10.35	10.35	5.88	0.84
Chinese	23.20	10.60	12.60	12.60	6.04	0.86

TABLE 9.3: Milk composition of different buffalo breeds from same place

Breed	Fat%	Solids-not fat %	Protein %	Ash %
Mehsana	7.4	9.31	3.91	0.72
Murrah	7.4	9.38	3.94	0.74
Zafarabaid	7.4	9.52	4.01	0.73
Non-descript	7.3	9.51	4.01	0.73

TABLE 9.4: Composition of milk during different stages of lactation (%)

Stage of lactation	Fat	Protein	Casein	Lactose
Early lactation	6.8	3.61	2.94	5.11
Mid lactation	7.0	3.67	3.01	5.09
Late lactation	8.4	3.91	3.15	4.84

TABLE 9.5: Montly variation in milk composition (%)

Month of Lactation	Egyptian Buffalo			Murrah Buffalo		
	Fat	Protein	Lactose	Fat	Protein	Lactose
1	6.16	3.69	5.30	6.19	4.61	4.66
2	5.73	3.75	5.03	5.80	4.20	4.66
3	6.59	3.59	5.18	6.12	4.13	4.66
4	5.57	3.51	5.00	6.46	4.06	4.76
5	6.11	3.88	5.16	6.56	4.08	4.63
6	7.20	3.73	4.86	6.86	4.08	4.63
7	7.05	3.59	4.68	7.00	4.09	4.85
8	7.98	4.34	5.00	7.53	4.26	4.69
9	7.01	3.53	5.11	8.06	4.39	4.72
10	-	-	-	8.16	4.45	4.75
11	7.18	4.05	4.64	-	-	-

3. **Variation due to parity:** Variable reports are available on the effect of parity on the chemical composition of milk. The various milk constituents are generally low (Table 9.6) in the first calvers of Egyptian and Indian buffaloes (Ragab et al., 1958, Asker et al., 1971; Pandey, 1981) whereas higher percentage of milk constituents has been observed in the Russian buffaloes (Akhundov, 1966; Dzafarov, 1969). The reason may be small sample size of Russian buffaloes.

TABLE 9.6: Variation in milk composition due to parity

Parity	Fat %	Protein %	Total Solids %	Solids-not fat %
Egyptian Buffalo				
First	6.21	3.81	16.17	9.96
Second	6.38	3.91	16.42	10.0
Third	6.41	3.86	16.43	10.2
Murrah Buffalo				
First	6.76	4.07	16.74	9.98
Second	6.84	4.19	16.83	9.99
Third	6.74	4.20	16.69	9.95
Fourth	6.95	4.35	16.96	10.01
Fifth	7.08	4.37	17.09	10.01
Russian Buffalo				
First	8.75	4.52	18.52	9.77
Second	8.71	4.47	18.49	9.78
Third	8.69	4.41	17.83	9.14

4. **Variation due to season:** Seasonal variation in milk composition is associated with the change in agro-climatic conditions affecting the chemical composition of the feeds and fodders. Significant seasonal variation in milk composition may be observed (Table 9.7), but the trend will differ due to breed and lacation (El-Sokkary and Hassan, 1949; Ghosh and Anantakrishnan, 1963; Khan et al., 1970, El-Ghandour et al., 1979).

TABLE 9.7: Seasonal variation in milk composition (%)

Season	Fat	Solids-not fat	Protein	Lactose + ash
Winter	6.75	9.67	3.97	5.69
Summer	6.49	9.67	3.88	5.79
South-West Monsoon	7.09	9.52	3.87	5.67
North-East Mansoon	6.81	9.66	3.95	5.70

5. **Variation due to pregnancy:** Pregnancy has significant effect on the milk composition probably due to demand of nutrients for foetal development. Pregnancy affected the various milk constituents and a definite trend of increase in lactose percentage and fall in ash percentage (Table 9.8) has been reported during the rising as well as declining phases of the lactation period (Parekh and Gangwar, 1968).

TABLE 9.8: Variation in milk composition due to pregnancy

Milk Composition (%)	Non-pregnant	Early pregnancy	Mid pregnancy	Late pregnancy
Rising phase of lactation period				
Fat	6.10	6.68	6.99	-
Total solids	16.50	17.01	17.39	-
Solids-not fat	10.40	10.33	10.99	-
Protein	4.57	4.46	4.79	-
Lactose	4.83	5.14	5.40	-
Ash	1.04	0.73	0.71	-
Declining phase of lactation period				
Fat	7.13	7.87	7.77	7.47
Total solids	17.45	18.54	18.24	18.25
Solids-not fat	10.32	10.65	10.47	10.78
Protein	4.74	4.76	4.53	4.76
Lactose	4.73	5.12	5.31	5.54
Ash	0.85	0.77	0.63	0.48

6. **Diurnal variation:** Diurnal variation in milk composition is frequently observed. Usually higher percentage of total solids and milk fat associated with lower milk yield at the evening milking than the morning milking is quite common in buffaloes (Fahmey, 1974; Dash and Basu, 1975; El-Ghandour et al.,1979). However, such variations are not consistent and differ between the farms (Table 9.9). Variation in milk fat percentage is normally highest amongst all the milk constituents (Pandey, 1981).

TABLE 9.9: Dirunal variation in milk composition (%)

Farm/Herd	Fat		Protein		Lactose		Total solids	
	M	E	M	E	M	E	M	E
Izatnagar	7.81	7.16	4.45	4.39	4.75	4.73	18.09	17.04
Pantnagar	7.25	7.29	4.39	4.35	4.64	4.65	17.27	17.27
Manjhra	6.39	6.24	4.03	4.04	4.77	4.74	16.32	16.20
Chak-Ganjaria	6.84	6.45	4.11	4.11	4.60	4.57	16.61	16.26
Pooled milk	6.94	6.60	4.19	4.16	4.68	4.66	16.87	16.49

*M = Morning milk, E = Evening milk

7. **Variation due to seson of calving:** Difference in milk composition is observed due to season of claving (Table 9.10). The percentage of various milk constituents of Egyptian buffaloes are higher in summer clavers than in winter calves (Ragab et al., 1974). In Murrah buffaloes, the milk of winter calvers is generally richer than the summer and monsoon calvers (Pandey, 1981).

TABLE 9.10: Variation in milk composition due to season of calving

Season of Calving	Fat %	Total Solids, %	Solids not fat, %	Protein %
Egyptian Buffaloes				
Winter	6.30	16.33	10.03	3.89
Summer	6.52	16.62	10.10	3.90
Murrah Buffaloes				
Winter	7.09	17.21	10.07	4.24
Summer	7.49	17.60	10.06	4.42
Monsoon	7.11	17.15	9.98	4.32

8. **Variation due to milking portion:** Significant variation occurs in the composition of different portiens of milk at a milking time and fat percentage is usually high in the last fraction of milk and the residual milk obtained after stripping at the end of milking (Olenov, 1954; El-Shazly et al., 1974; Hanna et al., 1979; Ludri, 1980). Fat percentage in different portions of milk may show more variation in the first month of lactation period (Table 9.11). Large variation occurs in the fat and total solids content of residual milk (Table 9.12).

TABLE 9.11: Difference in fat percentage of different portions of milk

Portion of milk	Month of lactation		
	1st	4th	7th
1	5.61	9.59	9.10
2	4.86	7.52	10.60
3	7.04	9.50	12.40
4	10.76	11.20	14.61

TABLE 9.12: Difference in the composition of normal and residual milk

Consituents (%)	Normal milk		Residual milk	
	Range	Mean	Range	Mean
Milk fat	3.7–7.6	5.9	4.8–22.0	12.15
Total Solids	13.2–18.3	16.0	14.2–32.4	22.20
Solids-not-fat	9.4–11.1	10.1	9.4–11.01	10.05

9. **Variation due to milking interval or frequency of daily milking:** Frequency of daily milking affects milk composition (Table 9.13) but the variation in composition does not show a definite trend (Dass et al., 1976; Kapoor and Ludri, 1984).

10. **Variation due to udder massage before milking:** Light massage of udder before milking increases milk yield as well as fat percentage in milk (Alim et al., 1977; Gotsiridze and Kitoshvili, 1981). The effect of udder massage on milk composition is quite variable (Table 9.14).

TABLE 9.13: Variation in milk composition due to milking interval

Milk constituents (%)	Milking Interval (hr)			
	4	8	12	16
Milk fat	6.82	7.04	6.87	7.06
Total solids	17.33	17.22	17.30	17.51
Solids-not fat	10.46	10.37	10.40	10.45
Protein	4.43	4.42	4.43	4.33
Lactose	4.58	4.64	4.61	4.75

TABLE 9.14: Variation in milk composition due to udder massage

Milk components (%)	Wet massage with warm cloth	Dry hand massage
Milk fat	6.88 ± 0.76	6.39 ± 0.75
Total solids	16.25 ± 0.98	15.78 ± 1.24
Solids-not fat	9.38 ± 0.42	9.39 ± 0.45

11. **Variation due to udder quarters:** Milk composition of different udder quarters of the same buffalo (Table 9.15) differs significantly (Polikhrovon and Tosev, 1970).

TABLE 9.15: Variation due to udder quarters

	Left fore	Right fore	Left rear	Right rear
Milk yield (%)	20.61	21.23	29.77	28.39
Fat in milk	8.38	8.27	8.34	8.38

12. **Variation due to lactation milk yield:** A negative correlation is normally found between the milk yield and percentage of fat, protein and total solids of the milk (El-Ghandour et al., 1980).

13. **Variation due to environmental cooling:** Arrangement of environmental cooling for the amelioration of heat stress significantly increases the daily milk yield. The increase in milk yield has been found to be associated with the fall in fat percentage and increase in lactose percentage of milk (Table 9.16). The effect of cooling arrangement is almost similar during the rising and declining phases of lactation period (Soni et al., 1980).

TABLE 9.16: Variation in milk composition due to environmental cooling

Treatments	Milk yield, kg/day	Fat %	Lactose %
Lactation phase–I			
Control	7.5	7.59	4.26
Shower bath	7.6	7.65	4.45
Wallowing	8.5	7.43	4.58
Lactation phase–II			
Control	6.8	7.96	4.40
Shower bath	7.0	7.98	4.52
Wallowing	7.3	7.70	4.77

14. **Variation due to individual, herd, families and lines of buffaloes:** Variation in the composition of milk due to individuals, herds or farms, families and lines is

not uncommon (El-Sokkary and Hassan 1949; Dzhafarov, 1971; and Pandey, 1981). The variation is greater due to individuality of the animals (Table 9.17).

TABLE 9.17: Variation due to individual, herd, families and lines

Factors	Fat %	Total solids %	Protein %
Individual	4.25–10.20 (6.64)		2.69–5.05
Herd	5.50–7.50 (6.60)		3.54–4.40 (3.96)
Family A	8.72	18.28	4.46
Family B	9.40	19.37	4.51
Line I	9.07	18.78	4.86
Line II	8.49	17.91	4.42
Line III	8.30	17.80	4.50

15. **Variation due to feeds:** The composition of rations and plane of nutrition may significantly affect the milk composition. Feeding of green leguminous fodders increases milk yield of less fat content (Patel et al., 1969). Additional feeding of concentrates over the requirement may not affect the milk composition (Touny et al., 1976; Kumar and Tripathi, 1978) but significant cut in concentrate feeds on a wheat bhoosa based diet may cause considerable fall in milk yield but increase in fat content (Shukla et al., 1972). Feeding of oil in diets affects the content and composition of fat in milk (Ahuja et al., 1972).

▶ **MILK DISTRIBUTION SYSTEMS**

One or more of the following activities are involved in the milk distribution systems:-
1. Milk production.
2. Purchase and collection of milk
3. Preservation and transportation of milk.
4. Sterilization/pasteurization of milk.
5. Packaging of milk.
6. Distribution of milk.

1. **Milk production:** The milk producers may be classified into three groups, i.e., (i) rural milk producers comprising farmers of different economic classes and landless farm families, (ii) urban and sub-urban dairy owners maintaining small to medium sized herds of lactating buffaloes, and (iii) organized dairy farms of Government Institutions, Cooperative Societies and Private organizations.

2. **Purchase and collection of milk:** The milk is purchased by retail comsumers, middleman, halwais, milk cooperatives and milk processing factories.
   The milk collection system differs in different areas. Mostly middleman or dudhias collect milk from door to door or at a common place according to convenience, while milk cooperatives establish milk collection centres with a small laboratory facility for milk testing, preferably milk fat percentage for the determination of milk price. Price of milk is normally paid in cash and/or kind at the milk collection centres according to fat percentage in the milk. The payment may be weekly, fornightly or monthly. Halwais in the Indian subcontinent mostly prefer to purchase milk on the basis of khoa recovery.

3. **Preservation and transportation of milk:** Milk is preserved by the use of common preservatives like hydrogen peroxide and cooling with the help of a water soaked

jute patti on the metallic milk continers and by chilling, if chilling plant is available. Normally milk is transported twice daily to market, milk collection centres and the milk processing plants. The mode of transport depends on the amount of milk, distance, transport facilities and local conditions. Milk may be transported by road, rail and water routes (Table 9.18).

TABLE 9.18: Modes of milk transportation

S.No.	Mode	Quantity of milk, kg	Distance km
		Road Transports	
1.	Head load	10–30	Up to 10
2.	Bahangi/Shoulder sling	10–50	Up to 10
3.	Pack animals		
	(a) Bullock	40–60	Up to 10
	(b) Pony	40–60	Up to 20
	(c) Camel	40–60	Up to 15
4.	Bullock cart	200–400	Up to 10
5.	Tonga/Ekk	200–300	Up to 20
6.	Bicycle	50–60	Up to 30
7.	Rikshaw	100–200	Up to 25
8.	Auto-rikshaw	300–500	Up to 50
9.	Truck/Tankers	1/2 –5 tons	More than 50
		Water routes	
1.	Boats		
2.	Steamers		
		Rail transport	
1.	Common containers	25–100	Up to 50
2.	Milk carriage	10 tons. cap	Long distance

Different types of containers are used for the transportation of fluid milk and their selection depends on the amount of milk, distance of transportation, initial cost of container, working life of the container, mode of transportation, easiness of cleaning and availability, etc. The following types of containers are commonly used for the transportation of milk:

1. Baked earthenwares
2. Wooden cans
3. Hollow bamboo cylinders
4. Aluminium cans
5. Galvanized iron cans
6. Empty tin containers available after the disposal of vegetable oils.
7. Aluminium cans
8. Plastic containers
9. Motor driven or rail tankers with arrangements of milk chilling.

4. **Sterilization and pasteurization:** For increasing the keeping quality of fluid milk it is essential to remove or reduce its microbial content. Milk is made free from microorganisms through sterilization and microbial count is significantly reduces and their multiplication is controlled through the pasteurization. The surplus fluid milk of evening milking is normally boiled and either kept for sale in next morning

or cultured for dahi making. This practice is followed by small milk producers of remote areas. The pasteurization of milk is practiced in the organized dairies.

5. **Packaging of fluid milk:** The pasteurized milk is filled in sterilized clean glass bottles or disposable paper/plastic containers of 0.5, 1, 2 and 5 liters capacity and packed in cartons for retail sale. Bulk milk packaging may be done in alloy or plastic containers.

6. **Distribution of milk:** The distribution of milk may be very simple like retails sale to consumers at the unorganized dairy farms of urban areas or a complex system of collection, processing, standardization, pasteurization, packaging and distribution processes of the organized dairies. Following are the common milk distribution system:

   i. Direct retail sale of fluid milk at the place of production. It is a daily routine sale for 1–2 hours in morning and eventing at the time of milking. The requirement of consumers varies from quarters liter to 4–5 liters daily.

   ii. **Door delivery:** Fresh fluid milk is sold from door to door within 1–3 hours of production. The vendors may be either producer or a middleman.

   iii. **Bulk supply to shops:** The milk collected by middleman from the rural areas is sold to shops in bulk. Average daily requirements of shops varies from 10 to 100 kg or more depending upon the market requirement of milk and milk products.

   iv. Supply of pasteurized milk through booth or sale agents. This system is common in cities and towns having organized dairies. The milk is available in a half or one litre sealed container. The mode of sale may be cash payment or coupan system. The third and most convenient system is the machine delivery where fixed quantity of milk is delivered by the automatic machine against pushing the cost of milk in definite coins. However, procurement of coins is a limiting factor in this system.

▶ MILK PRODUCTS

Various kinds of milk products are quite popular in the human dietary since ages. Buffalo milk is preferred over cows milk due to its high fat and total solids content for the preparation of several milk products of the tropical and other buffalo breeding countries. Approximately half of the total milk produced in India is believed to be utilized for the production of various dairy products which are more remunerative than the sale of fluid milk. The various milk products may be classified into the following six groups:

1. Fluid milk products.
2. Condensed milk products.
3. Dried or dehydrated milk products, and
4. Coagulated milk products.
5. Fermented or cultured milk products, and
6. Products of the cream, butter and ghee industry.

1. **Fluid milk products:** The milk products flavoured and sweetened for increasing the palatability and containing milk fat not less than the minimum legal requirement of market milk ar known as milks, while those with low fat content are known as drinks (milk drinks). The common examples are chocolate milk, frui flavoured milk, and vitaminised milk, etc. the most popular fluid milk drink is milk shake. These

products are normally coloured, sterilized and bottled in hygienic conditions and used as cold drinks during the summer season.

2. **Condensed milk products:** The milk products prepared by partial evaportation of water through the heating of whole milk, partially separated milk and skim milk are known as condensed milks. They may or may not contain added sugar (sucrose). The different kinds of condended milks are described as follows:

   i. *Unsweetened condensed milk/partial evaporated milk:* The milk product manufactured by the partial removal of water through heating is called unsweetened condensed milk or partial evaporated milk. It may contain not more than 0.3% of calcium chloride, citric acid, sodium citrate or sodium salt of orthophosphoric acid or polyphosphoric acid in the final product. Unsweetened condensed milk should contain not less thn 8% milk fat and 26% milk solids-not fat. Buffalo milk needs standardization of milk fat through the addition of skim for the manfacture of unsweetened condensed milk according to the legal standards.

   ii. *Unsweeteed condensed skim milk:* Unsweeted condensed skim milk is manufactured by partial evaporation of moisture of separated milk through heat treatment. The addition of calcium chloride, citric acid, sodium citrate and sodium salts of orthophosphoric acid or polyphosphoric acid should not exceed 0.3% by weight of the final product. It should not contain more than 0.5% milk fat and less than 20% total milk solids.

   iii. *Sweetened condensed milk:* The whole milk or stansrdized milk condensed through the partial evaporation of moisture content by heat treatment under a high vacuum after the addition of cane sugar should not contain less than 9% milk fat, 31% total milk solids and 40% added sugar (sucrose). The preservatives concentration as mentoned for the unsweetened condensed milk should not be more than 0.3% by weight of the finished product.

   iv. *Sweetened condensed skim milk:* It is prepared by partial evaporation of moisture of skimmed milk and addition of sugar (sucrose). The various preservatives as mentioned for unsweetened condensed milk should not exceed 0.3% by weight of the finished product. The milk fat should not be more than 0.5 percent, total milk solids less than 26% and cane sugar less than 40% by weight.

   The specifications for sweetened condensed milk approved by the Indian Standards Institution (IS: 1166 or 1973) are given in (Table 9.19).

TABLE 9.19: ISI (BIS) specification for sweetened condensed milks

Characteristics	Whole milk	Skimmed milk
Total milk solids, %, Min.	31.0	26.0
Milk fat, %, Min.	9.0	0.5 Max.
Sucrose, %, Min.	40.0	40.0
Acidity as lactic acid, %, Max.	0.35	0.35
Total bacterial count per g. Max.	500	500
Coliform count per g.	Nil	Nill
Yeast and mould count per g. Max.	10	10

Uses of condensed milk: Condensed milk is prepared mainly for use in the remote areas where regular supply of fluid milk is not assured. Condensation and other treatments increase its keeping quality and facilitate easy transportation when packed airtight after sterilization. The common uses are as follows:

  i.   Preparation of reconstituted milk.
  ii. Preparation of milk containing beverages like tea and coffee, etc.
  iii. Preparation of milk foods like kheer, ice cream, kulphi and other sweets.

3. **Dried milk products:** The milk products manufactured by the evaporation of moisture by heat treatment or other means are dried milks or milk powder. Milk powder contains less than 5% moisture by weight. It may be whole milk powder or skimmed milk powder. The content of various additives like calcium chloride, citric acid, sodium citrate and sodium salf of orthophosphoric or polyphosphoric acid should not be more than 0.3 percent and that of butylated hydroxyl anisole 0.01% by weight of the finished product. Whole milk powder should not contain less than 26% milk fat and skim milk powder may not contain higher than 1.5% milk fat. The total acidity expressed as lactic acid should be below 1.2% in whole milk powder and 1.5% in skim milk powder. The standard bacterial count (plate count) should not be more than 50,000 per g and coliform bacteria count higher than 90 per g. Maximum solubility index should be 15 and 2 for the roller dried and spray dried milk powders respectively as per the PFA Rules (1976) in India.

Uses of dried milk of milk powder
  i.   For the preparation of reconstituted milk.
  ii. For the preparation of tea and coffee.
  iii. For the preparation of cultured milk products and sweet dishes containing milk as an ingredient.

4. **Coagulated milk products:** Raw or heated milk is coagulated by the addition of citric acid, lemon juice, lactic acid or sour whey. The coagulum thus obtained is strained and processed for the preparation of chhana, paneer, cheese and their products.

5. **Fermented or cultured milk products:** The main products prepared from raw or heated milk with the help of natural or specific bacterial culture are known as fermented or cultured milk products. Common products are dahi (curd), yoghurt and chakka (Srikhand), etc.

6. **Concentrated butter fat products or the products of cream, butter and ghee industry:** Common milk products containing higher percentage of milk fat prepared through physical processing are cream, butter, makkhan and ghee/saman.

▶ COMMON MILK PRODUCTS OF DIFFERENT COUNTRIES

Various common milk products prepared from buffaloes milk in different countries are ghee or samna (clarified butter or butter oil), cream, butter, cheese and fermented milk products like dahi and yoghurt. Several varieties of cheese are prepared in different countries and some of the popular varieties are given in (Table 9.20).

Domiati Cheese

It is one of the most popular cheeses of Egypt and it is also known in other Arabian countries. Unlike other pickled cheesed the domiati cheese is prepared from the salted milk. Domiati cheese is prepared from whole milk of buffalo or cow or a mixture of whole and skim milk in different ratios. Howevers, buffalo milk is preferred due to its high fat content for the production of rich domiati cheese.

TABLE 9.20: Popular cheeses of buffalo milk in different countries

Name of cheese	Country	Milk used
Domiati	Egypt	Buffalo milk or mixture of cow milk
Karish	Egypt	Buffalo milk + Skimed cow milk or butter milk after acodification of cream.
Mis/Mish	Egypt	
Ras/Rahss	Egypt	
Roumy	Egypt	
Proviolone	Egypt, Italy	
Fres/Fresh Madhfoor Irage or Dhafayer	Italy	
Mozerella	Italy	
Ricott	Syria	
Shankalish	Greece	
Feta	Egypt. Greece	
Teleme	Bulgaria	
Salamora	Romenia	
Brandza de Braila, Vladeasa-Bucedis Homood cheese	India, Egypt, Italy etc.	
Cheddar	Italy	
Gouda	Dutch	

About 5–15% finely powdered salt is added directly in the raw milk. It is used to control the microbial growth during the manufacture of cheese at a relatively high temperature. The salted milk is strained through a piece of muslin or cheese cloth to clean it from visible impurities. The strained milk is heated before renneting by one of the following three methods:

1. Direct warming to 35–40°C or 95–105°F.
2. Heating for 15 minutes at 65°C (150°F) and then cooling to 35–40°C. This process is helpful in significant reduction of bacterial count, avoidance of gas holes in the cheese and improvement of texture and body of the cheese.
3. The told salf is added in two-third portion of the milk and remaining third of milk is heated to 77°C (170°F) for 5–10 minutes and them mixed with the salted milk. The final temperature 40–45°C (105–115°F) thus achieved is suitable for renneting. It also improves the texture and body of the cheese and slightly reduces the total bacterial count.

For the coagulation of milk about 20–25 ml good quality rennet is required for 100 kg milk and it takes about 2–3 hours at 40–46 temperature. The curd is ladled into metallic moulds or wooden frames and allowed to drain under adequate pressure to obtain a good firm cheese for easy handling. The pieces of fresh cheese are wrapped in cheese paper. Brine solution is usually prepared in whey available from the drainage of cheese. The cheese may be consumed fresh or ripened for 4–8 months in earthen pots.

The yield of Domiati cheese is dependent on the total solids content of milk and the concentration of salf added to milk (Table 9.21).

TABLE 9.21: Effect of salt quantity on the yield of Domiati cheese

Kind of milk	Salt content in milk (%)				
	0	*2.5*	*5.0*	*7.5*	*10.0*
Buffalo milk	17.25	20.33	28.49	32.72	36.50
Cow milk	11.18	13.08	18.4	24.71	27.75

The average values of total solids, fat and salt are 45 ± 4, 24 ± 3 and 4.5 ± 0.5 fresh; and 48 ± 4, 25.5 ± 3 and $4.8 \pm 0.5\%$ in the ripened domiati cheese.

Provolone Cheese

Provolone cheese is prepared in Egypt particularly in the small dairies of Alexandria. It is usually prepared from the raw mixed milk of cow and buffalo without addition of any starter. It is also prepared from raw milk of cow or buffalo. The raw milk is coagulated by adding a suitable quantity of rennet to obtain a good firm curd in one hour. The curd is cut and then allowed to remain in the whey for about 15 minutes. After this the whey is drained out and the curd is transferred into a cloth lined metallic hoop and left for 2–3 hours.

The curd is now cut into small pieces and left at room temperature of make it more elastic. It can be tested by dipping a piece of curd in hot water bath at about 79–80°C (175–176°F) for few seconds and then stretched slowly into a fine thread without the tendency to break. After this the curd pieces are dipped in hot water bath 79–80°C to make more elastic, so that small balls may be prepared. The curd balls are then dippen into a 20% salted whey solution for 24 hours and then placed in a rope net hanging from ceiling for 24 hours smoking with the smoke of burning wood in half-cut barrel.

The smoked cheese is then kept in ripening room at 10–12°C (50–54°F) for a period of 4 weeks and then used as a food item (El-Sokkary and Hassan, 1952; El-Soda et al., 1976a).

The difference in chemical composition of milk and provolone cheese (Table 9.22) prepared from the raw whole milk of buffalo and cow is significant.

TABLE 9.22: Composition of milk and provolone cheese of buffalo (B) and Cow (C) milk

Stepps in cheese making	pH		Fat %		Protein %		Salt %	
	B	*C*	*B*	*C*	*B*	*C*	*B*	*C*
Whole milk	6.6	6.7	6.15	3.70	4.29	3.40	-	-
Curd before shaping	5.2	5.2	30.50	24.50	17.39	19.53	-	-
Cheese before salting	5.4	5.4	29.00	24.00	15.67	22.39	-	-
Salted cheese	5.3	5.3	30.35	25.50	18.34	22.40	2.68	2.20
Smoked cheese	5.4	5.3	32.50	28.00	21.87	-	2.74	2.64
Ripened cheese	5.5	5.4	36.50	30.00	20.25	24.10	3.12	2.98

Formation of adequate concentration of desired volatile fatty acids is important for the development of characteristic flavour in the cheese. Acetic acid is found during all the stages of provolone cheese making. Butyric acid appears during the early stages of cheese manufacture and propionic, caproic and caprylic acids develop during the ripening period (El-Soda et al., 1976b).

In raw milk of buffalo, bacterial, yeast and mould counts are usually high, which significantly decreases in cheese (Table 9.23). This is due to formation of lactic acid, heating during smoking and increase of acidity during ripening stages (El-Soda et al., 1976c).

TABLE 9.23: Microbial condition of milk and provolone cheese

Microbial count	Raw buffalo milk	Provolone cheese
Total count X 106	0.0–14.0	4.00–6.00
Lactic acid bacterial X 106	0.02–1.0	1.60–12.00
Coliform bacterial X 103	10–1000	0.0
Enterococi X 103	2.30	0.0
Yeast and mould	Over count	0.0
Streptrococcus faecalis	83.4	66.7
Str. Lactis/Str. cremoric	16.6	22.9

Mish Cheese

Mish is a popular cheese of Egypt. It has yellowish-brow colour, sharp flavour and high salft content. The exact origin of mish cheese is not known but supposed to be similar to salted cheese found in the Egyptian tombs of king Horaha of the first dynasty about 3200 B.C. (Iskander, 1942). It is a popular dairy food of farmers and labourers of Egypt. Mish cheese can be prepared any time but large quantity is prepared during the winter season when large quantity of milk is available.

Mish cheese is prepared from karish cheese which is made of skim milk by latic fermentation. Process of mish cheese manufacture differes from one to another region, but various steps are almost similar (Hamdy and Taha, 1954). The cubes of karish cheese are packed under microaerophilic conditions in a large clean earthen pot known as 'ballas'. The space between cheese pieces are filled with whole milk, skim milk or butter milk containing about 10% salt which is known as 'Laban Khad'. The other additives used are sesame oil cake (kosba), residue of ghee or samna (Morta), oriental spices and medicinal plants and may be from 2 –7% of whole mixture. The ballas is covered by a plam leaf sheath and a piec of cloth and then tightly sealed with mud paste. The pores of ballas and mud seal keep the contents under partially anaerobic conditions during ripening period of about one year in a warm sunny place.

The moisture, fat, protein and salt content of mish cheese is about 55.76–74.14, 3.3–18.0. 12.64–14.16 and 10.3–18.0% in different samples. About 56.8–84.1% of the total nitrogen is present in the form of free amino nitrogen and arginine is almost absent (El-Erian et al., 1975).

The ripened mish cheese is yellowish-brown in colour with a characteristic sharp, pungent flavour and some what butyric adour. The old ripen pickling medium of mish cheese is called mish paste which resembles with the cheese in chemical composition, flavour and colour (El-Gendy, 1983). The various volatile fatty acids present in the ripened mish cheese are acetic, propionic, butyric, caproic, caprylic and valeric acids and the characteristic odour is imparted by the alpha-keto butyric acid (Amin and El-Kholy, 1979).

Shankalish Cheese

Shankalish is the native Syrian cheese almost similar to the mish cheese of Egypt (Abou-Donia and Abdel-Kader, 1979).

A coagulum of milk similar to karish cheese is prepared and collected in large containers. The curd is kneeded with 7.2% powdered salt and a mixture of oriental spices according to taste and then shaped into balls of 3–4 cm diameter. The cheese is ripened in a dark humid-hot room till the development of a characteristic sharp flavour. The surfaces of ripened cheese is cleand and then stored submerged in olive oil in glass containers, or sun dried for 2–3 days for preventing the over ripening. The average moisture, protein, fat, ash and salt content of shankalish cheese is 30.2, 46.4, 7.76, 7.02 and 5.5 per cent, and mean pH value is 4.5. The cheese is free from Enterobacteria and Staphylococci but contains proteolytic, lypolytic and aerobic spore forming bacteria.

Ricotta Cheese

Ricotta is a soft, fresh and unripened cheese of Italian origin. Ricotta cheese is prepared from the cheese whey in many Mediterranean and Scandinavean countries. Satisfactory ricotta cheese may be prepared from paneer whey. The paneer whey is first neuralized by mixing 1.0% solution of calcium hydroxide. After this whole milk and neutralized paneer whye are mixed in the ratio of 1: 9 and then heated to 95°C. A dilute solution (1.0%) of citric acid is added slowly while stirring the mixture for coagulation. Heating is stopped and coagulum is left in the whey for 45–60 minutes and then strained through a muslin cloth applying gentle pressure for squeezing the whey. The salt ricotta cheese, thus obtained is a rich source of protein, minerals and vitamins and consumed in different forms. Average yield of ricotta cheese is about 6% from the paneer whey of buffalo milk (Shukla and Brar, 1986).

Stracchino Type Cheese

It is a soft cheese from whole milk of buffalo. The technology of manufacture is quite simple (Mincione et al., 1984) and can be adopted easily. Lost of 100 kg whole milk of buffalo is filtered standardized to 6% fat by dilution with water or skimmed milk and pasteurized at 63°C for 30 minutes. A lactic starter culture (commercial yoghurt in milk) is added at the rate of 1.2% in the milk cooled to 43°C. After 10 minutes cultured milk is further cooled to 37°C for renneting (50 minutes total time). The curd is broken and separated from the whey and then cooked in moulds for about 5 hours, brined for 2 hours in 20% salt solution (4°C SH) and then dried and ripened at 6°C and 80% relative humidity for 21 days. The average yield of fresh cheese is about 23.6% but final yield is only 16.1% due to approximately 31.5% loss during the ripening of cheese. The blocks of mature cheese of normally 14 × 20 × 6 cm size had thin white to flesh colour skin, whitish colour, compact and soft pasty texture and delicate taste. It contains about 59% fat, 5.4% total nitrogen, 1.0–1.2% titrable acidity (equivalent to lactic acid) and 1.7: 1 ratio of calcium: Phosphorus on dry matter basis. Lactic acid bacteria count increases to maximum after about 14 days ripening and then declines. The ratio of lactobacilli to Streptococci also increases to maximum 9: 1 after 14 days but at the end of ripening period it is 1 to 1.5: 1.)

Cream

The high fat containing portion of milk obtained by either gravitational or mechnical sepration of whole milk is known as cream. According to the PFA Rules (1976) cream should not contain less than 25% milk fat.

Large variation occurs in the composition of cream. It is much richer in fat content than the milk and contains all the other milk constituents in lower proportion than in the whole milk. Cream may be classified into three types on the basis of fat percentage.

a. **Thin cream or light cream:** The cream containing less than 30% fat is called thin or light cream. The cream obtained by gravity method is usually thin and contains 10–25% milk fat. Thin cream my be also manufactured by centrifungal method for use in the preparation of coffee cream may be also manufactured by centrifungal method for use in the preparation of coffee cream, fruit cream and ice cream, etc.

b. **Medium cream or whipping cream:** It is prepared by centrifungal method and contains 30–40% milk fat. Market creams are normally medium type.

c. **Rich/heavy/plastic cream:** the cream containing more than 65% milk fat is known as rich, heavy or plastic cream. It is rarely manufactured for marketing.

Cream is a high energy milk product and used as human food as follows:-

  i. Direct consumption of fresh and pasteurized cream in coffee and other foods.

 ii. For the preparation of ice creams

iii. For the preparation of sweet cream butter from fresh cream or sour/ripened cream butter from cultured cream or aged cream. The latter is manufactured by fermentation of cream with a known culture of milk fermenting micro-organisms or natural dahi culture for the development of a characteristic aroma of ghee.

iv. For the manufacture of ghee either from sweet or ripened cream or the butter obtained from the churning of cream.

Composition of Buffalo Cream

The average chemical composition of different types of cream prepared from the whole milk of buffalo (Table 9.24) shows that various milk constituents separated in cream are negatively related with the percentage of milk fat.

TABLE 9.24: Composition of buffalo cream

Constituents (%)	Fat content in cream (%)			
	25	35	55	75
Total solids	32.6	41.5	59.5	82.0
Moisture	67.4	58.5	40.5	18.0
Solids-not fat	7.6	6.5	4.5	5.0
Milk fat	25.0	35.0	55.0	75.0
Protein	3.1	2.6	1.8	0.8
Lactose	3.9	3.4	2.3	1.0
Ash	0.6	0.5	0.4	0.2

Butter

The compact milk fat concentrate obtained by churning of sweet or ripened cream is known as butter. It may or may not contain salt and/or permitted colour.

According to PFA Rules (1976) butter should not contain less than 80% milk fat and more than 1.5% curd and colouring agents. Use of diacetyl as a flavour is permitted to maximum 4 ppm. Other additives for preservation like calcium hydroxide, sodium bicarbonate, sodium carbonate and sodium polyphosphate should not be more than 0.2%. These characteristics are also applicable to makkhan obtained from the churning of curd.

Various types of butters normally available in the market are: (i) Sweet cream butter: Butter prepared from sweet cream of less than 0.2% acidity. (ii) Salted sweet cream butter-Butter obtained from sweet cream of less than 0.2% acidity and containing about 3% added common salt. (iii) Ripend cream butter-Butter obtained from the churning of ripend cream. Normally *dahi* culture is used for the ripening of butter. Aging of cream to room temperature is also used for the development of a delicate butter aroma.

Fat globules of butter made from buffaloe's milk cream are larger and butter contains about 68.56% globular fat (Ismail and Sirry, 1966). Aging of buffalo cream for 12 hours at 10°C (50°F) helps in satisfactory crystallization of the fat (Nabar et al., 1969).

Butter is a popular dairy product in human dietary and used as follows:-

i. **Direct consumption:** Normally fresh or pasteurized butter is used as table butter for eating with bread, chapatti, dal and rice, etc.

ii. **Manufacture of ghee:** Butter obtained from ripend cream is preferably used for the preparation of ghee of pleasant characteristic aroma.

iii. Used as a cooking medium.

iv. Used for the preparation of sweet like butter samosa.

Butter Oil

Clarified milk fat obtained after the removal of moisture and solids-not fat from the cream or butter is known as butter oil. It is also known as dry milk fat, de-hydrated butter fat or anhydrous milk fat. This is similar to ghee of India and samna of Egypt.

Butter oil contains about 9.5–99.8% milk fat and traces of moisture. Acidity is nomally below 0.5% and peroxide value is less than 0.1 percent.

Butter oil is used as a cooking medium, preparation of sweets and reconstituted milk after mixing with powder and water.

▶ ICE CREAM

Ice cream is a frozen dairy product prepared from the mixture of sweet cream and common sugar (sucrose). It may or may not contain permissible flovour, colour and stabilizer.

According to the PFA Rules (1976) of India, ice cream should not contain less than 10% milk fat, 3.5% milk protein and 36% total milk solids. The concentration of permitted stabilizers and emulifiers must not exceed 0.5 percent. Special ice creams may be prepared by the addition of one or more edible additives like fruits, fruit juice, eggs, nuts, dry fruits and chocolate. These products must not contain less than 8% milk fat. Starch may be added up to 5% and must be declared prominently on the container of ice cream. Ice cream premix standard composition of ice cream fixed by the Indian Standards Institution vide its resolution number IS: 2802 to 1964 is given in Table 9.25.

TABLE 9.25: ISI specification of ice cream

Constituents	Content
Minimum weight, g/litre	525
Total solids, % minimum	36.0
Minimum milk fat, %	10.0
Maximum acidity as lactic acid, %	0.25
Maximum stabilizers/emulsifiers, %	0.5
Standard plate count per g.	Below 2,50,000
Coliform bacteria per g.	Below 90
Phosphatase test	Negative

Various types of ice creams are prepared in different countries but there appears to be no standard classification of ice creams for the international acceptance. Flavoured ice cream, chocolate ice cream, fruits cream or phaluda, nut cream and soft ice cream (softy) are quite popular in different countries. Demand of softy is more than the other kinds of ice creams and children are very fond of eating softy. It contains about 3–6% milk fat, 11–14% other milk soild, 12–15% added sugar, 0.4–0.5% stabilizers and emulsifiers and permitted flavour and colour. Softy is drawn at about –80C (18 0F) and served for eating in cones of starch and gelatin moulded in attractive shapes.

Good quality ice cream should be palatable and soft and it should not be rancid, bitter, coarse and sandy. Ice cream is generally eaten as a frozen dessert, while softy is taken during lunch break and pleasure trips to market, parks, cinema, circus and other places of recreation and relaxation.

▶ INDIAN MILK PRODUCTS

The nutritional contribution of milk of buffalo and other farm animals was recognized in ancient India thousands of years ago. The various milk products developed in the Indian subcontinent are referred as Indian milk products. Due to high fat and total milk solids percentage most of the Indian dairy products are preferably prepared from the buffalo milk. Dahi, ghee and paneer are most common dairy products of Indian subcontinent. Chhanna and khoa or Mava are coagulated and concentrated milk products respectively which are the base of a large variety of sweets prepared in the Indian sub-continent.

The common dairy products of Indian may be identified into the following three broad group:

1. Concentrated whole milk products like Kheer/Basundi/Tasmai/Havya, Khoa or Mawa, Rabri, Kulfi.
2. Coagulated milk products are paneer and Chhana.
3. Cultured milk products are Dahi and Srikhand or Chakka.
4. Products of concentrated butter fat industry are cream, makhan, ghee, lassi, and ghee residue.

Kheer

Kheer is prepared by the partial dehydration of whole milk in a pan by direct heating. Usually small quantity of rice and occasionally dry fruits and nuts are added and boiled to cook. Sufficient quantity of sugar is added in the last stage of boilig. Kheer prepared from milk standardized to 4% fat content and containing 2.5% washed rice and 5% sugar may contain about 67% moisture, 7.83% fat 6.34% protein, 8.45% lactose, 1.41% ash and 8.95% added sugar (De et al., 1976).

Rabri

A concentrated and sweetned whole milk product containing scattered clotted cream is known as rabri. Sugar is added at the rate of 5–6% of the original volume of milk. Rabri is nomally prepared by direct heating of milk in a shallow pan. The approximate content of moisture, fat, protein, added sugar, lactose and ash in rabri is 30, 20, 10, 20, 17 and 3% respectively (Singh et al., 1975)

Khurchan

Khurchan is prepared by simmering whole milk without stirring in a shallow pan on direct fire. This helps in slow evaporation of moisture. Finely powdered sugar is normally mixed at the time of eating. It contains about 27.9, 23.6, 15.4, 14.9, 15.2 and 3.0% moisture, milk fat, protein, lactose, added sugar and ash respectively (Gupta and Rao, 1972).

Malai or Sarhi or Sar

The upper layer of fat rich elastic layer (milk skin) removed from the boiled milk after cooling slowly at room temperature is called malai. It is available normally in home and also at the halwai shop. Drinking milk salers of Indian subcontinent invariably put a small piece of malai at the top of milk. Malai is also referred to the skin of curd and served at the top of sweet lassi commonly sold in summer.

Kulfi

It is a concentrated, sweetened, flavoured and frozen milk product. It may also contain pices of dry fruits and nut. The product is frozen in different shape to make it more attractive. Its composition is variable. Good quality Kulfi may be prepared from mixed cow and buffalo milk concentrated to contain about 26% total milk solids (Salooja, 1979).

Khoa or Mawa

The partially dehydrated whole milk prepared by direct heating in a pan is known as Khoa or Mawa. The milk is constantly stirred and scrapped from the sides of pan with the help of a khunti while heating till it becomes semi-solids. After this the content is cooled at room temperature and made in different shapes for marketing. It should not contain less than 20% milk fat (IS: 4883, 1968).

The chemical composition of khoa depends on the composition of raw milk and khoa prepared from buffalo milk may contain about 19.4, 37.1, 17.8, 22.1 and 3.6% moisture, milk fat, protein, lactose and ash respectively (Ray and De, 1952). Khoa of buffalo milk is dull white, soft, slightly greesy and rich. Its texture may be smooth or granular. Khoa is base material for the preparation of famous sweets like peda, burfi, gulabjamun, kalajam, kalakand, gujhia, etc.

Paneer

Paneer is prepared by the rennet coagulation of whole milk. It is an indigenous soft cheese of India. The different varieties of paneer are surati, bandal, and dacca.

Average yield of surati paneer of buffalo milk is 34%. The moisture, total solids and fat contents in surati paneer are 71.1, 28.9 and 13.1% respectively (Bhattacharya et al., 1971). Good quality paneer is prepared by coagulating the milk at about 80°C at pH 5 (Vishweshwaraiah, 1979).

Chhenna

Chhenna is prepared by the coagulation of boiled hot whole milk with lactic acid, citric acid, lemon juice or channa whey. According to PFA Rules (1976) it should not contain more than 70% moisture. The fat content should not be less than 50% of dry matter in chhenna. Average values of moisture, fat, protein, lactose and ash in chhenna of buffalo milk are 51.6, 29.6, 14.4, 2.3 and 2.0% respectively (Ray and De, 1953). Good quality chhenna may be prepared by coagulated whole milk citric acid at 700C (Kundu and De, 1972; Iyer, 1978; Ahmed et al., 1981).

In the process of chhenna making the heating of milk favours greater recovery of milk protein but loss of soluble nutrients remains unaffected (Table 9.26). A higher loss of fat occurs in the manufacture of chhenna frm buffalo milk (Ray and De, 1953). The yield of chhenna from buffalo milk is 22 to 24% of which about 50% is moisture. Homogenization of milk before coagulation resuits in higher yield die to more recovery of milk solids without affecting the quality of chhenna (Jagtap and Shukla, 1973). The chhenna of buffalo milk is whitish, slightly hard, coarse and greasy. Chhenna may be stored for several days at refrigeration temperature but not more than 2 days at the room temperature.

TABLE 9.26: Distribution of milk constituents in chhenna and chhenna-whey of buffalo milk (%)

Milk constituents	Chhenna	Chhenna-whey
Total milk solids	65	35
Solids-not fat	48	52
Milk fat	85	45
Milk protein	91	9
Lactose	12	88
Total ash	60	40

Good quality sweet chhenna is extensively used for the preparation of the famous Bengali sweets like rasgulla, pantoa, khirmohan, cham-cham and khurma, etc.

Dahi

Dahi or curd is a coagulated milk product obtained from boiled or pasteurized milk by acid fermentation with the help of natural lactic acid bacteria or specific harmless bacterial culture. Normally diluted curd is used as culture which is also known as starter or jaman.

Dahi may be prepared from whole as well as skim milk. The former is an intermediary step in the manufacture of makhan and ghee. Dahi may be classified into the following two types:

i. **Sweet or mildly sour dahi:** It is slightly acidic and lactic acid content (acidity) does not exceed 0.7% by weight. A mixed culture of Streptococcus lactis, Str. diacetilactis and Str. cremoris is used for the curdling of milk. Dahi is sweet or mildly sour with a pleasant characteristic aroma.

ii. **Sour dahi:** It has sharp acidic flavour. Starter for sour dahi preparation contains *Lactobacillus bulgaricus* or *Str. thermophillus* or both in addition to those responsible for the curdling of sweet dahi. The acidity as lactic acid should not be more than 1.0% by weight.

Both type of dahi should be negative for phosphatase test and should not contain more than 100 cells of yeast and mould and 10 cells of coliform bacteria per gramme of dahi. The milk solids in dahi are normally 5–10% higher than the original milk. Dahi prepared from whole milk of buffalo contains 6–8% milk fat, 18–20% total soilds and 0.8–1.0% acidity. In dahi of boiled milk about half of the total fat is present in one per cent top layer and less than 8% in the about half of the total fat is present in one percent top layer and less than 8% in the bottom layer. The difference may be still greater in a dahi of raw milk (Anantakrishnan and Kothavalla, 1946). Stirring of milk after 2–4 hours of inoculation with starter improves the uniformity of fat globules in dahi (Devengan et al., 1970). Use of higher level of starter (2.5 percent) produces more firm dahi than the low level and uneven distribution of fat globules is also reduced (Oommen, 1972).

Dahi has been found to be better milk food for lactose intolerant infants (Chandrasekaran et al., 1975). Buffalo milk dahi is a richer source of available nutrients than the cow's milk dahi (Khambatta and Dastur, 1950). Dahi eating help in the prevention of putrefactive processes and corrects various digestive disorders.

Sweetened Dahi/Lal dahi/Payodhi

This kind of dahi is prepared in the eastern part of India. Payodhi has characteristic brown colour, cooked flavour and firm texture. It contains 6–7% added sugar preferably before boiling. Sweetened dahi is normally set in earthenware known as nadi or kahantari and takes about 15–16 hours for proper setting (Ray and Srinivasan, 1972).

Chakka

The soild mass obtained from the partial straining of whole milk dahi through a maslin or cheese cloth is known as chakka. The composition of chakka is quite variable (Table 9.27) and depends on the composition of milk, degree of lactic fermentation and drainge of whey (Date and Mahajan, 1971). Chakka is the basic ingredient for the preparation of Srikhand and also prepared for easy transportation to long distance.

TABLE 9.27: Composition of Chakka (%)

Samples	Moisture	Fat	Protein	Ash	Lactic acid
1.	63.2	14.7	-	-	0.80
2.	59.6	22.4	10.3	1.03	2.32

Srikhand

Srikhand is a sweetened dairy product, prepared from the whey strained curd known s chakka. The chakka is thoroughly mixed with 30–50% powdered sugar. Flavouring agents and colour like saffron 20 ml of 0.6% solution, 2 g nutmegh powder and 1.5–2.0 g cardamom seeds are generally mixed in a 1 kg chakka (Ingle and Joglekar, 1974). An acceptable srikhand may contain 60% total solids, 42% sugar and 7% protein (Aneja et al., 1978). Srikhand is a popular dairy product of Gujarat, Maharashtra and Karnatak in India. It is also used for the preparation of Srikhandgolla. A dough prepared from chakka, maize flour and baking powder is made into small balls and fried in boiling ghee or edible oil and then soaked in sugar syrup for the preparation of srikhandgola (Waghmare, 1977). Srikhand and srikhand products have a short self life at room temperature in the tropical climatic conditions. Incorporation antioxidants, dehydration to less than 9% moisture content and storage below 10°C at a dry place may significantly increase the keeping quality and products may be stored for 4–6 weeks period without significant change in the taste and consistency.

Makhan

A concentrate milk fat product similar to butter and obtained from the churning of whole milk dahi by indigenous method is known as *makkhan* or *navneet* or *layanu*. According t the PFA Rules, 1976 it should not contain less than 76% milk fat. On an average makkhan contains 18–20 per cent moisture, 76–80% butter fat, 1–1.5% non-fat milk solids and acidity normally does not exceed 0.2%. Makkhan obtained from buffalo milk is light greenish-white in colour, hard and granular with a pleasant and slightly acid aroma when fresh. The recovery of makkhan is almost equal to fat percentage in the initial milk because the minor loss of fat in lassi or mattha is compensated for by the overrun in the makkhan.

Keeping quality of makkhan is relatively low and normally processed for ghee making after 7–10 days collection. Keeping quality may be significantly improved by storing the makkhan in butter milk which should be changed daily. It is further improved by storage in 0.8% lactic acid solution (Rangappa and Banerjee, 1948).

Fresh makkhan is used for direct consumption with cooked foods in the Indian sub-contient. Large quantity of makkhan is converted into ghee and a small amount is sometimes used for the preparation of indigenous tonics with other medicinal ingredients.

Ghee–Clarified Butter Fat

Ghee or clarified butter fat is a rich source of energy and produced by dehydration of makkhan, butter or cream by cooking at 110°C–120°C. Ghee has been used as an important food item since the Vedic period in the Indian sub-content (Yegna Narayana Aiyer, 1953). It is also a popular dairy product of the Arabic countries and commonly known as samna (El-Sokkary and Zaki, 1956).

Ghee is prepared by the following three methods, viz. desi method, creamery-butter method and direct cream method. Recovery of fat is significantly affected by the method of ghee preparation (Table 9.28) due to loss of fat in different fractions of processing (Misra and Kushwaha, 1970). Higher fat recovery is possible from the high fat and washed creams (De and Srinivasan, 1958; Madan Pal and Rajori 175). Similarly recovery of ghee from makkhan in desi method can be significantly increased by the use of improved technique of dahi churning (Jain et al., 1947).

TABLE 9.28: Average milk fat recovery of ghee by different methods

Method	Loss of fat (%)				Fat recovery (%)
	Skim milk	Lassi/butter milk	Ghee residue	Handling	
Deshi method	-	13.2	1.9	2.5	82.4
Creamary butter	1.4	0.8	1.4	4.5	91.6
Direct cream	1.4	-	9.0	1.7	87.7

Physical Qualities of Ghee

The colour of ghee is affected by the method of preparation and buffalo ghee is white with a greenish tinge when prepared by desi and creamery-butter methods but waxy-white on preparation by direct cream method (Lalitha and Dastur, 1956).

A pleasant, cooked and rich flavoured ghee of mildly sour acidity is preferred over the characteristic flat flavour of fresh milk fat. Large grains of uniform size are desired in good quality market ghee.

Good quality ghee should not be smoky and over cooked or under cooked. Rancidity, greasyness, burnt colour and high sediments are unwanted characteristics of ghee and reduces its market value.

The problem of adulteration of desi ghee with other fats and oils is frequently encountered. The common adultrants of ghee are:

a. Hydrogenated vegetable oils.
b. Refined vegetable oils.
c. Animal body fat like tallow and lard.

Some times small quantity of rice, smashed potato and banana are mixed in the adulterated ghee for improving the consistency.

Uses of Ghee

1. Direct consumption with chappati, cooked pulse soup and vegetable curry, etc.
2. Medium for cooking and frying.
3. In confectionary.

Lassi/Chhanchh/Mattha

The residual dahi left after the removal of makkhan by churning is known as lassi, chhanchh or mattha in different parts of the Indian sub-continent. Approximately 30–35 kg lassi is obtained for each kg of ghee production. The composition of mattha varies. Significantly and it depends on the rate of dilution during churning of dahi for the removal of makkhan. It contains about 90–96% water, 4–10% total solids and 0.4–0.6% lactic acid.

Uses

i. Direct consumption as a beverage. Sugar, salt and spice, ice and flavour are used according to taste and availability.
ii. As a starter for the setting of dahi by indigenous method.
iii. For the preparation of curry and dahiwada, etc.

Ghee–Residue

The semi-solid cooked residue obtained after the removal of ghee is called ghee residue. It may be light to dark brown in colour and contains 33–40% milk fat. Large variation occurs in the chemical composition of ghee residue (Table–29) obtained by different methods of ghee making has been reported. There is no standard for the ghee residue. (Prahlad, 1945).

Uses: It is nomally used for consumption mixed with sugar and may be also used for the preparation of sweets and milk toffees.

REFERENCES

Abd-El-Salam, M.H. and El-Shibiny, S. 1966. The chemical compostion of buffalo milk. I. General composition. Indian J. Dairy Sci. 19: 151–154.

Abu-Donia, Y.I. and Abdel-Kader, Y.I. 1979. Microbial flora and chemical composition of native Syrian hard cheese 'Mesanarah', 'Medaffarah' and 'Shankalish'. Egyptian J. Dairy Sci., 7: 211–229 (Fide Dairy Sci. Abst., 42: 3788).

Ahmed, A.R., Vyas, S.H., Upadhyay, K.G. and Thakar, P.N. 1981. Study on manufacture of chhana from buffalo milk. Gujrat Agril. Univ. Res. J., 7: 32–36.

Ahuja, S.P., Sukhija, P.S. and Bhatia, I.S. 1972. Utilization of fat by milch buffaloes (Bos bubalus): the effect of amount and type of dietary lipids on milk fat secretion in lactating buffaloes. Indian J. Anim. Sci., 42: 167–173.

Akhundov, D. 1958. Chemical composition of milk of Azerbaijan buffaloes. Sots. S-kh. Azarb., 8: 19–21 (Fide Dairy Sci. Abst., 22: 1708.

Adhundov, K.R. 1966. Changes in the composition of buffalo's milk depending upon season and calving period. Trudy. Azerb. Nanchno. issled. Vet. Inst., 20: 238–244 (Fide Dairy Sci. Abst. 30: 321 and 2505).

Alim, K.A. 1975. A report on general aspect of studies on animal production in buffalo and cattle in the Philippines. World Rev. Anim. Prod., 11: 69–70.

Alim, K.A., Barbari, A. and Badran, A. 1977. Management trails on milking technique and concentrate feeding with local cattle and buffalo. World Rev. Anim. Prod., 13: 27–32.

Alsafar, T. and Juma, K.H. 1970. Studies on Iraqui buffalo milk with reference t the effect of month of lactation. II. Composition and some properties. Tropic. Agric. Trinidab, 175–179.

Anantakrishnan, C.P. and Kothavalla, Z.R. 1946. Distribution of fat in dahi. Indian J. Vet. Sci. Anim. Husb., 16: 56–54.

Aneja, R.P., Vyas, M.N., Taneja, V.K. and Nanda, K. 1978. Development of an industrial process for the manufacture of shrikhand. Proc. Inter. Dairy Con., New Delhi, pp 992.

Asker, A.K., Bedeir, L.H. and Kamal, T.H. 1957. The effect of stage of lactation on the composition of the buffalo milk and correlation between milk constituents. Indian J. Dairy Sci., 10: 204–212.

Asker, A.A., Bedeir, L.H., El-Itriby, A.A., Ahmed, I.A. and Khishin, S.S. 1971. Factors affecting butter fat content in Egyptian buffaloes. Anim. Prod., U.A.R., 9: 181–187.

Basu, K.P., Paul, T.M. Shrof, H.B. and Rahman, M.A. 1948. Composition of milk and ghee. Final report of the scheme. Report Series No. 8, ICAR, New Delhi.

Basu, S.B., Sharma, P.A., Nagarcenkar, R. and Sadana, D.K. 1979. Buffalo breeding, studies on butter fat and S.N.F. percentage. Annual report. NDRI, Karnal, pp. 177–178.

Bhargava, R.K. and Murdia, C.K. 1980. Research project report (1978–80). All India coordinated Research Project on Buffaloes. Vallabhanagar, Udaipur.

Bhattacharya, D.C. Mathur, O.N., Srinivasan, M.R. and Samlik, O. 1971. Studies on the method of production and self life of paneer (cooking type of acid coagulated cottage cheese). J.Fd. Sci. Technol. 8: 117–120.

Bhimasena Rao, M. and Dastur, N.N. 1955. Hydrogen ion concentration of milk. I pH on milk of animal of different breeds and individuals. Indian J. Dairy Sci., 8: 158–172.

Chandrasekaran, R., Kumar, V., Walia, B.N.S. and Moorthy, B. 1975. Carbohydrate intolerance in infacts with acute diarrhea and its complications. Acta Paediatrica Scandinavica, 64: 483 –488.

Dalaly, B.K., Abd-El-Mottaleb, L., El-Shazly, A. and Abdallah, R. 1976. The compostion of buffaloes in Mosui area. Mesopatamia J. Agric., 11: 55–60 (Fide Dairy Sci. Abst., 39: 6709).

Dash, P.C. and Basu, S.B. 1975. Diurnal variation in milk secretion of Murrah buffaloes. Indian J. Dairy Sci., 28: 135–136.

Dass, P.C., Basu, S.B. and Sharma, K.N.S. 1976. Effect of frequency of milking on Murrah buffaloes. Indian J.Dairy Sci., 29: 113–116.

Date, W.B. and Bhatia, D.S. 1955. Preservation of Indian milk sweets-some preliminary studies on shrikhand wadi and milk burfee. Indian J. Dairy Sci., 8: 61–66.

De, S. and Srinivasan, M.R. 1958. Production and marketing of ghee. I. Production. Indian Dairyman, 10: 156–160 and 165.

De, S., Thompkinson, D.K., Gahlot, D.P. and Mathur, O.N. 1976. Studies on methods of preparation and preservation of kheer. Indian J. Dairy Sci., 29: 216–318.

Devangan, M.L., Ogra, J.L. and Rao, Y.S. 1970. Studies on fat globules. Balwant Vidyapeeth J. Agril. Sci. Res., 10: 19–22.

Dilanyan, Z., Agabadyan, I.A. and Aslanyan, E. 1971. Characteristics of protein in buffaloes milk and some products made from it. Proc. Inter. Unit. Dairy Conf., pp. 359–362, Baku. (Fide Dairy Sci. Abst., 34: 1856).

Dzafarov, T.V. 1969. The effect of age (in calvings) on the content of protein, fat and dry matter in buffalo milk. Uchen. Zap. Azeb. Sel'-Khoz, Inst. Ser. Zhivot. No. 1: 94–96 (Fide Dairy Sci. Abst., 39: 1544).

El-Erian, A.F.M., Farag, A.H. and El-Gindy, S.M. 1975. Chemical studies on mish cheese. Agril. Res. Rev., U.A.R., 53: 173–181.

El-Ghandour, M.A., El-Gazzar, H. and Youniss, N.A. 1979. Studies on the buffalo's and cow's milk in the upper part of Egypt. Res. Bull. Faculty Agric. Alin Shama Univ. 977, 978 and 979 (Fide Dairy Sci. Abst.m 41: 6294–96).

El-Soda, M.A., El-Hagarawy, I.S., Rakshy, S.E.S.E. and Abou-donia, S.A. 1976a. Studies on provolone cheese. Part I. Chemical composition. Indian J. Dairy Sci., 29: 18–21.

El-Soda, M.A., Abou-Dania, S.A., Rakshy, S.E.S.E. and El-Hagarwy, I.S. 1976b. Studies on provolone cheese. II. Changes in the volatile fatty acids during processing and ripening. Indian J. Dairy Sci., 29: 88–90.

El-Shazly, A.H. and Hassan H.A. 1949. The composition of the milk of Egyptian cows and buffaloes. J. Dairy Res., 16: 217–226.

El-Sokkary, A.H.and Hassan, H.R. 1952. Lactose and chloride content of Egyptian cows and buffaloes milk. Analyst., 75: 143–146 (fide Dairy Sci. Abst., 12: 191).

El-Sokkary, A.H. and Zaki, M.H. 1956. Effect of stage of lactation and individuality of animal on the stability of resultant samna. Anim. Agril. Sci., Cairo, 1 (1): 83–105 (Fide Anim. Breed. Abst., 27: 675).

Fahmy, A.H., and Sharara, H.A. and El-Shazly, A. 1974. Some factors affecting physical and chemical properties of Egyptian cow's and buffalo's milk. Milchwissenchaft, 29:599–601.

Ganguly, S., Boman, T.J., Dastur, N.N. and Vaccha, S.M. 1959. Chemical composition of chakka. Indian J. Dairy Sci., 12: 121–124.

Ghosh, S.N. and Ananta Krishan, C.P. 1963. Composition of milk. Part IV. Influence of season, breed and species, Indian J. Dairy Sci., 17: 190–202.

Gotsiridze, N. and Kitoshvili, I. 1981.The effectiveness of buffalo breeding. Zhivotnovodstov, No. 3: 37–38 (fide Anim. Breed Abst., 49: 5687).

Grigorov, H.Y. Shalichev, Ye. And Goranov, N. 1962. Composition and properties of buffaloe's milk. Proc. XVII Inter. Dairy Cong. A: 209.

Gupta, M.P. and Rao, Y.S. 1972. Chemical quality of khurchan. Indian J. Dairy Sci., 25: 70–72.

Hamdy, M.K. and Taha, S.M. 1954. Mish: a soft ripened Egyptian cheese. Milk Prod. J., 45 (II): 14–15 * 29–33 (fide Dairy Sci. Abst., 17: 116).

Hanna, A.K., Hassan, A., Yassen, A. and Badawy, A. 1979. The effectiveness of sub-cutaneously versus intramuscular administration of oxytocin upon removal of residual milk in buffaloes and cattle. Alexandria. J. Agril. Res., 27: 567–574. (Fide Dairy Sci. Abst., 42: 6554).

Ingle, U.M and Joglekar, N.V. 1974. Comparative performance of buffaloes and Sahiwal cows as diary animals. Agril. Pakistan, 26: 75–78 (fide Dairy Sci., Abst., 41: 569).

Ismail, A.A. and Sirry, I. 1966. Technological aspects of butter made from cow's and buffalo's milk. Alexandria J. Agril. Res., 13: 161–173 (fide Dairy Sci. Abst., 29: 2604).

Iyer, M. 1978. Physico-chemical studies on chhana from cow's and buffalo's milk. M.Sc. Thesis. Kurukshetra Uni. Khrukshetra.

Jagtap, G.E. and Shukla. P.C. 1973. A note on the factors affecting the yield and quality of chhana. J. Food Sci. Technol., 10: 73–74.

Jian, D.H., Srinivasan, M.R. 1984. Effect of different milking intervals in buffaloes on secretion rates of milk and some of its organic constituents. Indian J. Anim. Sci., 54: 153–157.

Khambatta, J.S. and Dastur, N.N. 1950. Nutritive value of dahi–rat feeding experiments. Indian J. Dairy Sci., 3: 87–93.

Khan, M.A., Choudhry, M.Z., Qureshi, M.J. and Dar, Z.I. 1970. Influence of season on butterfat and protein content in buffalo milk. W. Pakistan J. Agril. Sci., 8 313–317.

Kulkarni, P.S. and Dole, K.K. 1956. Investigations in viscosity of milk. Indian J. Dairy Sci., 9: 68–79.

Kumar, A. and Tripathi, V.N. 1978. Effects of levels and methods of pre-partum and post-partum feeding on the yield and composition of milk and cost of milk production of murrah buffaloes. Haryana Agril. Univ. J. Res., 8: 125–129.

Kumar, A., Singh, L.N., Yadav, P.L. and Pandey, H.S. 1980.Studies on buffalo milk constituents during complete lactation. Final Project Report I.V.R.I. Izatnagar.

Kundu, S.S. and De, S. 1972. Chhana production from buffalo milk. Indian J. Dairy Sc., 25: 159–163..

Lalitha, K.R. and Dastur, N.N. 1956. Colour development in desi ghee Indian J. Dairy Sci., 9: 143–156.

Ludri, R.S. 1980. Milk let down response and residual milk in buffaloes. Indian J.Dairy Sci., 50: 891–893.

Madan Pal and Rajoria, G.S. 1972. Studies on the production and seft life of spary dried shrikhand. M.Sc. thesis, Punjab University, Chandigarh.

Mahajan, B.M. 1971. Studies on the production and self life of spray died shrikhand. M.Sc. Thesis, Punjab University, Chandigarh.

Merzametov, M.M. 1965. Buffalo milk a valuable food. VOP. Pitan., 24: 76–78 (Fide Dairy Sci. Abst., 27: 3617).

Minieri, L., Franciscis, G. De. And Interieri, F. 1965. Relation between pH, acidity and composition of buffalo milk. Acta Med. Vet. Napali 11: 107- 114 (Fide Dairy Sci., Abst., 28 1676).

Minieri, L., Interieri, F. and Pane, G. 1967. Effect of lactation number on milk yield and composition in buffaloes. Acta Med. Vet., Napali, 13: 251–261 (Fide Dairy Sci. Abst., 30: 1053.

Mishra, R.C. and Kushwaha, N.S. 1970. Studies on methods of preparation of ghee. Indian J. Dairy Sci., 23: 115–117.

Nabar, A.B., Srinivasan, M.R. and Iya, K.K. 1969. Studies on the water insoluble acids of cream and butter from buffalo milk. Indian J.Dairy Sci., 22: 121–127.

Olenov, Yu. M. 1954. Causes for the differences between the butterfat content of portions of milk obtained after milking. Doki. Akad, Nauk. SSSR 97(2);: 361–364 (fide Dairy Sci. Abst., 17: 230).

Oommen, S,. 1972. the distribution of fat and fat globules in dahi. India J. Dairy Sci., 25: 184–188.

Pandey, H.S. 1981. Genetic studies on the milk constituents of buffalo and their association with related triats. Ph.D. Thesis, Rohilkhand University, Bareilly.

Parken, H.K.B. and Gangwar, P.C. 1968. Chemical composition of buffalo milk. Indian J. Dairy Sci., 21: 177–182.

Patel, B.M., Dharni, B.M. and Patel,C.A. 1969. Studies on the effect of partial green feeding over dry feeding to milch buffaloes. Indian J.Dairy Sci., 22: 17–20.

Polikhronov, D. and Tosev, A. 1970. Functional characters of udder quarters in local buffaloes. Zhivot. Nauk., 7(3): 11–15 (fide Anim. Breed. Abst., 40: 205).

Prahlad, S.N. 1954. Studies on the technological aspects of processing and storage of dairy by-products-ghee residue M.Sc. Thesis, Univ. of Bombay, Bombay.

Rangappa, K.S. and Banerjee, B.N. 194. Storge of indigenous butter. Indian J. Dairy Sci., 1: 45–47.

Ragab, M.T., Asker, A.A. and Kamal, T.H. 1958. The effect of age and season of calving on composition of Egyptian buffalo milk. Indian J. Dairy Sci., 11: 18–28.

Rao, M.K. and Nagarcenkar, R. 1977. Potentialities of the buffalo. World Rev. Anim. Prod., 13 (3) 53–62.

Ray, H.P. and Srinivasan, R.A. 1972. Use of microorganisms for production of indigenous fermented milk products (Sweatened dehi). J. Fd. Sci. Technol., 9: 63–65.

Ray, S.C. and De, S. 1952. Indigenous milk products of India. II Khoa. Indian Dairyman, 4: 27–29.

Ray, S.C. and De, S. 1953. Indigenous milk products of Indian. III Chhana, Indian Dairyman, 5: 14–17.

Salerno, A. 1967. Cited by H.S. Pandey in Ph.D. Thesis, Rohikhand University, Bareilly.

Salooja, M.K. 1979. Studies on standardization of techniques for kulfi production. M.Sc. thesis, Kurushetra University, Kurukshetra.

Schneder, B.H., Warner, J.N., Dharni, I.D., Agarwal, B.P., Sukhatme, P.V., Pendarkar, V.G. and Shankaran, A.N. 1948. The composition of milk. Misc. Bull., 61, ICAR, New Delhi.

Shalichev, Ye. And Polikhronov, D. 1969.Composition and properties of milk of Murrah buffaloes imported from India. Zhivotn. Nauki., Sofia, 6: 57- 62 (fide Dairy Sci. Abst., 33: 3135).

Shalichev, Ye, Tanev, G. and Polikhronov, D. 1975. Milk yield and compostion of purebred Murrah buffaloes and their crosses with Bulgarian buffaloes. Zhivotn. Nauki., Sofia, 12: 73 –77 (Fide Dairy Sci. Abst., 38:3976).

Sharma, U.P., Rao, S.K. and Zariwala, I.T. 1980. Composition of milk of different breeds of buffaloes. Indian J. Dairy Sci., 33 7–12.

Shukla, K.S., Ranjhan, S.K. and Netke, S.P. 1972. Effect of various rates of concentrate feeding on the efficiency of milk production in Murrah buffaloes. Indian J. Anim. Prod. 3: 57: 64.

Soni, P.L., Gangwar, P.C., Bahga, C.S., Srivastava, R.K. and Dhingra, D.P. 1980. Effect of environmental cooling on milk yield and certain milk constituents in buffaloes. Indian J. Nutr, Dieted., 17: 220–227.

Singh, R.P., Singh, M., Rao, Y.S. and Singh, S.N. 1961. Quantitative relations among the milk constituents. 1. Effect of breed, stage of lactation and age of animals. Indian J. Dairy Sci., 14: 119–129.

Singh, K., Ogra, J.L. and Rao, Y.S. 1975. Observations on the microbial quality of some indigenous concentrated milk products. Indain J. Dairy Sci., 28: 304–305.

Stewart, A.D. and Banerjee, 1930–31. Indian J. Med. Res., 18:57.

Tiwana, M.S., Bhullar, M.S. and Bhalaru, S.S. 1980. Progress report of Ludhiana Centre. 5th. Workshop, All India Coordinated Res. Project on Buffalo Breeding, University of Udaipur.

Touny, E.M., El-Shobokshy, A.S. and El-Demerdash, O.M. 1976. The productive performance of lactating buffaloes fed different levels of concentrate. Agril. Res. Rev., U.A.R., 54: 9–14 (Fide Dairy Sci. Abst., 40: 5465).

Trung, L.T. and Gonzales, R.R. 1978. Organoleptic acceptance of fresh carabao milk, Philippine J. Nutr., 31: 36–40 (fide Dairy Sci. Abst., 41: 2226).

Vishweshwaraiah, L. 1979. Studies on paneer, M.Sc. Thesis. University Agril. Sci. Bangalore.

Waghmare, P.S. 1977. Shrikhandgolla- a new milk based sweet meat. Indian Dairyman, 29: 759–760.

Yegna Narayana Aiyer, A.K. 1953. Indian Dairyman, 5: 63–77.

10

Buffalo Meat and Meat Products

The edible part of carcass is known as meat. It includes flesh alongwith adipose tissue, bones and kidney knob. Head, liver, pluck and knuckles as well as other buffalo are normally excluded despite use of considerate parts for human foods. In the markets of Indian subcontinert and many other countries almost al offals are sold as meat Buffalo metat (Buff, Buffen, Cara beaf or Bada meat) is consumed by a large population of India and other buffalo breeding countries like Pakistan, bangladesh, Nepal, Iran, Iraq, Mayannar, Thailand, Combalia, Loos, S R Vietnam, Singapore, Hong Kong, China, Korea, Taiwan, Japan, Philippines, Indonesia, Malayasia, Australia, Russia, Italy, Romania, Bulgaria, Egypt and other African countries, Brazil, Venezuela, West Indies and many other contries. In their native lands river buffaloes are primarily reared for milk production and swamp buffaloes for draught purpose. Subsequently buffaloes gained importance as multi purpose animal of significant economic importance and meat has emerged as a very good source of edible flesh of high nutritive value due to low cholesterol and richer in essential amino acids than most of th edible of mammalian species. Buffalo fattening is growing at a faster rate due to continuously increasing demand of edible meat not only in buffalo breeding countries but in other countries also.

This has helped in protection of calves from early mortality with the adoption of health protection measures, particularly in India where large number of buffalo calves used to be intensely eliminated from the early mortality with the adoption of health protection measures, particularly in India where large number of buffalo calves used to be intensely eliminated from the production system about a few years ago. Now greater number of these protected calves are better cared and being fattened to 300–400 kg body weight at 12 to 18 months of age. Even underfed calves weaned as a poor animal of 60 to 100 kg body (Baruah et al., 1982). Buffalo veal had a greater demand as this low fat and light colour meat is more acceptable (Ferrara, et al., 1963; De Franciscis et al., 1970). The larger proportion are found in the paddy dominated agriculture based Tropical countries of Asia due to the high adaptability in the agroclimatic conditions of humid tropical and sub tropical contries. Although sufficient informations on various aspects of buffalo production have been published since the early half of the twentieth century, indeed some misconcepts are carried by many people regarding the buffalo production that the animal can be fattened on fibrous crop residues of cereals without much supplemental feeding. Such views are totally baseless and it appears to baed on wheresay of locl people who do not account for grazing and feeding of grain processing by products available in home for the feeding of animals. In most of the rural house holds of India only purchased ingredients are accounted. For obtaining daily body weight gain more than 500 g in weaned buffalo calves of 8–10 months of age, a palatable diets of 12–13% crude protein and 60–65% total digestible nutrients TND) are required (Pathak et al., 1982; Baruah et al., 1983; Pathak, 1966). Such high levels of protein and energy could not be obtained by feeding inferior quality of feeds and fodder. Buffaloes of high growth potential are not uncommon and average growth rate of 0.7 to 1.2 kg had been obtained by feeding of high energy balanced diets (Avalisvili, 1956; Dzafarov, 1958; Kassir et al., 1969; Taha et al., 1980). Most of the recognized breeds of riverine and swamp buffaloes are heavy animals of high growth potential and buffalo. In countries like India and Paskistan the control of early calf mortality itself may provide large number of animals for fattening provided adequate nutritious feeds and fodder are available for feeding.

▶ GROWTH PERFORMANCE OF BUFFALOES ON NATIVE (NATURAL) AND IMPROVED PASTURES

The native pastures of buffalo tract are mostly unmanaged grass cover and provide inferior quality herbages for grazing during the longer span of dry season of the year. Sehima and cenchrus are the dominant grasses of tropical region and they also grow in the hostile climate of semi-arid some parts of arid zones. Great variation occurs in the herbage density during the different seasons being maximum during the humid season. The nutritional quality of pastures is also much better in humid-hot season than the dry-hot and cold season. Great variation has been reported in the growth response of buffaloes grazed on natural and improved pastures of India (Upadhyay et al., 1980; Siddiqui et al., 1982) and Australia (Ford, 1978; Robertson et al., 1982). Average growth rate of buffalo calves on natural pastures of mixed grasses in semi-arid climate has been 0.22 kg against the dry matter intake rate of 2% of body weight (Siddiqui et al., 1982). Significantly higher growth rates of 333 g on sehima dominant pasture and 439 g on cenchrus dominant pasture has been observed during the lush growth of rainy season in central part of India (Upadhyay et al., 1980). On the natural grass cover of Northern Australia very poor growth rate has been observed in feral swamp buffaloes during the long duration pasturing exceeding 3 years. Average of daily gain in body weight of swamp buffaloes after weaning was 0.16 to 0.17 kg (Ford, 1978). This growth improved to 0.24 to 0.32 kg when native pasture was improved by sowing of pangola and stylos (Robertson et al., 1982). Significant effect of quality and quantity of forage availability is reflected in body weight gain which ranged from –0.15 kg in dry season (July-December) to 0.58 kg in the wet season (October-March) I the Northern territory of Australia. Similarly and libitum feeding of chaffed elephant grass could support 0.26 kg daily gain in body weight which increased to about 0.54 kg daily on the feeding of rice bran to replace almost half of the dry matter supplied by the elephant grass. The CP content in grass was 7.5–12.1% on dry matter basis (Moran, 1983). About 300–500 g daily gain in body weight of riverine buffalo calves may be obtained on ad libitum feeding of good quality mixed fooder of cereal and legume crops (Agarwal, 1974; Naidu and Raghavan, 1985). The concept of buffalo rearing for meat production on unmanaged native pastures may be considered ill conceived and form the results of some studies it is apparent that adequate supply of nutritious feeds and fooder is an important component of buffalo fattening.

▶ BUFFALOES AVAILABLE FOR MEAT PRODUCTION

Meat production systems are quite different in the native lands of buffaloes and the translocated animals in other countries. In most of the native lands meat had been a by product and only during past 2–3 decades organized fattening systems have been taken up. Organized buffalo farming as a dual purpose animal for milk and meat in case of riverine type and for meat in case of swamp type is practiced in most of buffalo breeding countries of Euro-Asian region, Africa, Australia and South America. Following four types of buffaloes are available for meat production:

1. Young pre-ruminant calves of both sexes born at the buffalo dairy stalls of urban and periurban areas in the Indian sub continent ar considered economic burden and intensely starved to eliminate at very young age of 2–4 weeks. These are potential sources and in recent years some programmes have been taken up for utilizing these calves for fattening and replacement female production.
2. Growing male calves culled at the end of lactation period of 8–10 (rarely more than 15 months in the rural areas. These are mostly very poor animals of 60 to 100 kg body weight by still retaining the growth potential for finishing to 300–400 kg body weight on good feeding for 12–15 months.
3. Sterile heifers unable to conceive even up to 5 years of age and well grown body weight and infertile failed to conceive after 1 to 3 calvings.
4. Spent dairy buffalo females after more than 5 calvings, infertile bulls and retired males of more than 12–15 years of age. These animals are mostly poor in body condition and mostly require some recuperative feeding of high energy diets for few (2–4) months.

▶ PATTERN OF BODY WEIGHT GAIN

Effect of adequate feeding of good quality balanced diet is apparent and it has been demonstrated through several feeding trials that buffalo calves may be raised to produce excellent veal comparable with that buffalo calves may be raised to produce excellent veal comparable with that of cattle veal on feeding high level of whole milk, milk replacer, concentrate mixture alongwith good quality legume hay (Kalugin, 1933. Growing buffaloes have great inherent potential of grining 400 g to more than 1 kg daily during the active growth phase and canb e finished a 300 kg animals at 9 to 24 months of age depending on the breed, plane of nutrition and management (Arora and Gupta, 1962; Ragab et al., 1966; Chares and Johnson, 1972; Taha et al., 1980; Borghese et al., 1981; Buruah et al., 1982). Improvement in the meat quality of spent buffaloes and poor neglected buffalo calves through good feeding has been demonstrated (Avalisvili, 1956; Polikhronov et al., 1979). The growth pattern of buffaloes for meat production has been presented separately for different kinds of buffaloes.

Daily Weight Gain in Buffalo Veal Calves

The growth rate of pre-ruminant stage young buffalo calves is affected by body weight at birth, inherent growth potential, feeds, system of feeding and management practices. Normally buffalo calves for veal production are fed high level of whole milk for a period of 4 to 18 weeks. The buffalo veal calves are sacrificed at the body weight of 60 to 150 kg in 4 to 18 weeks of age (Badreldin, 1955; Ferrara et al., 1963; Zakhariev, 1973; Salerno et al., 1983). The frequency of feeding milk or milk replacer has significant effect on body weight gain which is higher on thrice daily feeding at about 8 hours interval (Verma and Tomer, 1984) > Replacement of whole milk of buffalo by whole milk of cow significantly reduces the body weight gain due to much lower content of protein and energy in cow milk (Abou Hussain and Rafat, 1962; Ferrara et al., 1967).

Daily Body Weight Gain in Growing Buffaloes

Great variation occurs in the growth pattern of weaned buffalo calves. The rate of gain in body weight is mainly affected by the plane of nutrition which varies with the feeding value of rations. The calves specially the male calves of dairy breeds suffer from the date of birth particularly at the commercial dairy buffalo stalls of the Indian sub continent. The surviving calves of such buffalo stalls and the neglected male calves of rural owners are the poor animals of 60 to 125 kg body weight at 9 to 14 months of age. Growth patter is dependent on feeding and management, and it ranges from negative growthon exclusive wheat straw and urea supplemented wheat straw (Johri et al., 1982). Average daily gain in body weight ranges from 0.16 to 0.26 kg on poor natural grassland of semi-arid regions of India, Australia and Malayasia (Ford, 1976; Robertson et al., 1982; Siddiqui et al., 1982; Moran, 1983). Higher daily body weight gain of 0.33 to 0.44 kg is obtained on relatively better pastures of Sri Lanka and central part of India during the wet season Imatasukawa et al., 1976; Upadhyay et al.,1980). It has been found difficult to rear the growing buffalo calves on the feeding of inferior roughages like wheat bhoosa as a sole diet. Supplementation of 2% or more urea alone or mixed with small amount (7 to 14%) of molasses with urea failed to maintain the buffalo calves (Johri et al., 1982). On the feeding of low quality diet of urea-molasses liquid didt (UMLD) alongwith small amount of conventional intact protein supplement and fodder gain in body weight may be 200 g to 300 g daily (Pathak et al., 1978; Pathak and Ranjhan, 1979). Good quality nutritious green fodder and hay (mixture of cereal fodder and leguminous fodder) support satisfactory growth on and libitum feeding (Agarwal, 1974; Naidu and Raghavan, 1985). On the feeding of conventional diets of good quality fooder and concentrates body weight gain from 0.4 kg to more than 1 kg daily may be obtained in different breeds Dasgupta, 1943; Tantawy, 1984; Cumburidze and Dalakisvilli, 1959; Sharma and Talapatra, 1963; Ivanov and Zahariev, 1966; Ragab et al., 1966; Kassir et al., 1969; Juma et al., 1972; Romita et al., 1978; Rosa and Crata, 1978; Taha et al., 1980; Borghese et al., 1981; Baruah et al., 1982; Pathak et al., 1982; Pathak, 1995).

Daily Body Weight Gain in Culled and Spent Buffaloes

The feeding of culled buffaloes for meat production depends on the body condition and age of animals, availability of good quality feeds at a reasonable price and return on capital inputs from the sale of animals or meat and by-products. A system of conditioning culled buffaloes through feeding of high energy diets is practiced in some countries fro the improvement of carcass quality. In a feeding trial of culled buffaloes of 7 to 11 years of age for recuperative fattening, 840g daily body weight gain has been recorded in Bulgaria. The rate of gain varies from 580 to 870 g in male and 790 to 1080 g in female buffaloes (Avalisvili, 1956). Feeding for compensatory growth not only support good body weight gain (> 700g) but also increases the ratio of fat in the carcass (Polikhronov et al., 1979).

▶ GROWTH PERFORMANCE OF BUFFALOES ON NATURAL AND IMPROVED PASTURES

The pastures commonly found in Asian buffalo land are mostly unmanaged natural grass cover grossly depleted of nutritious legumes due to selective grazing for several generations. These grass lands provide satisfactory herbage cover for grazing only during the wet season of 3 to 6 months. Doob is a very good grass distributed widely on scrub lands, canal bunds, road sides and fruit tree orchards but dominant grasses of natural tropical pasures are sehima, cenchrus, panics and guinea grass etc. Sehima and cenchrus also grow in dry semi arid region. The nutritional quality of natural tropical pastures is quite satisfactory during the humid-hot season than the hostile dry hot season. Large variation is observed in the growth performance of buffaloes grazing on natural and improved pastures of India (Upadhyay et al., 1980; Siddiqui et al., 1982) and Australia (Ford, 1978; Robertson et al., 1982). Average growth rate of weaned buffalo calves on natural patures of mixed grasses in semiarid climate has been 0.22 kg against the dry matter intake at the rate of 2% of body weight (Siddiqui et al., 1982). But higher growth rate of 333g daily on sehima rich pasture and 439 g daily on cenchrus dominated pasture are recorded during the lush growing pasture of rainy season in India (Upadhyay et al., 1980).

On the natural grass cover of northern Australia very poor growth rate has been observed during the long duration pasturing exceeding 3 years. Average of daily body weight gain after weaning has been about 160 g daily (Ford, 1978) which increased to about 240 g daily on improving the natural pasture by the sowing of pangola, calopo and stylos (Robertson et al., 1982). The growth rate is significantly affected by the qualitative and quantitative availability of forages, and it ranges from 0.15 kg daily in dry season (July-December) to more than 0.58 kg in the wet season) (October-May) in the northern territory of Australia. Similarly and libitum feeding of chaffed elephant grass could support about 0.26 kg daily gain which further increased to about 0.54 kg daily on the feeding of rice bran to replace almost half of the dry matter supply by the elephant grass. The elephant grass. The elephant grass contained 7.5–12.1% crude protein on dry matter basis durig the feedig period (Moran, 1982). About 300 to 500 g daily body weight gain in riverine buffalo calves may be obtained on and libitum feeding of palatable good quality fodder or cereal and leguminous crops (Agarwal, 1974; Naidu and Raghavan, 1985). The concept of buffalo rearing for meat production on unmanaged natural pastures may be considered ill conceived in a competitive situation for food between human and farm animals. Good feeding management is the appropriate anser for the fattening of buffaloes for meat production.

▶ FEED/NUTRIENTS CONVERSION EFFICIENCY

Considerable informations are now available on the feed and nutrients conversion efficiency of buffaloes for body weight gain. However, most of the studies were aimed at growth for replacement dairy and draught animals. Some data are also available on feeding for veal and buffen or carabeef production and also for the carcass improvement of spent buffaloes.

Average feed intake from whole milk and other feeds has been found equivalent to 4.29 Scandinavian feed units for 1 kg gain in live weight (Salerno, 1948). Similarly for 1 kg gain in body weight 6 kg and for 1 kg dressed veal production 9 kg whole milk is consumed (Badreldin, 1955). Cow milk and can replace buffalo milk but intake will increase by about 66% (Ferrara et al., 1967). Young calf production for high quality meat on milk and calf starter ration requires about 2.51 kg whole milk and 1.03 kg concentrate mixture per kg gain in body weight on finishing at 36 weeks of age. The animals are also offered good quality fodder for and libitum consumption (Borghese et al., 1981).

Dry matter intake per kg gain in the body weight of buffaloes during the post weaning period varies from 5 to 21 kg depending on the quality of feeds and duration of feeding (Agarwal, 1974; Tilakratne et al., 1976; Pathak and Ranjhan, 1979; Pathak et al., 1982; Baruah et al., 1983). The dry matter intake per unit gain in body weight decreases with the corresponding increase in th available energy content of rations.

Implantation of a oestradiol-progesterone implant (Synovex-S) significantly improves feed intake and body weight gain. Mean feed intake per kg gain in body weight 8.8 kg is significantly less than 9.63 kg consumed in non implant make buffalo calves (Ali et al., 1983).

Egyptian Fattened buffaloes of about 230, 360 and 450 kg mean body weight at 12, 18 and 24 months of age required 8.4 kg, 9.0 kg and 11.7 kg starch equivalent per kg gain in body weight respectively (Ragab et al., 1966).

Average requirement in terms of Scandenavian feed unit for mediterenian buffaloes for 1 kg gain in body weight ranges from 6 to 9.4 kg for fattening buffaloes gaining at the rate of 0.7 to 0.9 kg daily (Proto and Landi, 1965; Ivanov and Zahariev, 1966). The feed conversion efficiency is significantly less on pasture feeding (9.1 FU per kg body weight gain) due to lower energy content (Kasimov, 1971; Gadzhiev et al., 1973). Fattening Bulgarian, Murrah and their crosses required 7.24, 7.77 and 7.25 Oats Feed Unit (OFU) per kg gain in body weight for 1024, 951 and 1035 g average daily gain in body weight respectively (Ognjanovic et al., 1970); and mean body weight ranged from 374 to 401 kg at 11 to 11.6 months age.

Fattening on high plane of nutrition from birth to about 400 kg body weight required 4.71 to 5.2 kg total digestible nutrients (TND) for each kg gain in body weight (El-Naggar et al., 1972; Ahmed and El-Shazly, 1975). In case of poor weaned residual buffalo calves TDN consumption varies from 4.06 to 5.55 kg for each kg gain in body weight and 5.77 to 7.15 kg for each kg production of carcass on finishing at about 300 kg body weight and 450 to 550 g average daily gain in body weight (Baruah et al., 1982; Pathak et al., 1985).

For the improvement of carcass quality of spent buffaloes the requirement of energy is about 12.2 SFU per kg gain in body weight on feeding high plane of nutrition to support about 711 g daily gain in body weight (Polikhronov et al., 1979). In most of the Asian countries spent buffaloes are mostly aged retired animals in poor body condition and also the dry females available at the dairy stalls of urban and peri-urban areas disposed after hormonal extraction of milk at the cost of body tissue depletion.

▶ CARCASS CHARACTERISTICS

The characteristics of edible carcasses of bovine are usually presented as carcass yield, dressing percentage, carcass length, carcass composition and yield of edible and non edible offals, etc.

Carcass Yield and Dressing Percentage

The weight of carcass varies greatly due to body size and physical status of the buffaloes at the time of slaughter. Average weight of carcass including edible offals like liver, kidneys, heart, mesenteric fat and tail may be about 40.4 kg at about 30 to 40 days of age.

Average yield of edible parts, head, knuckles (feet) has been reported 65.75, 7.32 and 5.03% respectively (Badreldin, 1955). Average dressing percentage may be 55–72% for properly fed buffalo veal calves of 7 to 18 weeks of age (Ferrera et al., 1963; Ragab et al., 1966; Minieri et al., 1968; Rasheed, 1977). Average dressing percentage of males may be a little higher than the females veal calves of same group (Salerno, 1962). Carcass yield is normally low for the culled buffaloes and varies from 38 to 59% depending on the body condition of the animals (Maymone, 1945; Salerno, 1948; Dominguez, 1956; Kurbanov, 1961; ferrara, 1964; Rao, 1978). Feeding of culled buffaloes for 2–3 months on good quality palatable rations improves carcass grade and dressing percentage has been found to be 47.8 to 50.2% on 90–120 days finishing dits (Avalisvili, 1956, Polikhronov et al., 1979).

Dressing percentage may be affected by the age at slaughter, sex, plane of nutrition and quality of feeds etc. The effect of various factors except the plane of nutrition has been found quite variable in different studies. An increase in dressing percentage has been found quite variable in different studies. An increase in dressing percentage has been recorded with the corresponding increase in post weaning body weight (Table 10.1) of male and female buffaloes (Maymone, 1942, 1945; Salerno, 1948; Ragab

TABLE 10.1: Effect of age carcass yield of buffaloes

Age in months	Body weight, kg	Carcass weight, kg	Dressing %	Chilling loss %
15	407.4	195.5	48.1	3.0
18	441.3	220.8	50.3	1.5
24	486.5	249.8	51.4	1.6

TABLE 10.2: Effect of sex and age on dressing percentage of buffaloes

Sex	Age (months)	Body weight (kg)	Dressing (%)	Reference
Male	6–12		45	Maymone, 1945
	12–18		47	
	Adult		52	
Female	6–12		46	
	12–18		46	
	Adult		48	
Bulls	1.5	74	60	Ragab et al., 1960
	6	158	57.2	
	12	230	53.7	
	18	359	57.6	
	24	449	52.7	
Steers	12	236	53.3	
	18	360	54.5	
	24	450	54.3	
Entire	30	617	55.9	Zicarelli et al., 1975
	42	683	58.9	
Castrated	30	611	55.3	
	42	688	60.0	
Bulls	A	388	50.8	Valin et al., 1984
Steer I	A–0.5	387	51.4	
Steer II	A + 5.5	477	53.3	
Steer III	A + 7.0	541	53.1	

et al., 1966; Zakhariev, 1973; Afifi et al., 1974; Zeiden et al., 1976). Great variation may occur in dressing percentage due to sex (Table 10.2) of buffaloes reared under different management but little variation is observed in the animals of similar growth potential raised under same management. Mean dressing percentage in local Sinhalee buffalo and Murrah buffalo has been 49.7 and 53.4 respectively for the animals raised on a dry zone pasture of Sri Lanka (Matsukawa et al., 1976) but in Bulgarian, Murrah and their crosses was 53.7, 54.7 and 54.1 respectively for the animals fattened intensively for a period of 130 days (Ognjanovic et al., 1970).

Plane of nutrition and density of digestible energy in the rations significantly affect the carcass yield and dressing percentage. An increase in carcass yield and dressing percentage had been observed due to the level of feeding and composition of diets (Agarwal, 1974; Pathak and Ranjhan, 1979). Good feeding of even poor animals significantly improves growth, carcass yield and dressigng percentage (Table 10.3). The dietary energy concentration has recuperative effect (Baruah et al., 1982).

TABLE 10.3: Effect of dietary protein and energy levels on carcass yield

Plane of nutrition	Body weight (kg)	Dressed weight (kg)	Dressing %
Before feeding trial	75	35	46.8
Low protein × low energy	294	166	56.5
Low protein × medium energy	297	175	59.0
Low protein × high energy	309	178	57.6
High protein × low energy	293	161.6	55.2
High protein × medium energy	306	173.6	56.7
High protein × high energy	298	186.2	62.5

Dissectable Tissue Ratio of Buffalo Carcass

The acceptability of edible carcass for human consumption is determined by the ratio of lean, dissectable fat and bone in the carcass. There is large variation in the liking of people of different countries. People of high income group prefer to eat lean meat while those of low income group engaged in heavy physical works prefer fatty carcass. The eye muscle or loin eye are or cross section of longissimus dorsi muscle at 10th or 20th rib is considered a satisfactory index of muscle content in the carcass. The ratio of dissectable tissue in he carcass is mainly influenced by age, sex, plane of nutrition and energy content of diets (Ognjanovic et al., 1970; Zakhariev, 1973; Agarwal, 1974; Charles and Johnson, 1975; Zicarelli et al., 1975; Pathak et al., 1982; Vali et al., 1984). Since different carcass samples have been used in different studies (Table 10.4) the values may not be closely comparable, indeed they are informative and may be used for the assessment of carcass quality.

TABLE 10.4: Percent dissectable tissues in the carcass of buffaloes

Type of buffalo	Dissectable carcass tissues			Reference
	Muscle %	Fat%	Bone %	
Types/breeds				
Bulgarian	71.9	9.9	18.2	Ognjanovic et al., 1970
Murrah	70.1	9.9	20.0	
Murrah × Bulgarian F1 cross	69.4	11.4	19.2	

Contd.

TABLE 10.4: Percent dissectable tissues in the carcass of buffaloes (*Contd.*)

Type of buffalo	Dissectable carcass tissues			Reference
	Muscle %	Fat%	Bone %	
High concentrate diets:				
(a) High level feeding	55.0	26.2	17.6	Agarwal, 1974
(b) Medium level feeding	53.2	26.9	18.5	
High roughage rations				
(a) High level feeding	57.5	19.2	20.8	
(b) Medium level feeding	56.0	19.1	23.1	
At 30 month age:				
Entire	70.3	9.1	14.4	Zicarelli et al., 1975
Castrated	68.5	10.1	15.6	
At 40 months age				
Entire	69.6	10.9	13.6	
Castrated	65.5	13.2	14.0	
Plane of nutrition				Pathak et al., 1982
Low protein x low energy	62.9	15.8	21.3	
Low protein x high energy	63.2	17.0	19.8	
High protein x low energy	61.9	16.9	21.1	
High protein x high energy	62.4	16.6	21.0	
Sex and age				Valin et al., 1984
Bulls A months	54	24	22	
Steers A–0.5 months	52	29	19	
Steers A + 5.5 months	47	34	17	
Steers A + 7 months	53	29	18	
Buffalo veal and young calf (muscle includes bones also)				Zakhariev, 1973
At birth	66.1	0.7		
3 months	72.9	0.5		
6 months	76.0	3.5		
12 months	79.0	8.2		
18 months	81.5	9.0		

The carcass of spent buffaloes are generally differentiated into 3 grades, viz, good, fair and poor on the basis of the profile of hind quarters. The profile of shoulders and loin is also satisfactory (Kondaiah et al., 1981) Average meat percent is higher in the male than the female (Table 10.5). The ratio of bones increases with the decrease in conformation score of the carcass. Dissectable fat tissue is invariably higher in female than in the carcass of male buffaloes of same grade (Kondaiah et al., 1983).

TABLE 10.5: Ratio of dissectable tissues in the carcass of spent buffaloes

Carcass grade	Sex	Carcass wt. (kg)	Muscle (%)	Bones (%)	Fatty tissue (%)
Good carcass	Male	155.2	71.7	22.5	4.8
	Female	188.4	65.3	19.1	15.1
	Pooled	171.3	69.0	20.8	10.0

Contd.

TABLE 10.5: Ratio of dissectable tissues in the carcass of spent buffaloes *(Contd.)*

Carcass grade	Sex	Carcass wt. (kg)	Muscle (%)	Bones (%)	Fatty tissue (%)
Fair carcass	Male	157.5	68.1	26.5	5.4
	Female	178.7	67.5	22.7	9.8
	Pooled	168.1	67.8	24.6	7.6
Poor carcass	Male	142.6	66.0	28.9	5.1
	Female	139.2	63.7	29.5	6.8
	Pooled	140.9	64.8	29.2	6.0

Meat: Bone Ratio

Mucle and fat including fasciae are considered together in the edible part of the carcass although marrow of bones is also used fr the preparation of soup and other dishes. A wider meat: bone ratio indicates better finish and meatiness of the carcass. In addition on nutritional status the age, sex and conformation are the other factors affecting the carcass quality (Table 10.6). Flesh content is higher in the veal and young animals (Ferrera et al., 1963; Romita et al., 1978). A wider meat: bone ratio is normally observed in the carcasses of female and castrated buffaloes (Minieri et al., 1972; Kondaiah et al., 1983) and the buffaloes fed high level of energy (Agarwal, 1974; Charles and Johnson, 1975; Pathak et al., 1982).

TABLE 10.6: Effect of various factors on meat: bone ratio of buffen

S.No.	Factors	Meat: Bone ratio	Reference
1.	Age: 20 months	3.02	Romita et al., 1978
	28 months	3.54	
	36 months	3.54	
2.	Sex buffalo bull	3.97	Minieri et al., 1972
	Buff steer (Castrate)	4.01	
3.	Conformation score		Kondaiah et al., 1983
	(a) Good Male	3.46	
	Female	4.18	
	(b) Fair Male	2.78	
	Female	3.44	
	(c) Poor Male	2.47	
	Female	2.39	
4.	Feeding regime		Charles and Johnson, 1975
	(a) All hay	4.08	
	(b) All pellets	4.48	
5.	Feed energy level		Pathak et al., 1982
	(a) Low	3.69	
	(b) High	4.04	

Eye Muscle or Loin Eye Area

The area of eye (Longissimus dorsi) muscle or loin eye is a good indicator o meatiness of the carcass. It is area measured at cross section of eye muscle between the 12th and 13th ribs. The eye muscle area is affected by age, sex, breed and carcass conformation

(Table 10.7) but in aged retired and mostly depleted animals it may not be very useful (Kondaiah et al., 1983).

TABLE 10.7: Effect of different factors on eye muscle area (cm^2)

S.No.	Factors	Eye muscle area	Reference
1.	Age 50 days	24	Ragab et al., 1966
	6 month	37	
	12 months	45	
	18 months	66	
	24 months	85	
2.	Sex		
	Castrate 12 months	40	
	18 months	63	
	24 months	75	
3.	Breed Bulgarian	64.3	Ognjanovic et al., 1970
	Murrah	60.6	
	Murrah X Bulg, F1)	63.4	
4.	Plane of nutrition		Baruah, 1982
	Very poor weaned calf	11.3	
	Low protein and low energy	41.9	
	Do and medium energy	49.4	
	Do and high energy	50.6	
5.	Carcass grade: Good	23.5	Kondaiah et al., 1983
	Fair	21.9	
	Poor	20.4	

Carcass Cutability Characteristics

The carcass is normally cut into different defined cut for satisfying the demand of retail customers. The retail cuts of buffaloes are not yet standardized and varies from country to country. Various cuts are given different names in different country which vary significantly. Some information (Table 10.8) are available on cuts of buffalo carcass (Agarwal, 974; Baruah, 1982) following the method described by Ziegler (1964) for beef cattle.

TABLE 10.8: Cutability characteristics of buffalo carcass (% of eviscerated carcass)

Carcass cuts	High concentrate feeding	High fodder feeding
Neck	4.13	4.98
Chuck	17.43	18.22
Fore shank	5.25	5.11
Brisket	6.30	6.42
Plate	6.37	6.68
Rid	10.17	10.61
Loin	14.97	15.99
Rump	5.47	7.21
Round	22.35	20.33
Hind shank	5.03	5.49

▶ **EDIBLE OFFALS**

Different organs, head and tongue are also consumed by humans and these are sold in edible meat in many countries. The yield of edible offals mainly depends on the breed, body weight and general condition of the animal (Kassir et al., 1969, Ognjanovic et al., 1970, Agarwal, 1974, Baruah, 1982, Pathak et al., 1982, Lakshmanan et al., 1984). Buffalo offals may be placed in the following groups:

1. **Offal meat:** Meat of head, oesophagus, diaphragm, knuckles and tail.
2. Edible organs include liver, kidneys, brain, heart, udder, teats, tongue, testis, lungs with windpipe, spleen and gut.
3. Fatty tissue like caul, mesentery, etc
4. Whole blood, clot and serum

In addition to these skin of some specific body part specially the hips is also used for the preparation of special dishes in some Asian-Pacific regions. Yield of edible offals in different types of buffaloes is quite variable (Table 10.9). Buffaloe with long and massive horns had higher proportion of head in the body weight than the buffaloes of short horns similary ratio of many organs is higher in poor than in the healthy buffaloes.

TABLE 10.9: Proportion of edible offals in the live weight of different buffaloes

Attributes	Iraqui buffalo	Bulgarian buffalo	Murrah buffalo	Murrah X Bulgari, F1	Indian desi	Swamp buffalo	Buffalo veal
Bwt., kg	335	376	374	401	298–312	300	61
Offals % of body weight,							
Head	4.06	3.87	3.66	3.91	5.91–6.37	5.8	7.32
Feet (knuckles)	2.36	1.95	1.99	1.83	1.91–1.97	2.9	5.03
Liver	1.41	1.12	1.15	1.12	0.73–0.89	1.4	-
Kidneys	0.27	0.20	0.26	0.17	0.20–0.21	-	-
Heart	0.41	0.36	0.43	0.37	0.31–0.37	0.6	-
Tongue	-	0.23	0.27	0.19	-	-	-
Spleen	-	-	-	-	0.20–0.25	0.2	-
Lungs	-	0.52	0.56	0.49	-	-	1.26
Blood	-	-	-	-	3.83–4.02		

Some Characteristics of the Muscle Tissue

The structural units of muscles are the muscle fibres which are long slender cells containing several nuclei. Th diameter of muscle fibres is influenced by age, sex, breed, plane of nutrition and exercise. Variations in physical and chemical characteristics of muscle tissue (Tables 10.10 and 10.11) has been observed for some breeds (Orgnjanovic et al., 1970), body conditions (Rao, 1978), age (Yadav, 1982, body weight and sex at finishing (Vallu et al., 1984) and fibrs of the muscle (Soloman et al., 1985).

TABLE 10.10: Some chemical and physical characteristics of muscle fibers

Factors	Moisture (%)	Protein (%)	Lipids (%)	Myoglobin (%)	Oxyproline (%)	Muscle Number	Fibres Dia (u)
Poor animals, 60–69 kg	78.46	18.82	1.52	-	-		33.37

Contd.

TABLE 10.10: Some chemical and physical characteristics of muscle fibers *(Contd.)*

Factors	Moisture (%)	Protein (%)	Lipids (%)	Myoglobin (%)	Oxyproline (%)	Muscle number	Fibres dia (u)
100–139 kg	76.38	18.90	1.27	-	-	-	41.07
140–160 kg	78.27	18.59	1.24	-	-	-	28.89
Breeds							
Bulgarian	-	-	1.36	1.53	0.78	-	58.83
Murrah (Bulg)			0.64	1.40	0.74	-	57.14
Bulg × Murah			1.04	1.37	0.70	-	56.67
Fibre type							
At 14 month (372 kg Bwt.)							
(i) Red fiber						20.7	28.97
(ii) Intermediate fibre at 7 year (675 kg Bwt.)						79.3	38.29
(i) Red fiber						26.3	51.15
(ii) Intermediate fiber						73.7	58.34

Bwt. = Body weight

TABLE 10.11: Effect of age and finishing body weight (Bwt.) on physico-chemical characteristics of muscle tissue of buffaloes

Body wt. kg	Muscle name	Moisture %	Protein %	Lipid %	Glycogen %	Myoglobin, %	ph	Muscle fibre diameter, μ
Bull, 388	Longissimus dorsi	75.5	23.1	1.8	-	2.9	5.6	-
Steer, 387		75.4	22.7	1.7	-	2.7	5.6	-
477		74.3	22.6	1.6	-	3.8	5.8	-
541		74.9	23.0	1.5	-	3.7	5.9	-
Bulls,								
A 1 yr 160	Do	78.2	16.6	-	1.19	-	5.91	44.65
B 2 yr 289		77.5	17.0	-	1.28	-	5.95	57.16
C 3 yr 367		76.5	17.3	-	0.96	-	5.83	65.32
D > 5 yr 498		75.7	19.2	-	0.90	-	6.10	89.19
A	Biceps	78.8	16.70	-	1.11	-	5.95	42.56
B	Brachei	77.3	16.85	-	1.17	-	5.99	57.68
C		76.6	17.54	-	0.95	-	5.87	64.60
D		75.7	19.45	-	1.01	-	6.10	84.86
A	Semitendinosus	78.5	16.61	-	1.05	-	5.83	44.95
B		77.3	17.23	-	1.17	-	5.96	58.67
C		76.7	17.30	-	1.00	-	5.82	68.89
D		75.8	19.29	-	1.00	-	6.01	91.77

Chemical Composition of Buffen (Buffalo Meat)

Buffen contains relatively more protein and less lipids than the beef at same level of growth. Protein content is higher in lean meat and bones of the carcass than in the adipose (fatty) tissue (Agarwal, 1974). The chemical composition of meat is affected by the age, sex, breed, degree of fatness, composition of diet and the use of hormoses and other growth promoting biostimulators (Karbanov, 1961; Ferrenra et al., 1969; De Franciscis et al. 1970; Rao, 1978). Normally ratio of moisture decreases and that of fat increases with the increase in age and degree of fatness through the feeding of high energy diets (Table 10.12).

TABLE 10.12: Percent chemical composition of buffen (Buffalo meat)

Type of meat	Moisture	Protein	Fat	Total ash	GE (kcal/kg)
Buff veal	73.02	20.84	4.30	0.97	1230
Buff veal finished on					
(a) Buffalo milk	71.68	21.41	5.83	1.04	1400
(b) Cow	73.15	20.37	5.35	0.01	1300
Light weight	70.70	21.00	7.24	0.97	1515
Fatty carcass	64.42	19.18	15.40	1.00	2556
Medium carcass	68.87	20.50	9.60	1.03	2080
Lean carcass	73.35	22.40	1.15	1.08	1386
Poor carcass	77.70	18.77	1.43	-	-
High energy fed-					
Muscle tissue	68.20	24.34	6.06	1.56	1540
Bone tissue	36.73	22.74	11.85	28.68	2006
Fatty tissue	13.55	3.65	82.56	0.31	7783

▶ AMINO ACID COMPOSITION OF BUFFEN (BUFFALO MEAT)

Amino acid composition of buffen of some buffalo breeds (Table 10.13) shows th difference in protein quality (Ognjanovic et al., 1970).

TABLE 10.13: Amino acid content in fresh longissimus dorsi muscle (%)

Amino acids	Bulgarian buffalo	Murrah breed (Bulgaria bred)	Murrah X Bulgarian (F1 crossbred)
Alanine	1.416	1.571	1.488
Arginine	1.218	1.435	1.422
Aspartic acid	2.555	2.518	2.625
Cystine	0.363	0.523	0.544
Glycine	1.066	1.053	1.051
Glutamic acid	3.965	4.311	4.154
Histidine	0.767	0.868	0.835
Isoleucine	1.227	1.159	1.233
Leucine	1.878	1.825	1.952

Contd.

TABLE 10.13: Amino acid content in fresh longissimus dorsi muscle (%) *(Contd.)*

Amino acids	Bulgarian buffalo	Murrah breed (Bulgaria bred)	Murrah X Bulgarian (F1 crossbred)
Lysine	1.800	2.162	1.722
Methionine	0.646	0.660	0.659
Phenylalanine	0.904	0.955	0.966
Proline	1.185	0.194	0.928
Serine	.874	0.899	0.926
Thronine	1.172	1.186	1.231
Tyrosine	0.816	0.871	0.893
Valine	1.318	1.370	1.355

The amino acid content in F1 (Murrah X Bulgarian) crossbred buffalo meat shows variable genetic effect but for most of the amino acids the values fall between the values of the two breeds.

The amino acid composition of the skeletal muscle (Table 10.14) of water buffalo (*Bubalus bubalis*), African wild buffalo (*Syncerus caffer*) and ox (*Bos Taurus*) shows the nutritional superiority of buffalo meat (Cutinelli-Ambesi et al., 1975).

TABLE 10.14: Amino acids content of skeletal muscles of water buffalo, African buffalo and ox (A = mg per g dry meat; B = g per 100 g amino acids)

Amino acids	Water buffalo		African buffalo		Ox (Cattle)	
	A	B	A	B	A	B
Alanine	52.6	6.3	61.4	6.4	35.6	7.5
Arginine	56.8	6.8	69.7	7.1	27.9	5.9
Aspartic acid	89.4	10.7	82.5	8.4	47.9	10.2
Glutamic acid	142.8	17.1	132.4	13.5	70.6	15.2
Glycine	34.2	4.1	44.3	4.5	21.0	4.5
Histidine	29.2	3.5	29.5	3.0	15.5	3.3
Isoleucine	46.8	5.6	52.5	5.4	27.5	5.8
Leucine	76.0	9.1	102.3	10.4	42.0	8.9
Lysine	79.4	9.5	81.9	8.4	38.0	8.1
Methionine	23.4	2.8	35.8	3.7	14.9	3.2
Phenylalanine	34.2	4.1	46.3	4.7	24.8	5.3
Proline	27.6	3.3	41.4	4.2	16.1	3.4
Serine	35.1	4.2	45.2	4.6	21.0	4.5
Threonine	35.9	4.3	48.8	5.0	23.8	5.0
Tyrosine	29.2	3.5	48.9	5.0	21.7	4.6
Valine	42.6	5.1	55.1	5.6	23.4	5.0

The amino acids composition of the sarcoplasmic, myofibrillar and insoluble fractions of the skeletal muscle protein shows higher solubility of histidine, valine, leucine, tyrosine, phenylalanine and methionine (Table 10.15) in meat of domestic buffaloes (Colonna et al., 1975).

TABLE 10.15: Amino acids composition of different fractions of skeletal muscle Protein of domestic buffaloes (% per 100g protein)

Amino acid	Soluble muscle proteins		Insoluble muscle protein
	Sacroplamic	Myofibrillar	
Alanine	6.1	7.9	9.1
Arginine	4.9	6.7	7.6
Aspartic acid	9.0	10.4	9.8
Glutamic acid	11.9	18.4	17.5
Glycine	5.0	3.9	12.4
Histidine	7.8	2.5	1.8
Isoleucine	5.9	6.1	5.4
Leucine	12.1	10.8	7.9
Lysine	11.7	10.2	8.0
Methionine	3.9	3.8	2.8
Phenylalanine	5.8	4.8	4.1
Proline	3.0	2.7	7.5
Serine	4.2	4.8	3.1
Threonine	5.2	5.8	4.2
Tyrosine	4.3	3.5	3.7
Valine	7.4	5.2	5.7

▶ BY-PRODUCTS OF SLAUGHTERED BUFFALOES

Average carcass yield of buffaloes ranges from 40 to 60% of body weight depending on the condition of the animal and the remaining parts are the edible and non-edible slaughter by products. The edible slaughter by products are blood, liver, kidneys, hear, spleen, lungs including wind pipe, head, limb bones and washed and cleaned gut. The edible by products ranges from 10–20% of body slaughter weight. Non edible by products include hide, horns, hooves, hairs and gut fill. Yield of different byproducts are higher (Table 10.16) in the buffaloes of poor body condition mostly spared for slaughter in most of the Asian countries (Kondaiah et al., 1983).

TABLE 10.16: Yield of by products from slaughtered buffaloes

By-products	Range (kg)	Mean (kg)	% of body weight
Hide	34–70	47.0	13.62
Head	15–21	17.3 .	5.02
Blood	7–13	9.5	2.76
Pluck	4–9	6.3	1.83
Feet (knuckles)	5–7	6.1	1.76
Horns	0.9–3.2	1.9	0.55
Liver	2.7–5.8	4.3	1.26
Spleen	0.6–1.2	1.0	0.29
kidneys	0.8–1.1	1.0	0.29
Brain	0.4–0.5	0.5	0.13
Caul fat	2.3–7.3	4.7	1.37

Contd.

TABLE 10.16: Yield of by products from slaughtered buffaloes *(Contd.)*

By-products	Range (kg)	Mean (kg)	% of body weight
Empty rumen	5.4–10.2	7.5	2.18
Empty reticulum	1.1–2.1	1.6	0.47
Empty omasum	1.9–3.8	2.8	0.80
Empty intestines	0.9–1.8	1.3	0.37
Mesentry	8.0–21	15.5	4.49
Rumen contents	4.6–8	6.0	1.74
	20–67	42.4	12.28

▶ MEAT PRODUCTS

Edible buffalo meats include primal cuts, edible glands and edible offals. The primal cuts are used for the preparation of standard dishes according to liking and demand in different countries. Trimmed meat and meat in some offalas as well as meat of aged buffaloes is mostly used for the preparation of minced meat (keema). The primal cuts are sold at retail shops. Since availability of edible meat from different species is grossly short for human consumption in most of the buffalo raising countries, little serious attempt has been made for the development of preserved buffen products. Offal meat commonly called as variety meats include the meat separated from the head, feet, pluck, oesophagus, ruminoreticulum and upper half of the diaphragm. These are chpped fine and then minced to make 'keema'. Various recipe of keema ar quite popular in the Indian sub continent. Few examples are keema curry, pakoda, kofta, tikka, kabab etc. Most of the preparations ar spicy and hot due to excess use of dry chilli and black pepper. These are used baked, cooked on direct heat of coal or deep fried in boiling oil or fat for eating as snacks, and also for the preparation of different recipe of curry. Meat of glands like liver. Kidneys and testes are cut into small pieces and mostly consumed deep fried. The knuckle and other long bones are used for several hours (mostly over night) on slow heat to facilitate the extraction of greater part of minerals. Boiled preparations of liver, kidneys, testes and long bones are also recommeneded by physicians of different systems for the supporting treatment of many diseases.

▶ SOME LOCAL MEAT PRODUCTS OF DIFFERENT COUNTRIES

Although surplus meat is not available for preservation in most of the tropical countries, indeed some special preserved products are prepared in most of the countries for serving at special occasions.

Products of Indian Sub-continent

The system of cooking meat and preparation of meat products are almost similar in the people of Indian sub continent. Most of the meat products are hot due to excessive use of chilli, black pepper along with other spices and condiments.

1. **Dried salted meat:** Fresh meat is cut into strips of 1–2 cm thicknes and spread on a clean surface. After this powderd common salt is thoroughly rubbed with the meat strips. The salt is used at the of 3–5% of the raw meat. Now salted meat strips are spreas on a clean cloth or polyethylene sheet for Sun drying. In good sun light exposure of 8–10 hours daily in dry season it takes 3–5 days to reduce the moisture

content below 10 percent. Dried salted meat is used during the scarcity period and at remote places where meat is not available. The salted meat strips are washed in fresh water and cut into desired size before cooking by common methods.

2. **Dried masala meat:** Fresh meat is cleaned and cut into 13 to 23 cm size and then thoroughly mixed with a paste of spices and condiments and 2–3% fine powder of common salt. Now salted masala met cubes ar Sun dried by the method used for the drying of salted meat. Dried masala meat is a ready to cook products and served dry after deep frying in hot oil or cooled to prepare curry.

Both the dried meat products are stored in dry containers and arrangements are also made to protect form the humid air of rainy season.

3. **Pickled meat:** The meat cubes used for the preparation of dried masala meat are partially Sun dried to about 70–75% dry matter and then put in mustard oil or sesame oil or vinegar. After this the earthen or glass or ceramics jar containing pickles meat dipped in oil is put in Sun light for 6–7 days. Now pickled mean is ready for eating. Meat pickle is always taken out with the help of a dry fork or spoon. The container is weekly checked for the contamination because preserved meat products are susceptible for fungal contamination.

Products of Turkey

Steaks and stuffed products (sausages) are quite popular in Turkey.

Products of Philippines

'Chikarones' or cracklings are prepared from the fresh hide of hips removed with tail. The another common hide product is 'kari–kari'.

Products of Indonesia

Generally 3 types of buffen products are popular.

1. **Sun dried meat:** The strips of raw meat is rubbed with blood of the same animal and then Sun dried for use as 'Biltong' or jerked meat. The product is more popular in Bali island.
2. 'Kerupuk kulit' is prepared from the hide of hip region after scrapping and cleaning in boiling water.
3. 'Djingur' is prepared from the lips.

Products of Thailand

Three varieties of edible hide products quite popular in the northern region of Thailand are 'khab-kwai', 'nung-pong' and 'chui-pong'. These are prepared by boiling, salting and drying of the hide stripes. These are eaten after cooking as curry or deep fried in fat.

▶ MODERN MEAT PRODUCTS

Now buffalo meat is being used for the preparation of edible products of longer self life like meat ball, masala meat ball, meat tikka and sausases, etc.

REFERENCES

Abou Hussain, E R M and Raafat, M A 1962. J Anim Prod, UAR, 2; 27–33

Afifi, Y A, Shahin, M A, Omara, S F and Youssef, F M 1974. Agriculture Res Rev., 52 (7); 1–15

Agarwal, V P 1974. Ph. D thesis, Agra University,Agra

Ahmed, I A and El Shazly, K 1975. World Animal Rev., 14; 28–30

Ali, A, Cheema, A U, Mirza, I H and Alvi, A S 1983. Buffalo Bull., 4; 55

Arora, S P and Gupta, B S 1962. J Vet Sic Anim Husb Res, Mhou. 6; 19–21

Avalisvili, N 1956. Anim Breed Abstr., 25; 58

Badraldin, A L 1955. Indian J Vet Sci Anim Husb., 25; 61–64

Baruak, K K, Ranjhan, S K and Pathak, N N 1982. Proc 2nd Asian-Autralasian Assoc Anim prod Soc, PICC, Manila, Nov., 10 = 13

Baruah, K K, Ranjhan, S K and Pathak, N N 1983. Proc 5th World Conf Anim Prod, Tokyo, August 13–17

Borghese, A, Romita, A, Gigli, S and Marchini, S 1981. Anim Breed Abstr., 49; 44–48

Charles, D D and Johnson, E R 1972. Australian J agric Res., 23; 905–911

Charles, D D and Johnson, E R 1975. Australian J. Agric Res., 26; 407–413

Colonna, G, Irace, G, Balestrieri, C, Minieri, L and Salvatora, F. 1975. Comp Biochem Physiol., 51B; 197–200

Cunburidze, S and Dalakisvili, G 1959. Anim Breed Abstr., 28; 81

Cutinelli-Ambesi, N, Bocchini, V, Balestrieri, C and Salvatora, F 1975.Comp Biochem Physiol., 51B; 193–196

Das Gupta, N C 1943. Indian J. Vet Sci. Anim Husb., 13; 196–200

De Franciscis, G, Interieri, F, Rinaldi, G and Rendius, N 1970

Domingues, O 1956. Animal Agric., Bras, 3(9); 15–21

Dzafarov, S 1958. Anim Breed Abstr., 36; 1820

El-Naggar, A A, El-Shazly, K and Ahmed, L A 1972. Anim Breed Abst, 42; 925

Ivanov, P and Zaahariev, Z 1966. Anim Breed Abstr., 35; 33–47

Johri, C B, Ranjhan, S K and Pathak, N N 1982. Indian J. Anim. Sci., 42; 406–411

Kalugin, I 1933. Anim. Breed. Abst., 1; 89

Kasimov, M 1971. Anim Breed, Abst., 40; 130

Kassir, S M, Mc Fetridge, D G and Hansen, N G 1969. Anim Breed Abst., 38; 22–37

Kondaiah, N, Lakshmanan, V, Anjaneyulu, A S R and Sharma, N 1983. Indian J. Anim Sci., 53; 1208–1212.

Kondaiah, N, Lakshmanan, V, Eao, V K and Sharma, N 1981. Indian J. Anim. Res, 15; 107–111

Kurbanov, L 1961. Miasnala Industrija, SSSR, Mosk, 5; 47–49

Lakshmanan, V, Kondaiah, N and Anjaneyulu, A S R 1984. Buffalo Bull., 3; 6–8,

Matasukawa, T, Tilakratne, N and Buvanendran, V 1976. Tropical Animal Hlth Prod., 8; 155–162

Maymone, B 1942. Z. Tierzucht.Zuchtbiol., 52; 1–44

Maymone, B 1945. Annali Ist Spet Zootech Roma, 3; 5–65

Minieri, L, De Franciscis, G, Barbieri, V and Zicarelli, L 1972. Anim Breed Abstr, 41; 2500

Moran, J B 1983. J. Agric Sci., Camb., 100; 709–722

Naidu, M M and Raghavan, G B 1985. Indian Vet J, 62; 64–70

Ornjanovic, A, Polikhronov, D and Jaksimovic, J. 1970. Proc Meeting of Meat Res., Workers, Sofia, Bulgaria, September.

Pathak, N N 1985. Proc. National Symp. On use of Nuclear Tech in Animal Hlth Prod. P 15, IVRI, Izatnagar

Pathak, N N and Ranjhan, S K 1979. Proc. Protein and NPN Utilization in Ruminant p. 10/II, NDRI, Karnal

Pathak, N N, Krishna Mohan, DVG and Ranjhan, S K 1976. Indian J Anim Sci., 46; 451–453

Pathak, N N, Baruah, K K and Ranjhan, S K 1982.

Polikhronov, D, Boikovski, S and Pinkas A 1979. Anim. Breed. Abstr., 49; 24–88

Proto, V and Landi, F. Anim Breed Abstr., 34; 10–48

Ragab, M T, Darwish, M Yand Malak, A G A 1966 J Anim Prod, UAR, 6; 9–30

Rao, B R 1978. Indian Vet J, 55; 111–118

Rasheed, A A 1977. Anim Breed Abstr., 47; 3484

Robertson, J A, Ford, B D and Morris, C A 1982. Australian J agric Res., 33; 755–762

Romita, A, Borghese, A, Gigli, S and Giacomo, A Di 1978. Anim Breed Abstr., 47; 5331

Rosa, A and Creta, V 1978. Anim Breed Abstr, 47; 5910

Salerno, 1948. Annalu University Bari., 6; 51–96

Salem, M A I, Nigm, A A and Abdel-Aziz, A S 1983. Anim. Breed.Abstr., 52; 6337.

Sharma, K M and Talapatra, S K 1963. Indian J.Dairy Sci., 16;236–243

Sharma, N, Padda, G S and Kondaiah, N. 1982. Indian Food Packer, 50–52

Siddiqui, I A, Maheshwari, M L and Barsaul, C S 1982. Vet. Res., 5; 71–72

Solomon, M B, West, R L and Carpenter, J W 1985. Meat Science. 13; 129–135

11

Utilization of By-products of Buffalo

Different kinds of valuable by-products from the buffaloes available at the buffalo farms and processing of the main products, viz., milk and meat are utilized gainfully in different ways in various countries. A brief account of different ways of utilization of various by-products has been presented in this chapter.

▶ BUFFALO DUNG PRODUCTION

Buffalo dung is a daily product of buffalo farm and required daily disposal away from the farm or household in case of small holders. Buffalo dung possess species specific odour which shows very little variation due to composition and quality of diets. Dung disposal followed by cleaning and disinfection for th maintenance of hygienic condition is a routine daily operation in early morning and late evening. Hips of buffalo dung provides favourable conditions for the multiplication of different kinds of insects like flies, mosquitoes, beetles and white ants. For controlling the breeding of insects it is always advantageous to cover it with soil or ash.

The quantity of dung voided by the buffaloes depends on the body size, physiological state, activities, composition of the diet and level of feeding. About 10 gallon equivalent to kg daily dung production has been reported by Macgregor (1941) in the water buffaos. Average faecal output of Philippines buffaloes is about 18.8 kg daily or 6.86 tonnes annual, which contains about 73.86% moisture (Villegas, 1969). Average value of dung production in swamp buffaloes is about 18.10 kg per animal per day) Chaidet et al., 1983). Average daily fresh dung output in adult Murrah buffaloes is about 26.11 kg (20.78 to 31.52 kg) and 21.55 kg (20.29 to 22.81 kg) in the Vietnamese swamp buffaloes maintained on the standard farm conditions at the Buffalo Breeding Research Centre, Song Be, S R Vietnam (Pathak et al., 1985). Daily faecal void is about 0.79, 0.83 and 1.03% of the body weight in adult buffalo bulls, dry buffalo females and lactating buffaloes of Murrah breed respectively. The values for adult male and female Vietnamese swamp buffaloes are 1.01 and 1.05% of body weight. Annual fresh dung production varies from 7.41 to 11.50 tonnes equivalent to about 1.45 to 2.09 tonnes dry matter containing 80 to 85% organic matter, 1.5 to 3.0% nitrogen besibes minerals of agricultural values.

▶ CHEMICAL COMPOSITION OF BUFFALO DUNG

Influence of the chemical composition of diets and the digestibility of nutrients on the chemical composition of dung of normal healthy animals is well-known. The informations considered in this chapter represents the composition of composite dung of buffaloes reared in different countries of tropical Asia (Majumdar and Jung, 1963; Villegas, 1969; Baruah et al., 1983). The chemical composition of fresh buffalo dung (Table 11.1) still has potential for supplying nutrients to other animals and fishes after processing. The dung of buffaloes of Philippines contains about 26.14% total ash. In dried dung mean values of nitrogen, phosphorus, potassium and calcium are about 1.28, 0.57, 0.11 and 0.21% respectively.

TABLE 11.1: Chemical composition of buffalo dung (%)

Dung	Organic matter	Total ash	Nitrogen	Calcium	Phosphorus	Potassium
Fresh dung	16–17	3–4	0.25–0.30	0.12–0.14	0.06–0.08	0.09–0.13
Dried dung	80–85	15–20	1.35–1.42	0.60–0.70	0.30–0.40	0.48–0.56

▶ USES OF BUFFALO DUNG

Buffalo dung is one the important source of organic manure after composting and also fuel for cooking food in the rural area after Sun drying in different shape either alone after mixing some crop wastes in many tropical countries. The other uses are plastering of mud walls and flor of the houses and thach huts. For this purpose fresh dung is mixed with clay and water to make a slurry. It is quite popular in the rural areas of the Indian sub continent. The recent uses are fermentation of water diluted buffalo dung in biogas (gober gas) fermenter for the liberation of fuel gas, a mixture of methane. The fresh dung of buffaloes fed high concentrate or leguminous fodder rich diets may be utilized for the feeding of large bovines after ensiling with other feeds during the acute feed scarcity produced by failure of crops during the long drought period and also during the devastating floods washing off the standing crops and stored feedstuffs (Jakhmola et al., 1984).

Buffalo or catte dung cakes are known by various names like upla, kunda, gointha, chipari, gohra etc in different regions of India. The names often denote the shape and size of the dung cakes. The fuel efficiency of dung cake is increased by mixing different dry herbal wastes like soiled straw, fallen tree leaves, rice hull and wood savings etc. the surplus dung cake is sold is fuel deficit areas and a brick clines. During wet months of rainy season Sun dring becomes difficult and dung is diverted for manure preparation by composting. Educated, and economically sound families capable of arranging other fuels utilize all dung for composting. Compost manure made of buffalo dung mixed with soiled feed, beddings and urine make a very good compost. Compost is a very good organic manure for the improvement of soil health and crop production. Besides supplying nutrients to crops it also improves the water holding capacity of arable soil.

The development of gober gas (biogas) plant has helped in reducing the pollution problem and supply of both fuel in the form of biogas and manure in the form of biogas slurry. The slurry draining out of the biogas plant is a rich source of microbial protein and minerals resulting from the microbial decomposition of larger proportion of organic matter in the dung for the production of predominantly methane and carbon dioxide. In addition to the manorial use the biogas plant slurry may be also fed to supply about 20–30% of protein requirement for maintenance on cereal straw based diets (Pathak et al., 1982). Buffalo dung has been also used for making satisfactory silage (wastelage) in combination with chaffed cereal straw, green fodder and a small quantity (2–5%) molasses (Jakhmola et al., 1984; 1958, Singh et al., 1985). Use of wastelage may be helpful in mitigating the feed deficit during scarcity. However, farmers may required to be convinced for the life saving of their animals during extended duration of droughs and floods.

▶ **USES OF BUFFALO URINE**

Buffalo urine is a good source of non protein nitrogen of manorial value and it also contains minerals of manorial value. Each litre of buffalo urine contains 9.6–14.4 g nitrogen and 3.3 to 3.8 g potassium (Majumdar and Jung, 1963). Some proportion of urine is collected with dung, soiled fodder and soiled bedding but greater portion is hydrolysed releasing ammonia gas in the tropical climate. Buffalo urine can also be utilized for the nitrogen enrichment of low protein cereal straws by ensiling. The urine soaked staws are allowed reaction for 3–4 weeks in anaerobic environment of silo. The product this obtained is known as alkalage and nitrogen is unstable. Therefore, feeding management require some precaution for minimizing the nitrogen loss. This may be achieved by opening the silo just before offering feeds and mixing of quickly fermentable carbohydrates like molasses at the time of feeding. This approach is more a theoretical exercise and scope of practical uses is remote in the present mind set of most of the farmers specially that in India.

▶ **USES OF HORNS AND HOOVES**

Several cottage industries are engaged in the utilization of horns and hooves of buffaloes and cattle for the manufacture of beautiful decoration articles. Combs, coat buttons, hair pins, broaches, tie pin, walking stick, horn spoon for use in chemistry laboratories, handles, ear ringes, bengles, etc. In many tribal colonies of remote areas the large size horns are used after cleaning the marrow for keeping liquid items. The horns of buffloes of non Murrah group, swamp buffaloes and wild buffaloes are mostly long and massive, and their natual colour ranges from grey white to black. Normally both horns of an animal are identical in shape, size and colour, and it is a common practice in most of the countries to mount exceptionally large and massive horns alongwith skull embalmed head. These shields are used as decoration piece in the drawing rooms of hurters, heads of some tribal and ethnic groups and also in assembly halls of tribal groups. Such items can be seen in most of the tribal villages of tropical countries having domesticated and wild buffaloes.

The long horns become malleable on heating over the flame and can be moulded in desired manner for giving a shape of bird, animal, other fancy items, decoration items or household goods. Flute and bugle like pipe musical instruments of horns are quite common amongst the tribal communities of India and other countries. Handles of nives and hand hoe, hair decoration articles are quite popular in north-east Indian states, Bangladesh, Mayanmar, Thailand and other south-east asian countries. Buffalo hooves are less important and occasionally used for preparing low grade button but the fatty marrow in the hooves is used as lubricant. Refined oil of hooves is also used for lubricating machines and manure of hooves residue is preferredin tea and coffee plantations.

▶ **USES OF BUFFALO HAIRS**

Scanty body coat does not have much uses and idle family members some times use coat hairs for making cushions and brushes but long and coarse hairs of swich of the tail cut twice annually and used for the preparation of various useful items. Switch hairs are used for the spinning of beautiful ropes which are used as neck collar for hanging a bell and/or locket in the neck of buffaloes and other farm animals. It is also used by the ladies for the preparation of fancy goods for decoration, etc.

▶ USES OF GUT FILL

The rumini-reticular content and the digesta of lower digestive tract are collected daily from the slaughter houses in bulk and dumped in pits for composting. It is a very good organic manure. The liquid portion of gastrointestinal tract is also rich in many minerals and nitrogenous substances but greater proportion is wasted due to lack of provision in small and unorganized slaughter places. Such gut contents are left as such in open or drained into low lying area, and cause environmental pollution. The contents of rumino-recticulum are rich sources of microbial protein, undigested portion of feed, minerals and vitamins. These can be utilized in the food channel of livestock after ensiling with other fodder and a small amount of molasses or other source of easily fermentable carbohydrate and increasing the dry matter content 35 to 40 percent.

▶ USES OF BLOOD AND SERUM

Whole blood may be used for the manufacture of pharmaceuticals or dried to make blood meal for the feeding of pigs ansd poultry. Blood from small the sacrifice in local abbotoirs is largely consumed by the people in different form or left soiled in open. This is serious nuiscenc in manuy countries by attracting stray dogs and birds. Blood meal contains about 86–88% protein, 1.5–2% either extract and 4–5% nitrogen free extracts and 5–6% minerals on moisture free basis. Its digestibility is higher in simple stomach animals like pig and poultry than in the ruminants.

▶ MEAT MEAL, MEAT-CUM-BONE MEAL AND BONE MEAL

Rejecteed carcass unfit for human consumption and non autolyzed carcasses of dead buffaloes are used for the manufacture of meat meal and bone meal separately in big factories, meat-cum-bone meal or bone meal at the small scale carcass utilization centres. These are used in the diets of pigs and poutry for the supply of essential amino acids and minerals. The bones of dead animals left uncared are collected and used for the preparation of bone ash for use as manure or mineral supplement in the diets of farm animals. Meat meal contains 55–60% protein, 10–12 % fat, 4–5% non-nitrogenous organic matter and 24–27 % ash (minerals) on dry matter basis. The values in meat-cum-bone meal for the corresponding constituents are 50–55, 10–12, 4–5 and 37–35.

Steamed bone meal is fed in small quantity by mixing in concentrate mixtures as a source of dietary essential mineranls mostly deficient in common feeds of plant origin. It is a very rich source of calcium, phosphorus and other essential minerals, and contains 12–13% protein, almost equal amount of fat, 75–77% total ash, 30–32% calcium and 12–13% phosphorus on dry matter basis.

▶ USES OF GLANDS OF SLAUGHTERED ANIMALS

The fresh and healthy glands of slaughtered buffaloes are higly valuable and collected unspoiled fresh or frozen from the abbatoris. These are used for the manufacture of valuable pharmaceuticals like extract for the supply of vitamins, different hormones, enzymes, bile salts and serum proteins etc. the residue left after the extraction are used for the preparation of protein rich supplements for the simple stomach animals.

▶ BUFFALO HIDE

Buffalo hide is one of the most valuable by-product from fallen animals and slaughter houses. Approximately 19 million hides are available annually from the 120 million domesticated and feral buffaloes in the world. About 40% hides are obtained from the slaughtered buffaloes which are shifted to large processing factories for the manufacture of good quality leathers. The grearter proportion of the hide of fallen buffaloes is used in cottage industry for processing and manufacture of leather goods of farmers and agricultural uses. A simple method of hide preservation in remote areas of some countries is carried in the following manner:

1. Removal of traces of meat, blood and fatty tissue.
2. Application of concentrated solution of common salt.
3. Rubbing of fine salt powder on the inner wet surface of hide.
4. Air drying of hide for necessary drying so that moisture content is less than 20–30%.
5. Sun drying of hide is not desirered and it is damaging.
6. Application of a mixture of powdered common salt, washing, soda and naphthalene for preservation.

Two methods of tanning prevalent in the Indian sub continent are:

a. Tanning with bark extract of tannins rich plants abundantly found in the region. This method is called vegetable tanning and it is called vegetable tanning and it is a very old method.
b. The other method is tanning with synthetic chemicals like salt of chromium and the process is called chrome tanning and the leather is called chrome leather.

The hide of buffalo is significantly thicker than the hide of cattle and also less greasy. It is more porous but no way inferior of cattle hide for the manufature of leather. The leather manufacture from buffalo hide has rough and granular surface but it is stronger due to big bundles of collagen fibres with a well developed reticular sheath (Sarkar et al., 1964).

▶ USES OF BUFFALO HIDE

The greater proportion of buffalo hide is used for the manufacture of leather by different processes which is then utilizen for the manufacture of different kinds of household and industrial goods. A very quantity of soft skin from selected part of the body is utilized for the preparation of some kind of foods.

1. **Uses of buffalo hide in cottage industry:** This is an age old traditional family profession in many countries. The buffalo hide is treated in small number by different indigenous processes. Some of the things used for the manufacture of crude leather are the common salt solution and bark extract of some Acacia species and other tannis rich plants. The leather produced by this process is crude and hard. It is used for the preparation of water carrying large bags (masak) used for carrying water for washing of roads, streets, railway plateform and other pucca places, large bags (mot or pur) for drawing water from the well for irrigation. The other uses are preparation of local shoes, sandles and chapala, whips and ropes of different size for agricultular uses. In India, Khadi and Gramoudiyog Department is responsible for the development of cottage industry due to which use has been

diversified. The chaples, shoes, hand bags, purse, belt and other items are now popular and also finding export markets. Shoes for cattle and buffaloes are also prepared. Sole of such shoes is quite thick and made of hard leather. These shoes are used for draught animals only specialyfor those working on rough roads and also ploughing on dry and hard soils like black cotton soil which becomes sharp and damage hooves during ploughing.

2. **Medium scale industries:** These industries use only processed leather for the manufacture of leather goods. These are primarily responsible for the manufacture of leather goods and had linkage with business houses for marketing. These are also eligible for loan from the nationalized banks and other recognized financing organizations.

3. **Big industries:** Large size leather utilizing industries also manufacture almost all the goods manufactured b small industry but large factories are butter mechanized and capable of handling very large quantity of leather. They also manufature heavy items like horse saddles and camel saddles for riding animals and harnesses for draught animals used in different services and civilians maintaining the equines and camel.

▶ FOOD PREPARATION FROM FRESH BUFFALO HIDE

Some foods prepared from the hide of fresh sacrificed buffaloes are quite popular in some countries of east and south east Asia and the Asia-Pacific region particulary the island nations of Asia-Pacific region, Thailand, Philippines etc. The food items of buffalo hide are prepared after cleaning and boilding the hide in hot water. The boild hide pieces stripped in salt water are Sun dries to dehydrate almost completely for increasing the self life of the product. The hide foods are stored in moisture free sealed container for quite long period. The hide foods are deep fried in boiling fat or oil and serval hot as a delicious preparation. For this purpose soft hide pieces are selected from the specific region of the hide. This spoils the hide and sitgnificantly reduces the prices of hide byt the loss is compensated by the hide foods. Perhaps such kind of foods prepared from hide of buffalo or any other ruminant species is not known to large population in other countries.

▶ MILK PROCESSING BY-PRODUCTS

Substantial amount of milk processing by-products available from creamery and dehydrated (powder) and partly dehydrated milk (condensed milk) producing plant are the skim milk, whey, soiled milk powder and spilled condensed milk. These are rich sources of good quality protein, lactose and soluble minerals and used for the feeding of animals or washed off from the very small milk processing plants. Larger proportion of skim milk is used for the direct consumption either as such, as a diluent of whole milk for making tonned and double tonned milk. Skim milk is also utilized for the preparation of curd and sweets etc. the various industrial uses of skim milk are the manufacture of skim milk powder, casein and lactose.

REFERENCES

Chaldet, P, Pongpairoj, S and Khangkarn, R 1983. Buffalo Bulletin, 2 (2); 8 Jakhmola, R C, Kanra, D N, Rameshwar Singh and Pathak, N N 1984. Agricultural Waste, 10; 229–237.
Jakhmola, R C, Singh, R and Kamra, D N 1985. Agricultural Waste, 12; 23–28

Majumdar, B N and Jung, S 1963. Annals Biochem. Exptl. Med., 23; 91–94

Macgregor, R 1941. Veterinary Record, 53; 443–450.

Pathak, N N, Baruah, K K and Jakhmola, R C 1982. Indian J. Anim. Sci., 52; 435–436

Pathak, N N, Sharma, M C, Hung, N N and Vuc, N V 1985. Livestock Adviser, 10 (3); 39–42

Rameshwar Singh, Kamra, D N and Jakhmola, R C 1985. Agricultural Waste, 13; 127–133.

Sarkar, S K, Mitra, S K. and Nayudamma, Y 1964. Biological characteristics of Buffalo hide. A chaper in Fuller and Better Utilization of Hide, Editor P S Venkatachalam and K C Shivappa, Central Leather Research Institute, Mysore.

Villegas, V 1969. Animal Husbandry Agriculture Journal, January, 1969.

12

Economic Contribution of Domestic Buffaloes

The economic importance of buffaloes as a domesticated farm animal was recognized much later than the cattle because agro-climatic conditions in the buffalo dominant Asian countries there was plenty food of different varieties for the feeding of limited human population for the available natural resources. However, with the increase of pressure on the food resources buffaloes were domesticated in the Indian sub continent and tropical regions of other Asuan countries. Subsequently buffalo emerged s a multi purpose farm animal for the supply of nutritious milk and meat, draught power for agricultural oerations and agro-industrial haulage, valuable organic manure and valuable by products like hides, bones and fallen carcass. Due to heavy pressure of large human and livestock population the availabity of grazing land has shrunken to non productive rain fed waste lands with scantly herbage cover during greater part of year except the flush rainy season. However, buffaloes have well adopted for thriving and production on the diets containing greater proportion of low quality cereal crop residues like straws and stovers supplements with concentrates of celeals, pulses and oilseeds milling residues like cereal brans, dal chunnies and oilseed cakes. Supply of green fodder is highly variable and mostly seasonal. The economic contributions of farm buffaloes may be put under the following two classes and their subclasses.

1. **Direct economic contributions of buffaloes** like
   a. Milk production of high nutritive and market value
   b. Meat production of high nutritive and market value
   c. Dung supply for manure and preparation of dung cakes for fuel.
   d. Supply of hides for the manufacture of valuable leather and leather goods.
   e. Supply of glands from slaughtered buffaloes for the manufacture of hormones, enzymes, vitamins, other pharmaceuticals, and their residues for the supply of good quality animals proteins required for the balancing of essential amino acids in the diets of simple stomach animals, poultry birds and fishes.
   f. The non spoiled carcasses of fallen buffaloes are also used for the processing of hide for leather, horns for decoration pieces and fancy items, and flesh and bones for the manufacture of meat meal, meat-cum-bone meal and bone meal.
   g. The rumen content and other soiled wastes are used for composting.
   h. Draught power or work energy for traction.
2. **Indirect economic contributions** like
   a. Part or full time employment for many members of family according their skill, age, sex and working capacity.

  b. Employment in buffalo feed manufacturing and marketing industries.
  c. Development of dairy farm and dairy products manufacturing gadgets, appliances and instruments, etc.
  d. Employment in slaughter houses, retailmeat shops and meat products manufacturing and marketing businesses.

▶ BUFFALO, THE ANIMAL OF SUBSIDIARY INCOME FOR MANY SMALL HOLDERS IN MOST OF THE TROPICAL COUNTRIES

Unemployment and under employment causing large scale economic insufficiency is a chronic problem in most of the tropical countries causing large scale migration of human resources in the economically sound countries like USA, Europe, Gulp countries and Australia. The population unable to find other job or jobs of low earning for animal husbandry. In the Indian sub continent families engated in milk production and sale of liquid milk maintain 1 to 10 lactating buffaloes and their followers. Only small proportion of families keep more than 10 buffaloes for large scale coercial farming.

The most valuable recurring contribution of riverine dairy type buffaloes are the source of regular income with payment systems of daily, weekly and montly. The holders of very small units of 1 or 2 lactating buffaloes and to meet the require daily payment of milk price for the procurement of feeds for the buffaloes and to meet the requirements of households. The buffalo milk fetch higher price due to high milk fat and total solids content resulting in more yield of partially dehydrated products like Khoa, ruberi (rubdi) and Khurchan, milk solids precipitated products like chhenna and paneer, separated or churned products like cream, butter and ghee (Samna), and fermented products like dahi, shreekhand, yoghurt ad cheese of different varieties. In diary type buffaloes the heifer calves are more valuable being the future replacement stock and receive better care than the male calves. However, due to increase in demand of buffalo meat for local supply and export ttje male buffalo calves are now also given proper care due to payment of remunerative price by the meat producing commercial houses.

Both milk and meat are in deficit supply in almost all Asian and Asia-Pacific countries having largest number of buffaloes. A few decades earlier increase in mechanization of agriculture was considered a threat for the working buffaloes but increase in acceptance of buffen (buffalo meat) hs revived the importance of both male and female buffaloes. Due to its high adatability there is scope of further rise in buffalo production under the changing agro-climatic conditions. There is great variation in the feeding systems of dairy type buffaloes in different regions of Asia, Asia-Pacific, mediterenean region, African countries and Latin American countries. Now the famous milch animals is primarily a milch followed by power supply and meat in India, equally important for milk and meat in Pakistan, other countries of Asia, Island nations of Pacific region, middle east, European countries, Egypt and Wst Indies, but its main objective is meat production followed by limited use of milk or cheese and other products in Brazil and Venezuella. In the Latin American countries both riverien and swamp buffaloes have been placed on large natural pastures and marshes for free breedig and fattening only to harvest for meat when needed.

In the native lands of swamp buffaloes the calves are highly valuable animals and there is no discrimination in the rearing of male and female calves because both sexes are used for working in paddy fields. The only difference is the allotment of work load for the males is generally heavier and for strenuous works males are preferred over the females. Milking of swamp buffaloes is not common except in India. The calves are allowed full suckling as they move with their mother on pasture and also during working. In some of the east and south-east Asian countries a pair of working buffaloes may cost equal to the price of a power tiller or small tractor. The buffaloes are mostly reared on the natural grass lands and marshes. The grazing is supplemented with the baddy straw, rice milling byproducts (a mixture of polishing, embryos and tiny broken parts of rice. Some amount of oil seed cakes are also supplemented.

▶ COMMERCIAL BUFFALO DAIRY FARMS OF URBAN AND PERIURBAN AREAS IN THE INDIAN SUBCONTINENT FOR LUQUID MILK SUPPLY

Daily consumption of liquid milk is very high in the Indian sub continent and i.e. is increasing every day due to continent migration of people and families from rural areas to towns and cities. This has resulted in simultaneous increase of commercial dairy farms in and around the urban habitation. These dairies are buffalo based in the north, central and west parts of India and almost all over the Pakistan. The animals on such dairy stalls are mostly kept confined on stall feeding in limited areas without the provision of anu space or yard for free movement. The calves are the most neglected member of these buffalo (it is more appropriate to call stalls) and majority succumb in early life of 4–6 weeks due to starvation of various intensity, unhygienic crowded housing and neglected veterinary aids, this inhuman treatment is only for sparing milk for sale. It is much beneficial for such dairy stall owners to do away with the young calves to rear them for 3–4 years for replacement in limited space and high inputs. There is almost no consideration of hygiene and despite official ban oxytocin is extensively injected (almost twice daily) for the let down of milk in buffaloes without a living calf for stimulating let down of milk at the time of morning and evening milking. Most of the dry buffaloes of such dairy stalls. Terminate their life in slaughter houses and only a few fortunate buffaloes find a new owner for rearing till next calving. This practice has harmed so much to buffalo production in India that germ plasma of high yielding Murrah, Mehsana, Surti and other breeds of western part of India is highly depleted. Now many schemes have been initiated in the dairy buffalo breeding states for the protection and conservation of high milk yielding elite buffaloes.

▶ ORGANIZED DAIRY FARMS

The organized dairy farms with optimum management facilities are under the management of government, co-operative and a few Pinjrapoles and Ashrams in Gujarat. The main objective of such farms is the maintenance of elite herds under scientific management and production of good buffalo bulls, preferably progenutested for the multiplication of better productive buffaloes. Many of these organized buffalo breeding farms are the parts of research institutions engaged in the progress of crops and livestock production. Some of the buffalo breeding and reseach stations are the Central Institute for Research on Buffaloes for Murrah breeding at Hisar in Haryana and for Nili-Ravi breeding at Nabha in Punjab. Surti and Jaffarabadi are under the programmes of National Dairy Development Board, Anand in Gujarat. The other institutional farms of Murra breeding are the National Dairy Research Institute, Karnal and Government Livestock Farm, Hisar in Haryana, Punjab Agricultural University, Ludhiana in Punjab, Indian Veterinary Research Institute, Izatnagar and Narendradeo

University of Agriculture and Technology, Faizabad in Uttar Pradesh and one farm each in Andhra Pradesh and Tamil Nadu besides smaller units at other places. During past few decades many countries like Thailand, Combodia, Socialist Republic of Vietnam, Philippines and China etc have imported Murrah, Nili-Ravi and Surti buffaloes for the development of their own herds and also for the up grading of local swamp buffaloes s a multi purpose animal for milk, draught and meat.

During last few decades different National and international development programmes for the improvement of buffaloes through breeding (pure breeding and cross breeding), nutrition and health management have been taken up in several countries of the tropical region for the arugumenting the production of milk. Meat and draught power. The buffalo improvement programme in the Thailand had worked jointly with the Department of Livestock Development and Kasetsart University by assistance from the Rockfeller Foundation of United States of America. Another project worked at the Khon-kaan with the assistance from the World Bank Third Window loan. In Indonesia the Center of Animal Research and Development Board and the Department of Animal Husbandry are engaged with local Tarai breed of buffalo in Nepal. A cross breeding programme of local buffaloes with Murrah and Surti from India is running at Ridiuyagama in Sri Lanka for more than four decades. A multidisciplinary research project is working in malayasia with the collaboration between Agriculture University,Livestock Deparment, farmers organization and MARDI for enhancing the production of milk, meat and working buffaloes mainly through the up grading programme of local swamp buffaloes with Murrah buffaloes at the regional farm in the Trengganu state and small herds in the Ferak and Selangor states. In the Philippines the threee national research and development projects on the buffaloes are:

1. National beef/cara beef development programme
2. Barangay (Village) training for livestock production and
3. Dairy industry development act besides the internaltional UNDO/P/IAEA assisted buffalo development project at the Agriculture College, Los Banos, Laguna.

▶ INPUTS AND OUTPUT RATIO

The relationship between the capital investment on different aspects of production and the return form the sale of the products is known as input-output ratio and it is the balance of the success of an enterprise. Like other livestock industry the different inputs in buffalo production for milk, meat and draught power are:

i. cost of land and infra structure,
ii. cost of dairy farm instrument, appliances and gadgets, and recurring expenditure on feeding, veterinary aids and medicines, labout charges on routine activities like feeding, milking, electric charges, water charges, cleaning, washing of sheds, buffaloes and utensils, recording and marketing, etc.

Among all the recurring expenditure largest is on the feeding of buffaloes which may be 50 to 58% dpending on the circumstances and production. The cost of feeding is much less for milk production and it reduces with the increase in the milk yield when calculated on the basis of per kg milk yield. This is followed by labour charge and other expenses are generally less than 10% of total recurring expenditure. The cost of feeding of replacement heifers from birth to first calving and that of male calves fattening on standard feeding, raising of selected male calves for buffalo bull production and that of dry buffaloes from the date of drying to date of next calving is much higher because farmers do not receive any valuable return during the period. Being livestock the rearing period is highly risky and require special attention for the maintenance of health with the help of preventive vaccination and hygienic measures.

Relative Cost of Rearing of the Replacement Buffalo Heifers

The different expenses on the rearing of buffalo heifers from birth to date of first calving at about 42 months of age has shown the cost of feeding from 74.68 to 82.92% of the total expenditure arrhe organized farms in India (Gautam and Vimal, 1966). The expenditure on the feeding of concentrates is maximum and that on feeding of green fodder is minimum (Table 12.1). The cost of feeding dry fodder is more or les similar to concentrates. The draw back in this calculation is the consideration of the physical form of the feeds and not the nutritional contribution for the cost of feed.

TABLE 12.1: Percentage of different inputs on the rearing of buffalo heifers up to first calving at a farm in India

Age of heifer (months)	Feeds	Establishment	Labour charges	Miscelleneous	Depriciation	Interest	Morlatity
Birth–6	76.6	5.3	5.0	2.1	1.3	2.3	7.4
6–12	68.6	5.4	5.2	2.1	1.4	2.4	14.9
12–18	76.2	4.5	4.3	1.8	1.2	2.0	10.1
18–24	74.7	4.1	3.9	1.6	1.0	1.8	12.8
24–30	77.8	7.5	7.1	2.9	1.9	3.3	Nil
30–36	79.2	6.9	6.5	2.7	1.8	3.	Nil
36–42	82.9	5.6	5.3	2.2	1.4	2.5	Nil
Overall	77.3	5.7	5.4	2.2	1.4	2.5	6.5

The expenditure is maximum for the feeding of whole milk and milk replacer to young calves below 6 months of age. After this expenditure on the feeding of concentrate mixture varies from 40 to 55% at different age of the growing period, which is high during the first pregnancy (Table 12.2).

TABLE 12.2: Average expenditure (%) on different feeds during growing period

Age of buffalo heifer (months)	Milk	Concentrate mixture	Dry fodder	Green fodder
Birth–6	55.8	22.7	13.3	8.2
6–12		40	41	19
12–18		44	41	15
18–24		41	44	15
24–30		48	37	15
30–36		53	32	15
36 - 42		54	33	13

Relative Cost of Milk Production

Within the prevalent socioeconomic and agricultural system it will be very difficult for most of the farmers and other small holder buffalo owners to keep the buffaloes if he is not getting some return on the investment. In the prevalent socioeconomic conditions in the buffalo rearing areas of the Indian sub continent buffalo milk is preferred. The river buffaloes are kept in the urban and peri-urban areas with the primary objective of saling fluid milk to daily consumers. From remote rural areas the milk is either collected by the milk unions or by the local 'dudhia' (the persons or families mainly engaged in the business of milk saling, i.e. kind of middle man in milk marketing business). The economic consideration of most f the small holders many inputs including the cost of fodder collected by family members from the scrub lands and labour charges on the management of buffaloes. Expenditures on veterinary adis and artificial insemination are also excluded when provided free by the state veterinary service. Some earlier studies on the cost of milk production in India also excluded many inputs and worked out a reasonable cost of milk production, and most of the lactating zebu cows (Panse et al., 1961; Lall, 1963; Sharma and Senger, 1971; Bhatia and Gangwar, 1981). In the private commercial dairy farming under cluster system of only lactating buffaloes in crowded management of make shift for feeding, resting and milking the cost of feeding accounted about 70% of the total expenditure against 65% in the rural areas. However, the situation has significantly changes in many areas and cost of feeding has increased enormously due to use of chilling plants for the storage of milk before trsnsportation to dairy plants. The milk is also carried in refrigerated vans and rail transported to dairy plants. The milk is also carried in refrigerated vans and rail transported containers/ milk vans. There is great scope of improvent in the buffalo based dairy farming through the application of modern technology of clean milk production and processing of milk before marketing. There is also scope of breeding buffaloes for several lactation by following standard methods of buffalo herd management.

The economics of milk production at the organized and institutional dairy farms has shown about 44–57% expenditure on feeding, 14–24% on labour charges and 16–24% on the replacement of dairy buffaloes (Ram and Singh, 1976, Mudgal, 1981). The series of studies at the National Dairy Research Institute, Karnal, India have shown considerale variation in different inputs during different period (Table 12.3).

TABLE 12.3: Expenditure (%) on various inputs for milk production in Murrah buffalo

Inputs	1970–71	1974–75	1975–76	1977–78
Feedstuffs	46.5	57.0	44.4	45.9
Labour charges	13.9	16.1	21.8	23.7
Replacement	22.1	16.1	23.5	21.1
Supervision	2.3	1.0	1.8	1.6
Veterinary aid	0.7	3.1	0.2	1.9
Miscelleneous	14.4	6.7	8.3	5.9

The another study conducted at the dairy demonstration farm, Mathura, India gives a different picture of the cost of milk production. In this study expenditure on milk production has been worked out on the basis of the milk yield per day of inter calving period andit shows about 84.58% expenditure on the feeding of buffaloes followed by 12.78% on the labours and only 2.64% on other inputs (Kanchan and Tomar, 1984). The expenditure on inputs in the former studies appears to be an over estimatin on replacement and in later study it may be under estimation. Moreover, both the models of economic assessment need through revision for presenting a true economic picture of buffalo based dairy farming.

Expenditure (Inputs) on Buffen (Buffalo Meat Production)

It is well established that under intensive system of management the cost of meat production is much higher than the cost of milk production in bovines when calculated on the basis of feed conversion efficiency. The efficiency of conversion of feed nutrients decreases grandually with the increase in age and body size of the animal. This is due to increase in the maintenance requirement and also the loss in rumen fermentation of feeds after the development of functional rumen; but the animals are capable of utilizing larger quantity of fibrous fodder. The expenditure on feeding ranges between 50–60% of the total capital investment for meat production in buffaloes. The growth rate and the rations of different tissue growth are significantly influenced by the age, breed, composition of diets and source of dietary energy etc. (Sharma and Talapatra, 1963; Rosa et al., 1980; Buruah et al., 1983; Pathak et al., 1983). Feeding of high level of available energy significantly reduces the finishing period and thus, the expenditure on maintenance and increases the turn over rate of capital. However, it is not feasible to incorporate large quantity of high energy grains and proteinous oil cakes in many buffalo raising tropical countries either due to non availability or due to exorbitant cost in relation to return from the local sale of buffalo meat and by products. Export is remunerative but commercial houses do not pay to farmers.

In India, buffalo fattening for meat production is not an organized industry and buffen is largely produced from the surplus unserviceable stock. However, during last 2–3 decats buffalo fattening has been initiated in many parts and now more people are protecting and fattening the male buffalo calves for meat production. This is due to availability of inputs specially the balanced feed at easy terms and remunerative marketing of fattened buffaloes. The male buffalo calves are available at about 4 weeks of age from the buffalo dairy stalls of urban areas and weaned calves at 8–10 months of age in rural areas. Both groups of calves are mostly under fed but survival rate of calves of higher age is more. So far there appears to be no attempt of utilizing the unwanted pre-riminant calves but satisfactory feeding for fattening has started in areas supported by some commercial houses for the feeding and management of buffalo calves for finishing at about 12–15 months of age and 250 to 350 kg body weight. Even in areas not covered in the scheme, now some farmers has started the fattening of poor calves of 70–100 kg body weight spared after the dryig of buffaloes. Average feed requirement per kg gain in the body weight of such calves is aobut 10kg at the 50% concentrates feeding. Since price of fattened buffaloes in increasing with the cost of feding and management due to increasing demand of good quality bufen, this system of buffalo fattening is growing in many parts of India.

▶ INSTITUTIONAL FINANCE

1. Buffalo raising is a source of subsidiary income in most of the Indian households. It also provides gainful employment to aged family members, ladies and unemployed or under employed youth. In addition to some increase in family income, it is also a good engagement for the idle family members and significantly reduces the stress of negative thoughts of idleness specially for the aged retired persons seeking more attention from the busy family members.

2. Only lactating buffalo keeping with few or none buffalo calves is quite popular in the India sub continent with a sole objective of liquid milk sale to local consumers. The herd size mostly ranges from few (5 to 15) to 300 lactating buffaloes and in rare cases more than 500 buffaloes at the stalls near the cosmopolitan cities.

3. The number and type of buffaloes reared in rural families depends on several socio-econimic factors like economic status, domestic requirements, demand of milk in the area or availability of marketing facility, availability of feed at reasonable cost,

facility for institutional loan at low interest and easy terms and veterinary facility for the treatment of sick buffaloes and breeding, etc.

Small and marginal farmers and landless labourers of rural areas usually keep few (1–5) lactating buffaloes and their surviving followers for daily support income to meet the domestic requirement. Another group of families unable to keep lactating buffaloes out for rearing weaned buffalo heifers or dry buffaloes up to advance stage of pregnancy or the day of calving as per mutual contract on barter system. In this system they are not required to pay any price for the animals but they have to bear all the expenditure on rearing to desired stage. In most of the cases the productive heifer or buffalo is evaluated by a committee of farmers aware with market trend. On the basis of assessed price either party may retain the buffalo on payment of half of the assessed price. In case of unwillingness of retaining the buffalo is sold and money is equally divided between the two parties. Although rearing of replacement heifers and dry buffaloes is quite costly but it is opted mostly by economically weaker familes due to lack of resources for the purchase of lactating buffaloes. The cost of feeding is low because idle members of the family collect grasses and fodder from scrub land, road sides, aechards, canal bunds and river sides. Since regular job is not assured the labour input is considered as a recurring deposit in the form of growth of the animal.

4. In addition to regular income from the sale of milk the buffaloes excrete large quantity of 4–5 kg dry matter or 3.5–4.3 kg organic matter in dung, and about 80–100 g nitrogen in urine besides many minerals necessary for crop production. Although, buffalo ding is a very good organic manure but due to inadequate fuel availability a substantial proportion is used for the preparation of dung cakes for cooking foods and warming house during shivering cold months. Part of the dung cake is also sold to get small amount of money required for small household needs.

▶ OBJECTIVES OF FINANCING DAIRY FARMING

In order to meet the requirements of nutritious protein of animal origin in the diets of a predominantly vegetarian population of India a number of steps has been taken by different organizations. A few important programmes are the selectie breeding in good dairy breeds like Murrah, Surti, Mehsana, Nagpuri, Pandharpuri and Nili-Ravi, etc. up gradig of scattered so called non descript buffaloes with good breeds like Murrah, Mehsna and Surti, etc., development of nutritious fodder production, improvement in buffalo breeding by extensive use of artificial insemination and aso by providing good buffalo bulls in remote areas, improving veterinary services, providing facilities for the collection and marketing of milk at remunerative price against assured payment on daily, weekly, fortnightly or monthly basis. Inspite of all these facilities hard cash is required for many important purposes for starting, expansion and some times also for the maintenance of existing facilities.

▶ REQUIREMENT OF FINANCIAL SUPPORT

1. The applicant should have some backgroung of the profession. This may be a family profession for several generations or he/she has educational background imparting practical and theoretical training in buffalo/livestock management and fodder production.

2. The availability of initial inputs like shelter for the livestock, adequate water supply for drinking, cleaning and bathing or wallowing of buffaloes, assured regular supply of feed s and fooder at reasonable price and remunerative marketing facility for the sale of milk, milk products and by products (manure).
3. The approach of locale of farm from the financing institution.
4. Intergrity and socioeconomic reputation of the applicant in his village, neighbouring village and other financing agencies operating in the area.

▶ ELIGIBILITY FOR FINANCIAL ASSISTANCE

1. The applicant should have some background in the profession. This may be a family profession for several generation or he/she has educational background imparting practical and theoretical training in animal husbandry and fodder production.
2. The availability of initial inputs like shelter for the animals, assured water supply for drinking, bathing/wallowing and farm operations including irrigation of fodder crops. Veterinary services and marketing facility for milk and other products.
3. The approach of locale from the financial institution.
4. Integrity and socioeconomic status of the applicant in his village and some neighbouring villages, and other financing agencies operating in the area.

▶ MARGIN

Normally applicant is required to invest minimum 25% through his/her own resources in cash or king. In case of economically weaker classes like small and marginal farmers and landless farm families not included in subsidy scheme, 50% margin should be accepted. The margin is not a pre requirement in case of the Integrated Rural Development Programme because the applicant covered under the scheme is eligible for 50% subsidy. This class of farmers are required to route their application through the Block Development Officer of the area.

▶ BACKGROUND

The following points should be considered for financing the purchase of buffaloes for dairy farming in India.
1. The animal (buffalo) should be a recognized milch breed like Murrah, Mehsana, Surti, Nagpuri etc and their grades.
2. Animal should not have completed three lactations and should ordinarily be less than 5–6 year of age.
3. Milch buffaloes should be purchased in first month of calving to ensure considerable recovery of loan.
4. The dairy enterprise should follow scientifically regularized breeding programme for the maintenance of almost constant rate of daily milk supply.

▶ FINANCIAL INSTITUTIONS ADVANCING LOAN FOR ANIMAL HUSBANDRY

The various government, quasi government and private institutions providing financial support in the form of cash or kind. Many financial institutions make payment to suppliers against the approved supply of materials to the borrower. The financial institutions are:

1. All the nationalized banks
2. All the gramin banks
3. The prathma banks
4. The cooperative societies
5. The Cooperative banks
6. Registered money lenders
7. Registered financing companies
8. Economically sound large and medium farmers of the village
9. Local businessman (Lala or Baniya) of the locality.

▶ APPLICATION TO BANK FOR LOAN

An application is submitted to the bank on prescribed form of the bank. The application form usually contains the following enclosures:

1. Two recent photograph of the applicant.
2. Plan and estimates for the various inputs for which loan is required, viz, construction of animal sheds and feed store, purchase of dairy utensils and appliances, purchase of lactating buffaloes etc alongwith th proforma invoice or prevalent market rates.
3. A copy of record of land holding duly signed by the competent authority.
4. Valuation certificate of the property form the competent authority for security.
5. Agreement for the procurement of milk by the milk unions or milk cooperatives and the remittance of milk proceeds direct to bank under the tieup programme.
6. **Appraisal of the scheme:** The location and proposal for starting a dairy farm with the financial assistance from a bank is assessed by the Dairy Development Offices or Animal Husbandry Officer or Agricultural Development Officer of the bank. During the inspection of site following points are given special consideration:
    a. Suitability of the place for smooth running of the dairy farm.
    b. Sources of adequate feeds and fodder supply either produced by the farmer or available at reasonable rates in the local markets, and also the scope of cultivation or purchase of green fodder.
    c. Perennial water source to meet the requirement of daily farm and foder farm.
    d. Requirement of animal sheds and essential equipments and appliances.
    e. Cattle markets and other sources of purchasing milch buffaloes of recommended standard.
    f. Marketing facility for the assured disposal of milk at remunerative price and arrangements for the regular recovery of loan through some Govt. or quasi government organization.
    g. Distance of Veterinary hospital and facilities for breeding (A/I natural).
7. **Economic viability of the project:** The following three aspects of dairy farming are critically examined before sanctioning the loan for dairy farming:
    i. The cost estimate of the scheme.
    ii. Recurring expenditure for the maintenance of lactating buffaloes and their followers.
    iii. Return from the sale of milk.
    iv. Scope of pay back of loan from the savings of milk sale.

▶ DETERMINATION OF PAY BACK CAPACITY

Financial institutions invariably satisfy themselves for the capacity of generation of adequate income for sparing required money for the regular payment of loan instalments and interest. The repayment capacity may be worked out as follows:

Repayment capacity = Gross income–(Cost of maintenance + operational cost + instalment of loan)

▶ PREPARATION OF REPAYMENT SCHEME

Normally loans are sanctioned for the purchase of lactating buffaloes in the first month of calving and also for the essential infrastructures like animal sheds, utensils, dairy equipments and feeds etc. The common lactation period of dairy buffaloes is 9–10 months. This is followed by a lactational rest period of 3 to 6 months (average 4 months) and the next lactation period of 9–10 months. Repayment is normally fixed for two successive lactations and in the case of exceptionally poor borrower it is extended for the third lactation and in the case of exceptionally poor borrower it is extened for the third lactation period. The lactation curve of the buffalo is also considered for the calculation of repayment of instalments, which may be as follows:

1. Repayment at the rate of 15% of the loan during first 3 months of lactation.
2. The repayment rte is reduced to 10% for the next 3 months of lactation.
3. The rate is further reduced to only 5% during the next 3 months.

The 9 months repayment period is followed by the rest period of 4 months, and the repayment of balnce amount is again distributed in the previous order during 9 months of the successive lactation. In this system the borrower becomes owner of the milch buffalo and its progeny after about 22 to 24 months and may get another female heifer in production after 3–4 years from the date of start because the sex ratio in buffaloes is about 50: 50. Thus, out of the 2 calves born during the two lactations, 1 calf is expected to be female.

▶ LIVESTOCK INSURANCE

The death or disability of the livestock due to unforeseen disease or accident causes economic stress on the livestock owners. In order to provide protection from such economic distress to farmers a few insurance companies, viz, The New India Assurance Company, The Oriental Fire and General Insurance Company have provided several insurance schemes to cover the risk of economic loss from the permanent disability and death of the productive animal.

The age limit for lactating buffalo is minimum 3 year of the age at first calving and maximum 12 years, and for the working male buffalo the minimum and maximum age limit are 2 year and 8 years respectively.

The official financing institutions follow a well defined procedure and set terms and conditions besides low interest rate and convenient repayment programme.

Indeed private financing parties are operating and a considerable number of farmers still prefer them mostly for avoiding several barriers in their working with the official financing institutions.

The marginal farmers and landless farm families prefer to advance loan from the large and medium farmers whoprovide them short and long duration casual works during farming operations and also otherwise. This relation is working since generations.

There is wide variation in the rate of interest, terms of repayment and obligation to the financer. Most of the financing farmer advance loan in the form of kind. Generally non productive dry buffaloes and calves (preferably buffalo heifers) after weaning at 10–12 months of age are given by the large and medium farmers to a farm labouerer for rearing to reach the production stage. The prevalent terms and conditions in some parts of Indian sub continents are:

a. The animal is received without payment and current price of animal is decided a group of local experts of livestock marketing agreeable to both parties. After this an agreement of repayment with simple or compound interest is decided. Since most of the buffaloes take long time to achieve production stage, this system is rarely preferred.

b. The animals are received without payment, reared up to the last month of pregnancy or first few days of parturition and then evaluated according to current market ternd. After this it is open to both parties with the first preference to owner for taking the animal after the payment of half of the assessed price. In this system the investment of donor is the animal and that of borrower is the management up to production stage. There is no liability of casuality on the borrower and at many occasions donor provides financial assistance for the treatment during sickness. The regular daily gain against inputs to borrower is the dung which is highly needed for a landless farm family. The dung is made into cakes which are partly used for cooking food and partly sold for purchasing food grains and other necessary items. This system is quite popular in many areas.

REFERENCES

Agarwal, V P 1974. Ph.D. thesis, Agra University, Agra

Baruah, K K, Ranjhan, S K and Pathak, N N 1983. Buffalo Bulletin 2 (1) 10

Bhatia, H C and Gangwar, P C 1981. Indian. J. Dairy Sci., 34; 60–66 Borhami,

Gauam, J. P and Vimal, K R 1966. Indian Vet. J., 43; 1003–10

Kanchan, D K and Tomar, K R 1966. Indian Vet. J., 61; 1044–49

Lall, H.K 1963.Gosamvardhan, 10;7

Mudgal, V D 1981. Publication No. 101, National Dairy Res. Iust., Karnal

Panse, F G, Amble, V N and Puri, T R. 1961. Cost of milk production. Final report of ICAR scheme, New Delhi.

Pathak, N N and Ranjhan, S K 1976. Indian J. Anim. Sci., 46; 773–76

Pathak, N N and Rankjhan, S K 1979. Proc. Of All India Symp. On Protein and NPN Utilization in Riminants, NDRI, Karnal, May 21–23.

Pathak, N N, Baruah, K K And Ranjhan, S K 1983. Buffalo Bulletin, 2(1); 10.

Ram, Kuber and Singh, K. 1976. Murrah Buffalo, National Dairy Res. Inst., Karnal

Ranjhan, S K and Pathal, N N 1999. Text book of Buffalo Production, 4th Edition, Vikas Publishing House, New Delhi.

Rosa, A, Creta, V, Dzic, G and Fecior, R 1981. Lucrari Stiintifice ale Inst. De Ceretari Pentru Cresterea Taurinehor-Corbeanca, 7; 31–42.

Sharma, K M and Talapatra, S K 1963. Indian J. Dairy Sci., 16; 236–244.

Index